PHYSICAL ACTIVITY AND
THE AGING BRAIN

PHYSICAL ACTIVITY AND THE AGING BRAIN

EFFECTS OF EXERCISE ON NEUROLOGICAL FUNCTION

Edited by

RONALD ROSS WATSON

University of Arizona, Arizona Health Sciences Center, Tucson, AZ, USA

AMSTERDAM • BOSTON • HEIDELBERG • LONDON
NEW YORK • OXFORD • PARIS • SAN DIEGO
SAN FRANCISCO • SINGAPORE • SYDNEY • TOKYO
Academic Press is an imprint of Elsevier

Academic Press is an imprint of Elsevier
125 London Wall, London EC2Y 5AS, United Kingdom
525 B Street, Suite 1800, San Diego, CA 92101-4495, United States
50 Hampshire Street, 5th Floor, Cambridge, MA 02139, United States
The Boulevard, Langford Lane, Kidlington, Oxford OX5 1GB, United Kingdom

Notices
Knowledge and best practice in this field are constantly changing. As new research and experience broaden our understanding, changes in research methods, professional practices, or medical treatment may become necessary.

Practitioners and researchers must always rely on their own experience and knowledge in evaluating and using any information, methods, compounds, or experiments described herein. In using such information or methods they should be mindful of their own safety and the safety of others, including parties for whom they have a professional responsibility.

To the fullest extent of the law, neither the Publisher nor the authors, contributors, or editors, assume any liability for any injury and/or damage to persons or property as a matter of products liability, negligence or otherwise, or from any use or operation of any methods, products, instructions, or ideas contained in the material herein.

Library of Congress Cataloging-in-Publication Data
A catalog record for this book is available from the Library of Congress

British Library Cataloguing-in-Publication Data
A catalogue record for this book is available from the British Library

ISBN: 978-0-12-805094-1

For information on all Academic Press publications
visit our website at https://www.elsevier.com/

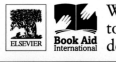

Working together
to grow libraries in
developing countries

www.elsevier.com • www.bookaid.org

Publisher: Mara Conner
Acquisition Editor: April Farr
Editorial Project Manager: Timothy Bennett
Production Project Manager: Edward Taylor
Designer: Mark Rogers

Typeset by TNQ Books and Journals

Contents

List of Contributors xi

Preface xiii

Acknowledgments xv

I OVERVIEW OF EXERCISE AND NEUROLOGICAL CHANGES

1. Effects of Physical Activity on the Cerebral Networks

A. BEGEGA, P. ALVAREZ-SUAREZ, P. SAMPEDRO-PIQUERO AND M. CUESTA

What Is Cognitive Ageing? 3
Physical Exercise and Health 4
Cognitive Ageing and Cerebral Networks 5
Physical Activity, Cognitive Reserve, and Neuroplasticity: Three Allies for Successful Ageing 7
Molecular Basis of Exercise and the Ageing Brain 8
Acknowledgments 8
References 9

2. Exercise and the Developing Brain in Children and Adolescents

M.M. HERTING AND M.F. KEENAN

Measuring Physical Activity Levels and Aerobic Fitness in Youth 13
Brain Development as Measured by Magnetic Resonance Imaging (MRI) 13
Aerobic Exercise and Brain Structure 14
Aerobic Exercise and Brain Activity 16
Aerobic Exercise and Cognition 17
Remaining Questions and Future Directions 17
Summary 18
References 18

3. Differential Expression of the Brain Proteome in Physical Training

T. RAVIKIRAN, R. VANI AND S. ANAND

Introduction 21
Methodology 22
Sample Preparation 22
Two-Dimensional Polyacrylamide Gel Electrophoresis (2D-PAGE) 23
Conclusion 26
Acknowledgments 26
References 26

4. Physical Exercise-Induced Changes in Brain Temperature

A.C. KUNSTETTER, W.C. DAMASCENO, C.G. FONSECA AND S.P. WANNER

Introduction 29
Measuring Brain Temperature During Exercise 30

Effects of Exercise on T$_{BRAIN}$..30
Final Remarks 37
References 37

II DRUGS OF ABUSE WITH EXERCISE TO MODIFY NEUROLOGICAL STRUCTURE AND FUNCTION

5. Physical Activity as a Therapeutic Intervention for Addictive Disorders: Interactions With Methamphetamine
S.S. SOMKUWAR, M.J. FANNON-PAVLICH AND C.D. MANDYAM

Introduction 41
Animal Models of Drug Reinforcement and Reward to Illicit Drugs 42
Animal Models of Sustained Physical Activity..43
Convergence Between Methamphetamine Self-Administration and Sustained Physical Activity in
    Animal Models 43
Neural Mechanisms Underlying Reinforcing Effects of Methamphetamine and Wheel Running....45
Neuroprotection by Wheel Running: Significant Interactions With Methamphetamine-Induced
    Neurotoxicity 45
Exercise as a Therapeutic Intervention for Methamphetamine Addiction 47
Acknowledgments 48
References 48

6. Pharmacological Intervention of Brain Neurotransmission Affects Exercise Capacity
X. ZHENG AND H. HASEGAWA

Introduction 53
The Structure and Function of the Nervous System 53
Physiological Properties of Monoamines 54
Monoamine and Exercise 57
Drugs Manipulating Brain Monoamine and Exercise Performance...59
Summary 62
References 63

7. The Endocannabinoid System and Chronic Disease: Opportunity for Innovative Therapies
A. YODER

Introduction 65
History of the Runner's High...65
Effects of Endocannabinoid System Stimulation 66
Possibilities of Therapeutic Uses of the Endocannabinoid System in Chronic
    Conditions...68
Brain Derived Neurotropic Factor and Depression 68
Chronic Pain 69
Epilepsy 69
Musculoskeletal Disorders 70
Alzheimer's Disease 70
Amyotrophic Lateral Sclerosis (ALS) 71
Stress-Related Disorders 71
Conclusion 72
References 72

III FACTORS MODULATING EXERCISE IN AGING AND NEUROLOGICAL CONSEQUENCES

8. Changes in Cerebral Blood Flow During Steady-State Exercise

M. HIURA AND T. NARIAI

Introduction 77
CBF Estimated by TCD Method 78
rCBF Measurement Using PET 79
Increased rCBF During Exercise: Underlying Possible Mechanisms 80
Increased rCBF During Exercise and Beneficial Effects of Brain 82
Conclusion 83
Acknowledgments 83
Disclosure/Conflict of Interest 83
References 83

9. Biochemical Mechanisms Associated With Exercise-Induced Neuroprotection in Aging Brains and Related Neurological Diseases

M.S. SHANMUGAM, W.M. TIERNEY, R.A. HERNANDEZ, A. CRUZ, T.L. UHLENDORF AND R.W. COHEN

Introduction 85
Exercise Effects: Neurotrophic Factors 86
Exercise Effects: Epigenetics 86
Exercise Effects: Apoptosis 87
Exercise Effects: Oxidative Stress 88
Exercise Effects: Neurogenesis 88
Exercise Effects: Synaptogenesis 89
Exercise Effects: Age-Related Neurodegenerative Diseases 90
Conclusions 91
References 91

10. Role of Melatonin Supplementation During Strenuous Exercise

J. DÍAZ-CASTRO, M. PULIDO-MORÁN, J. MORENO-FERNÁNDEZ, N. KAJARABILLE, S. HIJANO AND J.J. OCHOA

Melatonin: Sources, Biosynthesis, and Physiological Effects 95
Exercise: Oxidative Stress and Induced Inflammatory Signaling 96
Melatonin and Inflammatory Signaling 97
Effects of Melatonin in Strenuous Exercise 98
References 100

IV EXERCISE AS THERAPY FOR NEUROLOGICAL DISEASES

11. Mechanisms of Functional Recovery With Exercise and Rehabilitation in Spinal Cord Injuries

M. COWAN AND R.M. ICHIYAMA

Introduction 107
Mechanisms Underlying of Rehabilitation 108
Refining Rehabilitation Programs 112
Conclusions 115
References 116

12. Neural Structure, Connectivity, and Cognition Changes Associated to Physical Exercise

S. BONAVITA AND G. TEDESCHI

Introduction 121
References 129

13. The Effect of Exercise on Motor Function and Neuroplasticity in Parkinson's Disease

J. WATSON, K.E. WELMAN AND B. SEHM

Introduction 133
Parkinson's Disease 133
Exercise Interventions in Parkinson's Disease Patients 135
The Effects of Exercise on the Parkinsonian Brain—Animal Models 135
The Effects of Exercise on the Parkinsonian Brain—Human Studies 137
Conclusion 138
References 138

14. Physical Exercise and Its Effects on Alzheimer's Disease

A.M. STEIN AND R.V. PEDROSO

Introduction 141
Alzheimer's Disease and Level of Physical Activity 141
Alzheimer's Disease and Physical Activity Programs 142
Alzheimer's Disease, Physical Exercise, and Cognitive Functions 142
Alzheimer's Disease, Physical Exercise, and Neuropsychiatric Symptoms 145
Alzheimer's Disease, Physical Exercise, and Functional Capacity 145
Alzheimer's Disease, Physical Exercise, and Biomarkers 146
Final Considerations 148
References 148

15. Cortical Reorganization in Response to Exercise

P. STEPHANE

Introduction 151
The Exercising Brain 152
Fatigue-related Brain Reorganization 155
Brain Reorganization After Stroke 156
Conclusion 157
References 157

16. Exercise Enhances Cognitive Capacity in the Aging Brain

S. SNIGDHA AND G.A. PRIETO

Introduction 161
The Aging Brain 161
Making the Connection—Moving the Body Builds the Brain 162
Physical Exercise for Preventing Age-Related Cognitive Decline 162
Molecular and Cellular Building Blocks for Brain Remodeling by Exercise 165
Conclusion 168
References 168

V LIFESTYLE EXERCISE AFFECTING NEUROLOGICAL STRUCTURE AND FUNCTION IN OLDER ADULTS

17. Synergistic Effects of Combined Physical Activity and Brain Training on Neurological Functions

T.M. SHAH AND R.N. MARTINS

Introduction 175
Leisure Activities Improves Cognition and Reduces the Risk of Dementia and AD 176
Combined Physical and Cognitive Training Interventions Show Stronger Cognitive Benefits 176
Mechanisms Underlying the Synergistic Effects of Combined Physical and Mental Activities for Healthy
    Brain Aging 178
Future Directions 180
References 181

18. Physical Activity: Effects of Exercise on Neurological Function

R. BEURSKENS AND M. DALECKI

Introduction 185
Age-related Functional and Structural Changes in the Human Brain 185
Theories of Neural Plasticity in Older Adults 188
Exercise and Neurological Changes 190
Exercise as Therapy for Neurological Diseases 193
Conclusion 195
References 195

19. Update of Nutritional Antioxidants and Antinociceptives on Improving Exercise-Induced Muscle Soreness

N. LEELAYUWAT

Introduction 199
Mechanisms Responsible for the DOMS 199
Endogenous Antioxidants and Exercise-Induced Muscle Soreness 201
Nutritional Antioxidants and Exercise-Induced Muscle Soreness 201
Antioxidant Supplements 201
Functional Foods With High Antioxidant Concentrations 204
Antinociceptive Supplements and Exercise-Induced Muscle Soreness 205
References 206

20. Effects of Exercise-Altered Immune Functions on Neuroplasticity

A.L. ARAL AND L. PINAR

Introduction 209
Effects of Exercise on Immune Function 209
Role of Exercise in Enhancing Brain Capacity Through Neuroplasticity 211
Immunity of the CNS 212
Effects of Exercise-Altered Immune Function on Neuroplasticity 213
References 215

Index 219

List of Contributors

P. Alvarez-Suarez Institute of Neuroscience, Asturias, Spain

S. Anand Bangalore University, Bengaluru, India

A.L. Aral Gazi University Faculty of Medicine, Ankara, Turkey

A. Begega Institute of Neuroscience, Asturias, Spain

R. Beurskens Geriatric Center at the University of Heidelberg, Bethanien Hospital, Heidelberg, Germany; University of Potsdam, Germany

S. Bonavita Ist Clinic of Neurology, Second University of Naples, Naples, Italy

R.W. Cohen California State University Northridge, Northridge, CA, United States

M. Cowan University of Leeds, Leeds, United Kingdom; Imperial College London, London, United Kingdom

A. Cruz California State University Northridge, Northridge, CA, United States

M. Cuesta Institute of Neuroscience, Asturias, Spain

M. Dalecki York University, Toronto, ON, Canada

W.C. Damasceno Federal University of Minas Gerais, Belo Horizonte, MG, Brazil

J. Díaz-Castro University of Granada, Granada, Spain

M.J. Fannon-Pavlich Committee on the Neurobiology of Addictive Disorders, La Jolla, CA, United States

C.G. Fonseca Federal University of Minas Gerais, Belo Horizonte, MG, Brazil

H. Hasegawa Hiroshima University, Higashihiroshima, Japan

R.A. Hernandez California State University Northridge, Northridge, CA, United States

M.M. Herting Children's Hospital Los Angeles, Los Angeles, CA, United States

S. Hijano University of Granada, Granada, Spain

M. Hiura Hosei University, Tokyo, Japan

R.M. Ichiyama University of Leeds, Leeds, United Kingdom

N. Kajarabille University of Granada, Granada, Spain

M.F. Keenan Children's Hospital Los Angeles, Los Angeles, CA, United States

A.C. Kunstetter Federal University of Minas Gerais, Belo Horizonte, MG, Brazil

N. Leelayuwat Exercise and Sport Sciences Development and Research Group, and Department of Physiology, Faculty of Medicine, Khon Kaen University, Khon Kaen, Thailand

C.D. Mandyam Committee on the Neurobiology of Addictive Disorders, La Jolla, CA, United States

R.N. Martins McCusker Alzheimer's Research Foundation, Hollywood Medical Centre, Nedlands, WA, Australia; Edith Cowan University, Joondalup, WA, Australia; University of Western Australia, Crawley, WA, Australia

J. Moreno-Fernández University of Granada, Granada, Spain

T. Nariai Tokyo Medical and Dental University, Tokyo, Japan

J.J. Ochoa University of Granada, Granada, Spain

R.V. Pedroso Univ Estadual Paulista, Rio Claro, São Paulo, Brazil

L. Pinar Gazi University Faculty of Medicine, Ankara, Turkey

G.A. Prieto University of California-Irvine, Irvine, CA, United States

M. Pulido-Morán University of Granada, Granada, Spain

T. Ravikiran Bangalore University, Bengaluru, India

P. Sampedro-Piquero Institute of Neuroscience, Asturias, Spain

B. Sehm Max Planck Institute for Human Cognitive and Brain Sciences, Leipzig, Germany; University of Leipzig, Leipzig, Germany

T.M. Shah McCusker Alzheimer's Research Foundation, Hollywood Medical Centre, Nedlands, WA, Australia; Edith Cowan University, Joondalup, WA, Australia

M.S. Shanmugam California State University Northridge, Northridge, CA, United States

S. Snigdha University of California-Irvine, Irvine, CA, United States

S.S. Somkuwar Committee on the Neurobiology of Addictive Disorders, La Jolla, CA, United States

A.M. Stein Univ Estadual Paulista, Rio Claro, São Paulo, Brazil

P. Stephane University of Montpellier, Montpellier, France

G. Tedeschi Ist Clinic of Neurology, Second University of Naples, Naples, Italy

W.M. Tierney California State University Northridge, Northridge, CA, United States

T.L. Uhlendorf California State University Northridge, Northridge, CA, United States

R. Vani Jain University, Bengaluru, India

S.P. Wanner Federal University of Minas Gerais, Belo Horizonte, MG, Brazil

J. Watson Stellenbosch University, Stellenbosch, South Africa

K.E. Welman Stellenbosch University, Stellenbosch, South Africa

A. Yoder University of Arizona, Tucson, AZ, United States

X. Zheng Shanghai University of Sport, Shanghai, China

Preface

Physical activity including planned exercise in prevention and modification of neurological complications due to advancing age is beginning to be explored and will be described.

I. Overview of Exercise and Neurological Changes. Begega starts with the basics of physical exercise and its effects on nerves and their growth and function. In particular she reviews neurological networks as modified by activity or lack thereof. Neurological changes in infants and youth are subject to physical activity as described by Herting and Keenan. Such effects are the building components for the aged neurological system and changes in structure and function induced by exercise. Ravikiran, Vani and Anand describe changes in the brain proteome during planned exercise as an example. Damasceno, Fonseca, and Wanner describe the actions of exercise on brain temperature, as exercise can increase temperature and may affect brain functions.

II. Drugs of Abuse With Exercise to Modify Neurological Structure and Function. Currently the last decade or two of life result in many chronic, frequently incurable diseases with huge medical costs and health problems. Understanding the biology of chronic degenerative diseases of adults opens the way for therapies at hand for the aging adults. Mandyam, Somkuwar, and Fannon review the neurological effects of a drug of abuse and methamphetamine. Then they describe the potential of exercise to act as a therapy for this addictive substance. Brain transmission affects exercise and physical activity. Zheng and Hasegawa review pharmacological methods to change brain neurotransmission and how these can affect exercise and physical capacity and activity. The endocannabinoid system is modified by exercise-induced molecules similar in structural binding capacity to cannabinoids from marijuana. Yoder and Watson review this system affected by exercise as an opportunity for innovative therapies.

III. Factors Modulating Exercise in Aging and Neurological Consequences Hiura and Nariai review blood flow during exercise in athletes which affects the movement of modulators to the brain including nutrients. This review serves as a model for exercise in changing nutrient needs by building muscle and preventing major loss of food consumption with old age. Uhlendorf and her group review neuroprotection in growing and especially aging brains in protection from neurological disease. Seniors are getting progressively older and more numerous with each generation. The number and percentage of the population of many developing countries are continuing to increase. For example the front cover of *Time Magazine* (February 23, 2015) shows a child with the headline "*This baby could live to be 142 years old.*" This book looks at a tool at hand for seniors and their medical advisors to protect the brain and treat neurological diseases using physical activity. Díaz-Castro and his group of expert authors and researchers review the role of a well-known natural hormone that affects the brain and regulates sleep. They review the role of melatonin on the brain and body during strenuous exercise.

IV. Exercise as Therapy for Neurological Diseases. Exercise and physical activity has the potential to treat and overcome a variety of neurological diseases and especially damage. For examples Cowan and Ichiyama review spinal cord neurological injuries. They focus on the actions of exercise in spinal cord rehabilitation and recovery. Bonavita and Tedeschi describe the changes in a variety of brain organs and functions due to physical activity. Neural structure, cognition changes, and connectivity are modified by exercise and reviewed by this group. Parkinson's disease is susceptible to exercise modulation. Watson, Welman, and Sehm describe neuroplasticity and motor function changes during exercise therapy. Another significant neurological disease is Alzheimer's disease. Stein and Pedroso describe physical activity in Alzheimer's disease and its effects on the brain and neurological function. Hormones such as corticosteroids change structure and function. Perrey describes corticoid-induced reorganization in response to physical activity and exercise. Snigdha reviews the role of exercise in enhancing memory activity in the aging brain.

V. Lifestyle Exercise Affecting Neurological Structure and Function in Older Adults. Shah and Martin describe the role of exercise synergistic actions of exercise and physical activity during brain training on the actions of nerves and neurological functions. Beurskens and Dalecki provide an overview and description of exercise on neurological functions. Leelayuwat discusses the actions of nutritional antioxidants and antinociceptives on improving exercise-induced muscle damage. Aral and Pinar finally describe the immune systems and their changes on neuroplasticity.

Acknowledgments

The work of Dr. Watson's editorial assistant, Bethany L. Stevens, in communicating with authors and working on the manuscripts was critical to the successful completion of the book. The support of Kristi L. Anderson is also very much appreciated. Support for Ms. Stevens' and Dr. Watson's work was graciously provided by Natural Health Research Institute www.naturalhealthresearch.org. It is an independent, nonprofit organization that supports science-based research on natural health and wellness. It is committed to informing about scientific evidence on the usefulness and cost-effectiveness of diet, supplements, and a healthy lifestyle to improve health and wellness and reduce disease. Finally, the work of the librarian of the Arizona Health Science Library, Mari Stoddard, was vital and very helpful in identifying key researchers who participated in the book.

PART I

OVERVIEW OF EXERCISE AND NEUROLOGICAL CHANGES

1

Effects of Physical Activity on the Cerebral Networks

A. Begega, P. Alvarez-Suarez, P. Sampedro-Piquero, M. Cuesta
Institute of Neuroscience, Asturias, Spain

Abstract

It is well documented that ageing is accompanied by a decline in cognitive functions such as, memory, attention, and speed of information processing. Different nonpharmacological approaches have been proposed for the purpose of promoting health, such as, mental training, mediterranean diet, and physical exercise. This is because their benefits on both cognitive and cerebral function have been proven. Numerous studies have targeted the design of intervention programmes favoring these neuroplasticity processes such as exercise programmes. This intervention type have been shown, both in humans and rodents studies, to have benefits on neuroplasticity, neurogenesis, and levels of brain-derived neurotrophic factor, among others. Hence, any physical activity must be accomplished in order to maintain them as long as possible.

WHAT IS COGNITIVE AGEING?

In the past few decades, research in ageing and ageing-related cognitive changes have experimented a great breakthrough. It is well documented that ageing is accompanied by a decline in cognitive functions such as, memory, attention, and speed of information processing (Salthouse, 2012, 2000; Swain et al., 2012). Speed of information processing is defined as "the amount of information that can be processed per time unit or the speed at which a series of cognitive operations can be done". This difficulty reduces as how fast we process the information from the environment and affects other processes like short-term memory and information interference, which favors a higher distractibility in elderly people. Elders' attentional capacity is reduced and is accompanied by more distractibility and proactive interference.

In this case, proactive interference refers to the process by which we are not able to reduce the influence of previous-learned information so we can successfully perform the new-information required task (Bartko et al., 2010). Namely, besides difficulties in memory processes (Bamidis et al., 2014), executive functions were also affected in the elderly people. In light to this situation, it seems obvious that life quality is diminished as independence is compromised in everyday-activities (Vance et al., 2012), leading to emotional impairments which have been related to ageing, such as major depression and anxiety. This is a discouraging scenario for elderly population, but in recent years the field of Neuroscience has developed numerous ageing-related studies in order to know how to intervene and achieve the maintenance of these basic cognitive functions or, at least, delay their deterioration. Thus, different nonpharmacological approaches have been proposed for the purpose of promoting health, such as, mental training, mediterranean diet, and physical exercise. This is because their benefits on both cognitive and cerebral function have been proven (Ballesteros et al., 2015).

Regarding to this research, cognitive reserve acquires a special relevance and has been studied by Yaakov Stern's research team, among others. They define cognitive reserve as the ability to make flexible and efficient use of available brain reserve when performing tasks (Stern, 2002). Cognitive reserve has been related to lifestyle and how different circumstances, activities, and habits can positively influence independence and life quality during the ageing process. It has been most often estimated using education and IQ, although other variables have also been used including literacy, occupational complexity, participation in leisure activities, as well as the cohesion of social networks. Cognitive reserve can also be related to neurobiological mechanisms like neural compensation and neuronal reserve (Barulli and Stern, 2013), which refer to a subject's ability to use cognitive processes and, therefore, neuronal networks in an effective way, leading to a lower impact of ageing-related functional changes. Neural compensation by Stern (2002) is defined as the use of alternative neuronal networks due to an incapability to use the task-related impaired one, which is a common mechanism in the ageing process. On the other hand, neural reserve is associated with the functional use of the task-related neuronal network, which produces an increase in its activity, or to a functional support of secondary-related networks, which favors task efficacy. As both the processes seem to occur frequently during ageing, cognitive reserve continues to be influenced by circumstances throughout the lifespan. The cognitive reserve could subserve a delay in cognitive deterioration and in age-related dementia. Among the activities, aerobic exercise is seem to have a beneficial effects on cognitive reserve (Ballesteros et al., 2015).

PHYSICAL EXERCISE AND HEALTH

Exercise is commonly known by its wide benefits on health, especially in the muscle strengthening and the prevention of cardiovascular diseases (CVD). However, it positively affects many different aspects of the organism physiology, both in healthy individuals and those at risk of developing a disease or aggravating it. For example, it seems to increase the probability of normal delivery among healthy pregnant women, which means less caesarean cases (Domenjoz et al., 2014). As a matter of fact, exercised mothers and their children have shorter hospital stays, less complications, shorter labor, and less preterm labor than nonexercisers (May, 2012).

Ageing is characterized by a progressive reduction of the regeneration potential, determined by both genetic and environmental factors that lead to an imbalance between repair and accumulation of cellular damage. The decline of cellular function is accompanied by ageing-related, harmless phenotypes like grey hair and wrinkles (Ludlow et al., 2013), also by a loss of physiological integrity and higher vulnerability to death, the main cause for most of the major pathological human diseases such as Alzheimer's and other neurodegenerative diseases, diabetes, certain kinds of cancer, and CVD (López-Otín et al., 2013). Here, we number the benefits of exercise in some main human pathologies.

Several studies have demonstrated associations between active behaviors and age-related health outcomes. For example, it has been documented an inverse relationship between physical activity and all-cause mortality, just the same as a direct relationship between low-cardiorespiratory fitness and disease. On the basis of this, exercise has been included in most of the guidelines for prevention or reduction of CVD mortality, advising at least 30 min of moderate-intensity aerobic activity 5 days per week to gain even years in life expectancy (Schuler et al., 2013). Together with an appropriate diet, this simple recommendations are in order to reduce low-density lipoprotein cholesterol and blood pressure (Wenger, 2014).

It has been demonstrated that exercise stimulates mitochondria biogenesis in the skeletal muscle through oxidative stress, leading to a deceleration of age-related diseases caused by a loss of mitochondria or an impairment in their function, like sarcopenia, cancer, or neurodegenerative diseases (Sun et al., 2015). Physical exercise can be used as a therapy in many different muscle-affected disorders. It can potentially prevent muscle atrophy caused by muscle inflammation, physical inactivity, and systemic glucocorticoid treatments in patients with idiopathic inflammatory myositis (Munters et al., 2014). Moreover, it has been proposed to counteract many of the symptoms in multiple sclerosis, improving and/or maintaining functional ability, aerobic fitness, muscle strength, fatigue, and so on (Latimer-Cheung et al., 2013).

Type 2 diabetes prevalence has been increased in the recent years as it arises from a combination of genetic susceptibility and environmental factors like sedentary life and an unsuitable diet, which nowadays affect a wide range of the population, who become obese as a result of their lifestyle (Stanford and Goodyear, 2014). Therefore, the avoidance of this disease goes through the prevention of muscle atrophy and the reduction of CVD risk by the agency of regular physical activity. Exercise has also shown to reduce tumor incidence, tumor multiplicity, and tumor growth across numerous different transplantable, chemically induced, or genetic tumor models (Pedersen et al., 2015).

Finally, there is a large evidence about exercise benefits on cognitive reserve, as has been thoroughly reviewed by Franco-Martin et al. (2013). This aspect gains importance in the ageing process, in which the total brain weight is reduced from 10% to 20% as well as blood flow decreases about 30–40%, which leads to an impairment of learning and memory, attention, and cognitive functions. Physical endurance and aerobic exercise has been associated with successful cognitive ageing, as it delays or reduces the effects of ageing in the central nervous system (Franco-Martin et al., 2013; Cassilhas et al., 2015). For example, there is an inverse relationship between levels of brain-derived neurotrophic factor (BDNF) as a direct measure of the amount of exercise performed and the severity of cognitive decline due to Alzheimer's disease (Piepmeier and Etnier, 2014). There are strong proofs of the neuroprotective effects of vigorous exercise on Parkinson's disease as well, because it not only reduces the risk of developing the disease, but also slows the progression once it has already showed up and lengthens life expectancy (Ahlskog, 2011).

COGNITIVE AGEING AND CEREBRAL NETWORKS

Cognitive neuroscience addresses age effect on different cognitive functions (Antonenko and Flöel, 2013). Nowadays, the breakthrough in this field is related to the aim of establishing the extremely complex network of brain regions implicated and how they are modified by the ageing process, the type of task and pathologies like dementia. For this purpose, integrity and deterioration of functional connectivity between brain regions associated to processes like language, attention, or memory are assessed. Several authors have studied structural connectivity in white matter pathways in order to assess the integrity of anatomical connections, which underlies the communication between the nodes of these functional networks. It has been observed that numerous networks support different functions such as, sensory, motor, executive, memory, or language functions (Charroud et al., 2015). Neuroimaging techniques like functional magnetic resonance (fMRI) and magnetoencephalography allow the assessment of these cerebral networks in specific tasks and the characterization of age-related changes.

Recent studies showed how episodic memory is associated to, besides regions from the medial temporal lobe (MTL), a whole system of brain regions related to the default mode network (DMN) (Jeong et al., 2015). In the same way, attention studies in elderly population showed that this cognitive function is damaged, as they found a decrease in visual precision and a higher vulnerability to distraction from relevant information (Zhou et al., 2011). Three different networks have been described in attention: alerting network, orienting network, and executive control network (Petersen and Posner, 2012). The alerting network allows to maintain an alert state and to express a particular response facing a specific stimulus. The underlying neurobiological substrates are parietal and frontal areas. The orienting network refers to the selection of information from different sensory modalities, where parietal superior lobe and frontal eyes fields are involved. Finally, the executive network includes the prefrontal cortex and the cingulate anterior cortex. Taking this whole functional connectivity into account, Zhou et al. (2011) show that there are significant differences between young, middle-aged, and older Chinese adults, especially in the executive control network. However, the age effect on alerting and orienting networks is subtle or nonexistent, respectively. It has been observed that prefrontal cortex, anterior cingulate cortex, and hippocampal regions are severely damaged in ageing, so it seems that both executive control and alerting networks are vulnerable to the ageing process.

One of the brain networks that has received most attention in the recent years is the so-called DMN (Jeong et al., 2015; Raichle, 2015), defined as the group of brain regions that are active during resting states and inactive during the execution of any goal-directed task (Sala-Llonch et al., 2015). The resting state occurs experimentally when the subject is asked to avoid falling asleep and think about something in particular. Most of the times, these studies of functional connectivity are based on neuroimaging techniques like fMRI, which have shown that the DMN includes the medial prefrontal cortex, the posterior cingulate cortex, the retrosplenial cortex, and several hippocampal areas (Persson et al., 2014).

A variety of changes have been observed in ageing-related functional connectivity. The loss of contacts induces disconnection between DMN nodes, which is related to cognitive decline, which in turn has been associated to an impairment in functional connectivity throughout the main brain networks (Andrews-Hanna et al., 2014; Gozzi and Schwarz, 2015; Vidal-Piñeiro et al., 2014). Nevertheless, Campbell et al. (2013) consider that, during ageing, there is a maintenance of the connectivity between the main DMN brain regions. No differences were found between older and younger subjects on medial temporal lobe (MTL) regions, but elderly subjects showed a weaker connectivity in subsystems such as ventral posterior cingulate cortex and dorsomedial prefrontal cortex, but a stronger connectivity in the dorsal posterior cingulate cortex. These authors sustain the idea that this higher functional connectivity could be due to a bigger inflow of information from sensory areas to MTL areas, which could be producing more difficulties to delete irrelevant information in aged people. This would favor interference and impair memorization of new information. When performing a task, elders show hyperactivation of prefrontal areas, associated to functional compensation responses that allow a successful task execution (Campbell et al., 2013).

Regarding data analysis, multivariate analysis techniques are one of the best tools in assessing and determining functional connectivity (Jeong et al., 2015; Raineki et al., 2014). Functional connectivity is established through the relationship between different brain regions participating in a specific moment facing a specific situation. Thereby, when our interests are focused on detecting differences between groups submitted to different treatments, ANOVA-derived techniques (analysis of variance) in its different versions (intrafactor, interfactor, mixed) are a classic useful tool. In this context, and taking into account that we usually manage multiple measured variables, we can go a little

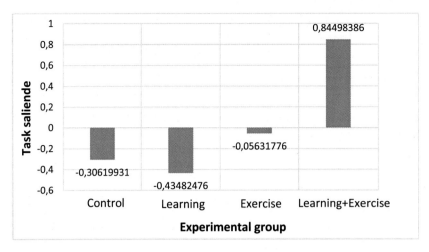

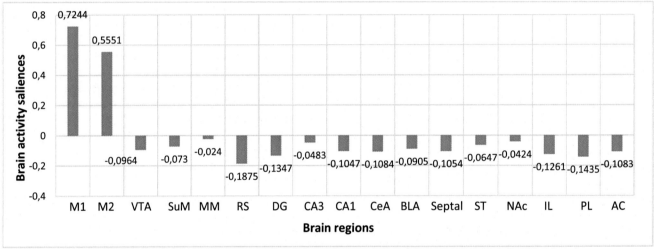

FIGURE 1.1   These figures represent the type of information that mean-centered task partial least squares correlation analysis can provide us. Through this analysis technique, we can obtain latent variables common to brain activity and the different experimental groups. As an example, a latent variable that allows the essential discrimination between learning + exercise group and control and learning groups is showed in graph 1. Graph 2 also shows saliences of the different considered brain structures, being the motor cortices the most important areas in this discrimination.

further in the analysis by using a multivariate perspective and incorporating techniques such as the multivariate analysis of variance (MANOVA) or the Discriminant analysis. Most of the studies about brain ageing consider that we should focus not only in a few particular brain regions, but in establishing functional networks by looking for the regions of which activity covariates during a specific task (Friston, 1994; Gerstein et al., 1978). Correlation-based techniques are the most commonly used and, as we usually work with a high number of brain regions implicated, the multivariate approach is preferable again. We can use applications of the structural equation modelling, like principal component analysis, multiple regression and canonical correlation (McIntosh and Gonzalez-Lima, 1994), or partial component analysis. In the last decades, the application of partial least squares (PLS) analysis of neuro-imaging data has gained a lot of popularity (Krishnan et al., 2011; McIntosh et al., 1996; Van Roon et al., 2014). PLS also form a part of structural equation modelling, but they avoid some of the typical issues associated to this field, such as collinearity, small sample size, high number of variables, or the presence of lost values. Because of that, they allow us to study associations between treatment groups and brain activity (Fig. 1.1). These analysis techniques have been spreading lately to animal model-based studies, in which early-expression markers of neuronal activation such as c-Fos or functional activity mapping are used (Sampedro-Piquero et al., 2014; Wheeler et al., 2013). Studies by Sampedro-Piquero et al. (2013) showed the benefits in neuronal metabolic activity of forced exercise in aged rats using Rotarod apparatus. Rats subjected to a 6-week exercise programme showed less energy consumption in brain regions associated to spatial reference memory, which has been related to a better performance in a spatial task (Sampedro-Piquero et al., 2013).

PHYSICAL ACTIVITY, COGNITIVE RESERVE, AND NEUROPLASTICITY: THREE ALLIES FOR SUCCESSFUL AGEING

Taking into account that loss of functional connectivity is a phenomenon attached to successful ageing, one wonders about possible interventions in elderly population in order to improve and maintain their brain health. Progress in the knowledge of Neurobiology of plasticity and in the maintenance of this process even in advanced ages has provoked a huge interest. Numerous studies target the design of intervention programmes favoring these neuroplasticity processes. For example, a single year of walking exercise caused an increase in the hippocampal volume (Erickson et al., 2013) as well as a shorter exercise programme (three 1-h sessions per week for 12 weeks) with a moderate intensity produced a cognitive improvement performance in an active old group versus the sedentary old group (Chapman et al., 2013). Exercise effects can impact cognitive functioning both in a global and in a specific manner, although executive functions are more positively affected after an exercise programme than other cognitive functions (Erickson et al., 2013).

Recent studies showed an improvement in functions such as working memory, processing speed, verbal fluency, and cognitive inhibition after an acute vigorous exercise programme (50 min on a stationary bicycle) (Basso et al., 2015). Nanda et al. (2013) established beneficial effects of exercise (30-min session of cycling on a stationary bicycle) in various cognitive domains like memory, planning or reasoning, but no concentration in an adult sample. Erickson et al. (2013) mentioned an improvement in executive functions in elderly people after an aerobic exercise programme. These executive functions encompass planning, scheduling, working memory, and inhibitory processes (Berchicci et al., 2013; Foster et al., 2011) and have special relevance in dairy activities. Therefore, their improvement make an impact in a positive way on aged population's life quality.

Ageing and ageing-related neuroplasticity phenomena have also been a prominent topic of interest in recent years, as positive neuroplasticity (Vance et al., 2012) can be observed during successful ageing (Bherer et al., 2013). Positive neuroplasticity is defined as an adaptive response to complex situations and contexts which avoids atrophy and functional loss of brain regions. Among the responses associated to this plasticity process are growth of stronger connections between neurons, axons elongation, and collateral ramifications growth (Foster et al., 2011). Naturally, positive neuroplasticity facilitates and promotes a bigger cognitive reserve, which in conclusion induces a maintenance or, at least, a delay in cognitive impairment and a better life quality.

Related to this type of plasticity, the study of neurogenesis becomes relevant. Neurogenesis is defined as the formation of new neurons from neural stem and progenitor cells which occurs in various brain regions such as the subgranular zone of dentate gyrus in the hippocampus and the subventricular zone of lateral ventricles. It has been observed that this neurogenetic process is favored by running programmes (Kempermann et al., 2010). Initially, one could guess that neurogenesis disappears in advanced ages, because there is a reduction in cognitive function. Nevertheless, studies in rodents have detected an increase in neurogenesis after exercise in the dentate gyrus both in aged and adult rats, which has been related to higher levels of BDNF in the hippocampus (Kempermann et al., 2010). Nouchi et al. (2014) found an enhancement in executive functions, episodic memory, and speed processing in successful ageing after a short exercise programme (4 week-long). Voss et al. (2010) assessed changes in functional connectivity after walking exercise for 12 months with functional magnetic resonance imaging (fMRI), and could distinguish three different networks: DMN, executive frontal network, and frontoparietal networks. In this study, they analyse the relationship between these changes in connectivity and performance in different tasks such as verbal short-term and executive functions, including task-switching, set-shifting, inhibition, and spatial working memory. After an aerobic exercise programme in older subjects, more efficiency has been observed in DMN and frontal executive network. This higher efficiency has positive repercussions in cognitive functioning, as DMN function is considered as an index of healthy cognitive ageing (Voss et al., 2010). Along these lines, work of Prakash et al. (2011) assesses the effects of cardiorespiratory fitness in the performance in a version of the Stroop task and in the recruitment of different brain regions. In this case, elders with higher fitness level showed an appropriate performance related to the recruitment of prefrontal and parietal areas. Moreover, it seems that fitness has more influence over anterior attentional control-related brain regions versus posterior processing areas (Prakash et al., 2011). Even imaginary exercise programmes based on, for example, imaging cycling uphill, induce activity in brain regions associated to movement, besides the activation of prefrontal regions related to executive control (Foster et al., 2011).

Finally, studies about different modalities of physical activity and their effects on cognitive functioning has been carried out in elderly population. Recent work establishes benefits of tango versus other dance styles in Parkinson's patients, although this study is performed in a small sample of people with moderate levels of Parkinson's disease-related impairments. It has been observed that a dance programme offers more benefits in march and balance, and even more if this dance style is tango (McNeely et al., 2015). It has also been shown that the previous performance of vigorous exercise leads to a reduction of Parkinson's disease symptoms emergence (Ahlskog, 2011), as happens with mild cognitive impairment and Alzheimer's disease (Foster et al., 2011; Swain et al., 2012). More recent studies about Tai Chi Chuan effects also indicated that this mind–body type of exercise could have beneficial outcomes in elders (Wei et al., 2014).Thus, most of the research in elderly population supports that promoting physical activity can have protective effects against cognitive deterioration. In conclusion, these results suggest that cognitive reserve and cerebral plasticity continue to be influenced by circumstances throughout the lifespan. Hence, any physical activity must be accomplished in order to maintain them as long as possible (Erickson et al., 2012; Llamas-Velasco et al., 2015).

MOLECULAR BASIS OF EXERCISE AND THE AGEING BRAIN

Regular physical activity is considered as an environmental stressor with positive effects on health as it increases the antioxidant genes expression, reduces inflammation, delays ageing, and protects against several ageing-related diseases (Ludlow et al., 2013). The molecular mechanisms that underlie the effects of exercise on the ageing process have become an issue of interest in recent years. The understanding of them may contribute to developing more specific and directed therapies in order to alleviate the symptoms of regular and pathological ageing.

Oxidative stress is a common cause of neurodegeneration because the high metabolic rates in the brain, so that neural tissues have higher levels than others of harmful agents result of cell metabolism, such as reactive oxygen species and reactive nitrogen species (Lee et al., 2015). Although exercise causes a moderate oxidative stress in cardiac and skeletal muscle due to an increased demand of energy and the consequent increased rate of mitochondrial activity (Sun et al., 2015), it also has positive systemic effects through neurogenesis; this happens by modulating neurotrophins like BDNF or nerve growth factor, elevating the angiogenesis rate and reducing the damage caused by oxidative stress (Lee et al., 2015). The expression of BDNF and circulating levels of BDNF are augmented in different brain regions in voluntary exercised individuals and cognitive impairment appears when BDNF action is artificially blocked (Huang et al., 2014). Thus, this neurotrophin seems to play a major role in the exercise effects on brain health, including proliferation, synaptic plasticity, cognitive reserve, and cell survival.

Telomeres are structural DNA elements located at the ends of linear chromosomes of which length is a hallmark of the ageing process (López-Otín et al., 2013). Their progressive shortening is implicated in regular ageing as a result of the combination of progressive cell replication and DNA-damaging agents such as ultraviolet radiation, inflammation, and oxidative stress, which promote the activation of cell senescence programmes (Blasco, 2007). Several studies have found a direct relationship between leukocyte telomere length and total brain volume (King et al., 2014) and hippocampal volume (Jacobs et al., 2014). Telomeres shortening has been associated to white matter hyperintensity and brain atrophy as well, two major hallmarks of neurodegeneration in ageing (Wikgren et al., 2014). A moderate amount of exercise throughout life plays a neuroprotective role through the stimulation (increased expression or activation) of telomere-associated proteins in immune cells, like telomerase and shelterin, which ultimately maintain telomeres length (Ludlow et al., 2013).

Regarding the immune function, exercise has an age-dependent effect on the inflammatory response, promoting antiinflammatory cytokines in young individuals and counteracting proinflammatory effects in the aged ones. Specifically, it has been observed in the hippocampus of 20-month-old rats an increase in TNF-α and IL-1β levels (proinflammatory cytokines associated with cognitive deficit) and a decrease in antiinflammatory cytokines, like IL-4. Physical activity could be blocking the inflammatory cascade in aged individuals, which ultimately leads to a higher susceptibility to changes in metabolism and cell death (Lovatel et al., 2013).

Another potential underlying mechanism of exercise benefits is the resilience to anxiety and stress. In relation to this, the hippocampus plays again a key role, because the exercise-associated modulation of glucocorticoid receptors (GRs) may be crucial to confront stressful events. Regular, moderate physical exercise seems to influence on stress response through increasing levels of GRs in the hippocampus, leading to an augmented inhibition on hypothalamus-pituitary-adrenal axis. These changes on stress response could be mediated via epigenetics, like downregulation of miR-124, an epigenetic inhibitor of the expression of GR gene, *Nr3c1* (Pan-Vazquez et al., 2015).

Acknowledgments

This work was supported by a grant from the National Ministry of Economy and Competitiveness of Spain PSI2013-42704P and by grants from NEUROCON (Excellence Group of Principality of Asturias).

References

Ahlskog, J.E., 2011. Does vigorous exercise have a neuroprotective effect in Parkinson disease? Neurology 77 (3), 288–294. http://dx.doi.org/10.1212/WNL.0b013e318225ab66.

Andrews-Hanna, J.R., Smallwood, J., Spreng, R.N., 2014. The default network and self-generated thought: component processes, dynamic control, and clinical relevance. Annals of the New York Academy of Sciences 1316 (1), 29–52. http://dx.doi.org/10.1111/nyas.12360.

Antonenko, D., Flöel, A., 2013. Healthy aging by staying selectively connected: a mini-review. Gerontology 60 (1), 3–9. http://dx.doi.org/10.1159/000354376.

Ballesteros, S., Kraft, E., Santana, S., Tziraki, C., 2015. Maintaining older brain functionality: a targeted review. Neuroscience & Biobehavioral Reviews 55, 453–477. http://dx.doi.org/10.1016/j.neubiorev.2015.06.008.

Bamidis, P.D., Vivas, A.B., Styliadis, C., Frantzidis, C., Klados, M., Schlee, W., et al., 2014. A review of physical and cognitive interventions in aging. Neuroscience & Biobehavioral Reviews 44, 206–220. http://dx.doi.org/10.1016/j.neubiorev.2014.03.019.

Bartko, S.J., Cowell, R.A., Winters, B.D., Bussey, T.J., Saksida, L.M., 2010. Heightened susceptibility to interference in an animal model of amnesia: impairment in encoding, storage, retrieval—or all three? Neuropsychologia 48 (10), 2987–2997. http://dx.doi.org/10.1016/j.neuropsychologia.2010.06.007.

Barulli, D., Stern, Y., 2013. Efficiency, capacity, compensation, maintenance, plasticity: emerging concepts in cognitive reserve. Trends in Cognitive Sciences 17 (10), 502–509. http://dx.doi.org/10.1016/j.tics.2013.08.012.

Basso, J.C., Shang, A., Elman, M., Karmouta, R., Suzuki, W.A., 2015. Acute exercise improves prefrontal cortex but not hippocampal function in healthy adults. Journal of the International Neuropsychological Society 21 (10), 791–801. http://dx.doi.org/10.1017/S135561771500106X.

Berchicci, M., Lucci, G., Di Russo, F., 2013. Benefits of physical exercise on the aging brain: the role of the prefrontal cortex. The Journals of Gerontology. Series A, Biological Sciences and Medical Sciences 68 (11), 1337–1341. http://dx.doi.org/10.1093/gerona/glt094.

Bherer, L., Erickson, K.I., Liu-Ambrose, T., 2013. A review of the effects of physical activity and exercise on cognitive and brain functions in older adults. Journal of Aging Research 2013 (657508). http://dx.doi.org/10.1155/2013/657508.

Blasco, M.A., 2007. Telomere length, stem cells and aging. Nature Chemical Biology 3 (10), 640–649. http://dx.doi.org/10.1038/nchembio.2007.38.

Campbell, K.L., Grigg, O., Saverino, C., Churchill, N., Grady, C.L., November 2013. Age differences in the intrinsic functional connectivity of default network subsystems. Frontiers in Aging Neuroscience 5, 1–12. http://dx.doi.org/10.3389/fnagi.2013.00073.

Cassilhas, R.C., Tufik, S., de Mello, M.T., 2015. Physical exercise, neuroplasticity, spatial learning and memory. Cellular and Molecular Life Sciences. http://dx.doi.org/10.1007/s00018-015-2102-0.

Chapman, S.B., Aslan, S., Spence, J.S., DeFina, L.F., Keebler, M.W., Didehbani, N., Lu, H., November 2013. Shorter term aerobic exercise improves brain, cognition, and cardiovascular fitness in aging. Frontiers in Aging Neuroscience 5, 1–9. http://dx.doi.org/10.3389/fnagi.2013.00075.

Charroud, C., Steffener, J., Le Bars, E., Deverdun, J., Bonafe, A., Abdennour, M., et al., 2015. Working memory activation of neural networks in the elderly as a function of information processing phase and task complexity. Neurobiology of Learning and Memory 125, 211–223. http://dx.doi.org/10.1016/j.nlm.2015.10.002.

Domenjoz, I., Kayser, B., Boulvain, M., 2014. Effect of physical activity during pregnancy on mode of delivery. American Journal of Obstetrics and Gynecology 211 (4), 401.e1–401.e11. http://dx.doi.org/10.1016/j.ajog.2014.03.030.

Erickson, K.I., Gildengers, A.G., Butters, M.A., 2013. Physical activity and brain plasticity in late adulthood. Dialogues in Clinical Neuroscience 15 (1), 99–108. http://dx.doi.org/10.4081/ar.2012.e6.

Erickson, K.I., Miller, D.L., Roecklein, K.A., 2012. The aging hippocampus: interactions between exercise, depression, and BDNF. Neuroscientist: A Review Journal Bringing Neurobiology, Neurology and Psychiatry 18 (1), 82–97. http://dx.doi.org/10.1177/1073858410397054.

Foster, P.P., Rosenblatt, K.P., Kulji, R.O., May 2011. Exercise-induced cognitive plasticity, implications for mild cognitive impairment and Alzheimer's disease. Frontiers in Neurology 1–15. http://dx.doi.org/10.3389/fneur.2011.00028.

Franco-Martin, M., Parra-Vidales, E., Gonzalez-Palau, F., Bernate-Navarro, M., Solis, A., 2013. Influencia del ejercicio físico en la prevención del deterioro cognitivo en las personas mayores: revisión sistemática. Revista de Neurologia 56 (11), 545–554. Retrieved from: http://www.ncbi.nlm.nih.gov/pubmed/23703056.

Friston, K.J., 1994. Functional and effective connectivity in neuroimaging: a synthesis. Human Brain Mapping 2 (1–2), 56–78.

Gerstein, G.L., Perkel, D.H., Subramanian, K.N., 1978. Identification of functionally related neural assemblies. Brain Research 140 (1), 43–62.

Gozzi, A., Schwarz, A.J., 2015. Large-scale functional connectivity networks in the rodent brain. NeuroImage. http://dx.doi.org/10.1016/j.neuroimage.2015.12.017.

Huang, T., Larsen, K.T., Ried-Larsen, M., Møller, N.C., Andersen, L.B., 2014. The effects of physical activity and exercise on brain-derived neurotrophic factor in healthy humans: a review. Scandinavian Journal of Medicine & Science in Sports 24 (1), 1–10. http://dx.doi.org/10.1111/sms.12069.

Jacobs, E.G., Epel, E.S., Lin, J., Blackburn, E.H., Rasgon, N.L., 2014. Relationship between leukocyte telomere length, telomerase activity, and hippocampal volume in early aging. JAMA Neurology 71 (7), 921–923. http://dx.doi.org/10.1001/jamaneurol.2014.870.

Jeong, W., Chung, C.K., Kim, J.S., August 2015. Episodic memory in aspects of large-scale brain networks. Frontiers in Human Neuroscience 9, 1–15. http://dx.doi.org/10.3389/fnhum.2015.00454.

Kempermann, G., Fabel, K., Ehninger, D., Babu, H., Leal-Galicia, P., Garthe, A., Wolf, S.A., December 2010. Why and how physical activity promotes experience-induced brain plasticity. Frontiers in Neuroscience 4, 1–9. http://dx.doi.org/10.3389/fnins.2010.00189.

King, K.S., Kozlitina, J., Rosenberg, R.N., Peshock, R.M., McColl, R.W., Garcia, C.K., 2014. Effect of leukocyte telomere length on total and regional brain volumes in a large population-based cohort. JAMA Neurology 71 (10), 1247–1254.

Krishnan, A., Williams, L.J., McIntosh, A.R., Abdi, H., 2011. Partial Least Squares (PLS) methods for neuroimaging: a tutorial and review. Neuroimage 56 (2), 455–475.

Latimer-Cheung, A.E., Pilutti, L.A., Hicks, A.L., Martin Ginis, K.A., Fenuta, A.M., MacKibbon, K.A., Motl, R.W., 2013. Effects of exercise training on fitness, mobility, fatigue, and health-related quality of life among adults with multiple sclerosis: a systematic review to inform guideline development. Archives of Physical Medicine and Rehabilitation 94 (9), 1800–1828.e3. http://dx.doi.org/10.1016/j.apmr.2013.04.020.

Lee, S., Park, S., Won, J., Lee, S., 2015. The incremental induction of neuroprotective properties by multiple therapeutic strategies for primary and secondary neural injury. International Journal of Molecular Sciences 16 (8), 19657–19670. http://dx.doi.org/10.3390/ijms160819657.

Llamas-Velasco, S., Contador, I., Villarejo-Galende, A., Lora-Pablos, D., Bermejo-Pareja, F., 2015. Physical activity as protective factor against Dementia: a prospective population-based study (NEDICES). Journal of the International Neuropsychological Society 21 (10), 861–867. http://dx.doi.org/10.1017/S1355617715000831.

López-Otín, C., Blasco, M.A., Partridge, L., Serrano, M., 2013. The hallmarks of aging. Cell 153(6), 1194–1217. http://dx.doi.org/10.1016/j.cell.2013.05.039.

Lovatel, G.A., Elsner, V.R., Bertoldi, K., Vanzella, C., Moysés, F., dos, S., Vizuete, A., et al., 2013. Treadmill exercise induces age-related changes in aversive memory, neuroinflammatory and epigenetic processes in the rat hippocampus. Neurobiology of Learning and Memory 101, 94–102. http://dx.doi.org/10.1016/j.nlm.2013.01.007.

Ludlow, A.T., Ludlow, L.W., Roth, S.M., 2013. Do telomeres adapt to physiological stress? Exploring the effect of exercise on telomere length and telomere-related proteins. BioMed Research International 2013. http://dx.doi.org/10.1155/2013/601368.

May, L.E., 2012. Effects of maternal exercise on labor and delivery. In: Physiology of Prenatal Exercise and Fetal Development. SpringerBriefs in Physiology, pp. 11–15. http://dx.doi.org/10.1007/978-1-4614-3408-5.

McIntosh, A.R., Bookstein, F.L., Haxby, J.V., Grady, C.L., 1996. Spatial pattern analysis of functional brain images using partial least squares. Neuroimage 3 (1), 143–157.

McIntosh, A.R., Gonzalez-Lima, F., 1994. Network interactions among limbic cortices, basal forebrain, and cerebellum differentiate a tone conditioned as a Pavlovian excitor or inhibitor: fluorodeoxyglucose mapping and covariance structural modeling. Journal of Neurophysiology 4, 1717–1733.

McNeely, M.E., Mai, M.M., Duncan, R.P., Earhart, G.M., December 2015. Differential effects of tango versus dance for PD in Parkinson disease. Frontiers in Aging Neuroscience 7, 1–8. http://dx.doi.org/10.3389/fnagi.2015.00239.

Munters, L.A., Alexanderson, H., Crofford, L.J., Lundberg, I.E., 2014. New insights into the benefits of exercise for muscle health in patients with idiopathic inflammatory myositis. Current Rheumatology Reports 16 (7), 1199–1216. http://dx.doi.org/10.1016/j.micinf.2011.07.011.Innate.

Nanda, B., Balde, J., Manjunatha, S., 2013. The acute effects of a single bout of moderate-intensity aerobic exercise on cognitive functions in healthy adult males. Journal of Clinical and Diagnostic Research 7 (9), 1883–1885.

Nouchi, R., Taki, Y., Takeuchi, H., Sekiguchi, A., Hashizume, H., Nozawa, T., Kawashima, R., 2014. Four weeks of combination exercise training improved executive functions, episodic memory, and processing speed in healthy elderly people: evidence from a randomized controlled trial. Age 36 (2), 787–799. http://dx.doi.org/10.1007/s11357-013-9588-x.

Pan-Vazquez, A., Rye, N., Ameri, M., McSparron, B., Smallwood, G., Bickerdyke, J., et al., 2015. Impact of voluntary exercise and housing conditions on hippocampal glucocorticoid receptor, miR-124 and anxiety. Molecular Brain 8 (1), 40. http://dx.doi.org/10.1186/s13041-015-0128-8.

Pedersen, L., Christensen, J.F., Hojman, P., 2015. Effects of exercise on tumor physiology and metabolism. Cancer Journal 21 (2), 111–116.

Persson, J., Pudas, S., Nilsson, L.-G., Nyberg, L., 2014. Longitudinal assessment of default-mode brain function in aging. Neurobiology of Aging 35 (9), 2107–2117. http://dx.doi.org/10.1016/j.neurobiolaging.2014.03.012.

Petersen, S., Posner, M., 2012. NIH public access. Annual Review of Neuroscience 21 (35), 73–89. http://dx.doi.org/10.1146/annurev-neuro-062111-150525.

Piepmeier, A.T., Etnier, J.L., 2014. Brain-derived neurotrophic factor (BDNF) as a potential mechanism of the effects of acute exercise on cognitive performance. Journal of Sport and Health Science 4 (1), 14–23. http://dx.doi.org/10.1016/j.jshs.2014.11.001.

Prakash, R.S., Voss, M.W., Erickson, K.I., Lewis, J.M., Chaddock, L., Malkowski, E., et al., January 2011. Cardiorespiratory fitness and attentional control in the aging brain. Frontiers in Human Neuroscience 4, 229. http://dx.doi.org/10.3389/fnhum.2010.00229.

Raichle, M.E., April 2015. The brain's default mode network. Annual Review of Neuroscience 413–427. http://dx.doi.org/10.1146/annurev-neuro-071013-014030.

Raineki, C., Hellemans, K.G.C., Bodnar, T., Lavigne, K.M., Ellis, L., Woodward, T.S., Weinberg, J., February 2014. Neurocircuitry underlying stress and emotional regulation in animals prenatally exposed to alcohol and subjected to chronic mild stress in adulthood. Frontiers in Endocrinology 5, 5. http://dx.doi.org/10.3389/fendo.2014.00005.

Sala-Llonch, R., Bartrés-Faz, D., Junqué, C., May 2015. Reorganization of brain networks in aging: a review of functional connectivity studies. Frontiers in Psychology 6, 663. http://dx.doi.org/10.3389/fpsyg.2015.00663.

Salthouse, T., 2012. Consequences of age-related cognitive declines. Annual Review of Psychology 63 (1), 201–226. http://dx.doi.org/10.1146/annurev-psych-120710-100328.

Salthouse, T.A., 2000. Aging and measures of processing speed. Biological Psychology 54 (1–3), 35–54. http://dx.doi.org/10.1016/S0301-0511(00)00052-1.

Sampedro-Piquero, P., Zancada-Menendez, C., Begega, A., Mendez, M., Arias, J.L., 2013. Effects of forced exercise on spatial memory and cytochrome c oxidase activity in aged rats. Brain Research 1502, 20–29. http://dx.doi.org/10.1016/j.brainres.2012.12.036.

Sampedro-Piquero, P., Zancada-Menendez, C., Cuesta, M., Arias, J.L., Begega, A., 2014. Metabolic brain activity underlying behavioral performance and spatial strategy choice in sedentary and exercised Wistar rats. Neuroscience 281C, 110–123. http://dx.doi.org/10.1016/j.neuroscience.2014.09.054.

Schuler, G., Adams, V., Goto, Y., 2013. Role of exercise in the prevention of cardiovascular disease: results, mechanisms, and new perspectives. European Heart Journal 34, 1790–1799. http://dx.doi.org/10.1093/eurheartj/eht111.

Stanford, K.I., Goodyear, L.J., 2014. Exercise and type 2 diabetes: molecular mechanisms regulating glucose uptake in skeletal muscle. Advances in Physiology Education 38 (4), 308–314. http://dx.doi.org/10.1152/advan.00080.2014.

Stern, Y., 2002. What is cognitive reserve? Theory and research application of the reserve concept. Journal of the International Neuropsychological Society: JINS 8 (3), 448–460. http://dx.doi.org/10.1017/S1355617702813248.

Sun, Y., Qi, Z., He, Q., Cui, D., Qian, S., Ji, L., Ding, S., 2015. The effect of treadmill training and N-acetyl-l-cysteine intervention on biogenesis of cytochrome c oxidase (COX). Free Radical Biology and Medicine 87, 326–335. http://dx.doi.org/10.1016/j.freeradbiomed.2015.06.035.

Swain, R., Berggren, K., Kerr, A., Patel, A., Peplinski, C., Sikorski, A., 2012. On aerobic exercise and behavioral and neural plasticity. Brain Sciences 2. http://dx.doi.org/10.3390/brainsci2040709.

Van Roon, P., Zakizadeh, J., Chartier, S., 2014. Partial Least Squares tutorial for analyzing neuroimaging data. The Quantitative Methods for Psychology 10 (2), 200–215.

Vance, D.E., Kaur, J., Fazeli, P.L., Talley, M.H., Yuen, H.K., Kitchin, B., Lin, F., 2012. Neuroplasticity and successful cognitive aging: a brief overview for nursing. The Journal of Neuroscience Nursing: Journal of the American Association of Neuroscience Nurses 44 (4). http://dx.doi.org/10.1097/JNN.0b013e3182527571.

Vidal-Piñeiro, D., Valls-Pedret, C., Fernandez-Cabello, S., Arenaza-Urquijo, E.M., Sala-Llonch, R., Solana, E., et al., September 2014. Decreased Default Mode Network connectivity correlates with age-associated structural and cognitive changes. Frontiers in Aging Neuroscience 6, 1–17. http://dx.doi.org/10.3389/fnagi.2014.00256.

Voss, M.W., Prakash, R.S., Erickson, K.I., Basak, C., Chaddock, L., Kim, J.S., et al., August 2010. Plasticity of brain networks in a randomized intervention trial of exercise training in older adults. Frontiers in Aging Neuroscience 2, 1–17. http://dx.doi.org/10.3389/fnagi.2010.00032.

Wei, G.-X., Dong, H.-M., Yang, Z., Luo, J., Zuo, X.-N., April 2014. Tai Chi Chuan optimizes the functional organization of the intrinsic human brain architecture in older adults. Frontiers in Aging Neuroscience 6, 1–10. http://dx.doi.org/10.3389/fnagi.2014.00074.

Wenger, N.K., 2014. Prevention of cardiovascular disease: highlights for the clinician of the 2013 American College of Cardiology/American Heart Association guidelines. Clinical Cardiology 37 (4), 239–251. http://dx.doi.org/10.1002/clc.22264.

Wheeler, A.L., Teixeira, C.M., Wang, A.H., Xiong, X., Kovacevic, N., Lerch, J.P., et al., 2013. Identification of a functional connectome for long-term fear memory in mice. PLoS Computational Biology 9 (1). http://dx.doi.org/10.1371/journal.pcbi.1002853.

Wikgren, M., Karlsson, T., Soderlund, H., Nordin, A., Roos, G., Nilsson, L.-G., et al., 2014. Shorter telomere length is linked to brain atrophy and white matter hyperintensities. Age and Ageing 43 (2), 212–217. http://dx.doi.org/10.1093/ageing/aft172.

Zhou, S., Fan, J., Lee, T.M.C., Wang, C., Wang, K., 2011. Age-related differences in attentional networks of alerting and executive control in young, middle-aged, and older Chinese adults. Brain and Cognition 75 (2), 205–210. http://dx.doi.org/10.1016/j.bandc.2010.12.003.

2

Exercise and the Developing Brain in Children and Adolescents

M.M. Herting, M.F. Keenan

Children's Hospital Los Angeles, Los Angeles, CA, United States

Abstract

Using the advances of magnetic resonance imaging, it is now known that the brain continues to undergo foundational development across childhood and adolescence. Critically, it seems that exercise, especially earlier on in this period of growth, may be an asset in building healthier brains. Here we review the studies that have examined how exercise relates to neurodevelopment in children and adolescents, as well as discuss the remaining questions regarding how to build a better brain through exercise.

MEASURING PHYSICAL ACTIVITY LEVELS AND AEROBIC FITNESS IN YOUTH

Assessing aerobic fitness in humans can be challenging. One common way to assess exercise in humans is to use self-report methods, such as a questionnaire, to determine the type and frequency of exercise (Armstrong and van Mechelen, 2008). The strengths of this method are that it is low in cost and subject burden; however, this method is limited by its subjective nature and that it may be influenced by the opinion and perception of the participant. Qualitatively speaking, young children are not always great at estimating time (e.g., estimating how many hours they may have walked or played this week). Thus, while self-reports of frequency and duration of aerobic activity levels can be used to assess the amount of exercise a subject may have performed over a given period of time, self-report of exercise tends to only modestly predict aerobic fitness level in children and adolescents (Morrow and Freedson, 1994). To this end, an objective method of exercise is also necessary when studying the effects of exercise. Two commonly used methods include actigraphy and maximal oxygen uptake during aerobic testing (known as VO_2max). Actigraphy is a noninvasive approach to measure active and resting periods of an individual. It usually includes wearing a 3D accelerometer or actimetry sensor on the body (nondominant arm or waist) for approximately 1 week. Wake-time estimates can then be used to gage activity levels in the individual. However, one limitation of this technique is that the type of physical activity (aerobic, nonaerobic, etc.) cannot be inferred from this data. On the other hand, maximal oxygen uptake (VO_2max) testing measures an individual's aerobic capacity. VO_2max testing assesses the highest rate of oxygen consumption by an individual during exercise and can ultimately determine an individual's ability to perform aerobic exercise (Armstrong and van Mechelen, 2008). This method is conceived as a relatively strong indicator of one's aerobic fitness because VO_2max values are seen to increase with aerobic training. Thus, much of the current literature in the field relies on this measure of aerobic fitness. In the current chapter, we review a number of studies that have shown how aerobic exercise relates to brain structure, white matter connectivity, brain function, and cognition in children and adolescents.

BRAIN DEVELOPMENT AS MEASURED BY MAGNETIC RESONANCE IMAGING (MRI)

With the advances of MRI, it is now possible to examine the shape, size, and even brain activity patterns to assess how the brain functions. Structural and functional MRI, as their names imply, examines tissue composition and brain activation in response to stimuli, respectively. In addition, white matter tractography and diffusion tensor imaging (DTI) examine connections (and the coherence of those connections) between different brain regions. Using these techniques, it is currently known that both the structure and function of the brain continues to mature well into the third decade of life. During childhood and adolescence, there are dynamic changes in both gray and white matter volumes (Giedd et al., 1999; Sowell et al., 2004), reflecting changes in cell bodies, cell number, and the amount of myelination coating cellular axons, respectively. Structural MRI studies have shown that gray matter volumes and the thickness of the cortical ribbon demonstrate an inverted U-shape pattern throughout development. Both the volume and thickness values increase during childhood, peak in early adolescence, and then decrease before stabilizing in adulthood (Giedd et al., 1999; Giedd, 2004). Subcortical limbic regions are important for emotion, such as the amygdala and hippocampus, also undergo significant development during this time (Giedd et al., 1996).

Patterns of brain activation also change with age across development. DTI examines the microstructural properties of white matter by measuring the restriction of water diffusion (Basser, 1995). This method is used to study the coherency of a tract, as measured by variables known as fractional anisotropy (FA), as well as estimation of white matter fiber tracts using tractography. DTI studies in children and adolescence show that the microstructural properties of white matter continue to develop, as indexed by higher FA values with age. These findings are thought to reflect the increases in myelination and/or larger neuronal axon diameters, allowing for faster processing of information along the axon of the brain cells and between the brain cells.

Lastly, brain activity can be assessed using functional MRI, which measures the changes in the use of oxygenated blood by brain regions (e.g., the magnitude and the extent of brain activation) across various task conditions (Huettel et al., 2009). Task examples include reading and math, holding information in memory and manipulating that information (known as working memory), and inhibiting responses. Overall, the changes that occur both structurally and functionally during development are thought to contribute to a more productive and efficient brain, underlying the cognitive milestones that are seen from childhood to adulthood (e.g., improvements in cognitive abilities, such as working memory, attention, and inhibition) (Casey et al., 2000).

Given that the brain is undergoing significant neurodevelopment, it is thought that the brain may be especially sensitive to internal and external conditions of the rearing environment. From a number of initial studies, it seems that physical activity, and especially a child's aerobic fitness, may be a particularly important factor in brain development across childhood and adolescence.

AEROBIC EXERCISE AND BRAIN STRUCTURE

Gray Matter

The main metrics for studying gray matter using MRI are cortical thickness, surface area, and volumes of cortical and subcortical brain regions. Cortical thickness is a measurement of the cortical ribbon, as defined as the distance between white matter and pial surfaces at each voxel; surface area, on the other hand, is defined as the area of the exposed cortical pial surface and hidden area of cortex within the sulci (Dale, 1999; Fischl et al., 2002; Fischl et al., 2004). While related, cortical volume, thickness, and surface area are unique metrics, showing distinct relationships with cellular, biological, and evolutionary (Raznahan et al., 2011). Early MRI studies of aging adults found increases in regional gray matter volume in the frontal, parietal, and temporal lobes following a 6-month aerobic exercise intervention in older adults (ages 60–79 years) (Colcombe et al., 2006). The frontal and parietal regions are shown to undergo significant maturation during late childhood and adolescence and are vital for attention, cognitive control, and learning and memory (Casey et al., 2000). Thus, it was thought likely that physical activity and aerobic fitness may also influence gray matter development in these brain regions in children and adolescents. To date, only two studies have examined exercise and cortical gray matter development in children and adolescents. Chaddock and colleagues examined 25 high-fit (defined as >70th percentile VO_2max) and 30-lower-fit (<30th percentile VO_2max) children. Despite differences in subcortical volumes (see below), higher- and lower-fit children were surprisingly found to have similar total gray matter volumes (Chaddock et al., 2010a). However, we have completed a more recent study in examining how aerobic exercise is measured by VO_2max related to gray matter volume and cortical surface area in adolescent males. We found that greater aerobic fitness (VO_2max) predicted larger left middle prefrontal cortex volumes. In addition, higher-fit adolescents had larger left precuneus and right occipital surface areas compared to their lower aerobically fit peers.

Subcortical Gray Matter

Beyond cortical gray matter, exercise-related brain research in all age ranges has largely focused on the basal ganglia and hippocampal volumes. These subcortical brain regions lie ventral to cortical gray and white matter, within the midbrain region. The basal ganglia is a set of structures at the base of the forebrain associated with procedural learning, emotions, voluntary movement, and cognition. Within the basal ganglia is the caudate nucleus, also known as the dorsal striatum; this structure is known for its association with voluntary movement, but has recently also been linked with learning. Located within the medial temporal lobe, the hippocampus is known to control emotion and memory functions. This focus of the influence of exercise on these subcortical regions has largely stemmed from a number of rodent studies showing that aerobic exercise (from wheel-running) leads to a new cell growth in the hippocampus (Uysal et al., 2005) and changes in the motor systems which includes portions of the basal ganglia (Black et al., 1990). Interestingly, translational studies in humans have been able to replicate these associations. For example, Chaddock et al. (2010b) examined a cohort of 9–10-year-old-boys and girls and grouped them into higher-fit and lower-fit categories (again based on VO_2max). Both groups completed structural MRIs to compare relative ventral (nucleus accumbens and olfactory tubercle) and dorsal (caudate and putamen) striatum volumes, as well as performance on a flanker task, which measures the selective attention, interference control, and action monitoring. Both ventral and dorsal striatum volumes and task performance were different between the groups. High-fit children demonstrated superior flanker task performance and had larger dorsal striatum volumes and globus pallidus volumes, which negatively correlated with interference control (Chaddock et al., 2010b).

Two similar types of studies have also shown the association between exercise and hippocampus translates to human children and adolescents. In a similar study design, Chaddock et al. examined 10-year-old preadolescent youths, the high-fit group (VO_2max) demonstrated larger bilateral hippocampal volumes as well as superior performance on a relational memory task (Chaddock et al., 2010a). Herting and Nagel (2012) later found similar results among adolescent males (15–18 years). Greater aerobic fitness (VO_2max) was found to predict better performance on a spatial learning and visuospatial memory task (virtual Morris Water maze) as well as larger bilateral hippocampal volume (Herting and Nagel, 2012). However, no relationship was found between aerobic fitness and memory recall on the water maze task, suggesting aerobic fitness may contribute more to the encoding of new memories rather than simply improving the recollection of memories.

White Matter Microstructure Using DTI

Properties of white matter may also be impacted by aerobic exercise in youth. To our knowledge, three studies have examined how aerobic fitness relates to white matter microstructure. Using tractography, lower aerobic fitness was found to relate to higher FA values in a left motor tract known as the corticospinal tract (Herting et al., 2014). In addition, lower-fit teen boys showed fewer streamlines, especially in this motor pathway, as well as an additional pathway that connects to the prefrontal cortex. Together, smaller streamlines, but high FA values, for the corticospinal white matter pathway may suggest lower aerobic fitness levels during adolescence may lead to less structural connectivity (i.e., axonal connections), ultimately requiring increased myelin or axonal caliber in order to compensate. Longitudinal studies are warranted to confirm such cause and effect hypotheses. However, these findings provide support that aerobic exercise relates to white matter structural connectivity in motor and prefrontal circuitry in adolescents.

The second DTI study published on aerobic fitness and white matter in youth examined FA in higher- versus lower-fit 9- and 10-year-old children. In contrast to the adolescent data, higher-fit children were found to have higher FA values in sections of the corpus callosum, corona radiata, and superior longitudinal fasciculus compared to lower-fit children (Chaddock-Heyman et al., 2014). A third study performed an 8-month-long longitudinal intervention in overweight 8–11-year-old children (Schaeffer et al., 2014). Among the 10 children who completed the intervention, increases were found in FA in the white matter pathway connecting the prefrontal cortex and temporal lobes. The descrepancy between high versus low FA values in higher-fit children and adolescents may be due to a number of reasons, including different methodology. However, given that white matter pathways continue to undergo developmental changes (such as increased myelination between childhood, adolescence, and in the 20s), it is feasible that the results from these cross-sectional studies reflect the possibility that exercise may influence the brain in a unique way(s) based on the individual's stage of development. That is, the influence of exercise on the brain may be largest for those regions undergoing the most substantial changes at the time in which the exercising occurs. Alternatively, it is also feasible that the effects of exercise are additive, such that the associations between exercise and the adolescent brain may reflect previous effects of exercise during childhood as well as exercise's current effects during the teenage years. Again, the few studies that have been completed were either in just children or just adolescents, and therefore, that cannot address these possibilities. Further longitudinal studies are needed following children and their exercise habits from childhood through adolescence and into adulthood. Nonetheless, taken together, these DTI studies suggest that white matter microstructure may be an additional mechanism as to which aerobic exercise may benefit the brain efficiency and function in children and adolescents.

AEROBIC EXERCISE AND BRAIN ACTIVITY

Executive Functions

In addition to the influencing brain structure, many studies have found a relationship between aerobic exercise and brain function, such as improved executive functioning or memory. To compare executive function, studies can use tasks that measure an individual's ability to inhibit certain responses or manipulate information to solve problems. One such study examined inhibition of responses in higher-fit and lower-fit children (9 and 10-years-old) (Chaddock et al., 2012a). They found that the higher-fit children maintained accuracy on more demanding inhibition trials across the entire task, whereas the lower-fit children showed poorer performance in the latter part of the task. In addition, the higher-fit children exhibited increased activation in prefrontal and parietal brain regions at the beginning of the task, but this activity was reduced as the task went on. In contrast, lower-fit children activated prefrontal and parietal regions to the same degree across the entire task. These findings suggest that higher-fit children are able to better modulate their brain activity to maintain their ability to do well on challenging tasks as compared to their lower-fit peers. Another study that included a 3-month exercise intervention in overweight 7–10-year-old found increases in math performance and executive control, measured by a Planning scale (Davis et al., 2011). In addition, the children who underwent the 3-month exercise program exhibited increased activation of the left and right prefrontal cortex and decreased posterior parietal cortex activation. Similar findings were also seen in children following a 9-month physical activity intervention with better performance on an attentional inhibition task and decreased prefrontal cortex activity while completing the task as compared to children who did not receive the physical fitness intervention (Hillman et al., 2014). Lastly, a third exercise intervention study in 8–11-year-old overweight children found decreased patterns of brain activation on one inhibition task known as the antisaccade task, but increased activation to the anterior cingulate cortex and the superior frontal cortex on another inhibition task (Krafft et al., 2014). The differences to what degree of exercise relates to increase or decrease in brain activation suggests more research is needed to clarify why and how exercise is influencing the brain to process these various cognitive tasks.

Learning and Memory

The link between exercise and hippocampal structure generated a great interest in determining a possible association between aerobic fitness and hippocampal activation while learning new memories in youth. One way to assess the role of the hippocampus in learning and memory is using the "subsequent memory effect paradigm"(Kim, 2011). This task requires the subjects to learn random word-pairings in the scanner and then complete a subsequent memory task after a delay. Higher- and lower-fit adolescent male youth completed this paradigm while their brains were scanned (Herting and Nagel, 2013). The imaging results were analyzed to compare brain activation when word pairs were learned correctly versus when learning was unsuccessful (i.e., later forgotten). The results showed that despite equivalent task performance lower-fit adolescent boys showed greater hippocampal activity as compared to their high-active peers, suggesting the hippocampus might have to work harder to learn new information in the lower-fit group. Moreover, the lower-fit adolescents also failed to turn-off "default" brain regions that are essential for the brain to more easily focus on goal-directed tasks, such as learning something new (Herting and Nagel, 2013). These findings suggest that aerobic activity during adolescence may be necessary to allow efficient brain function while learning something new.

Together, both the executive control and learning-related fMRI studies suggest that aerobic exercise may influence the modulation of neural circuitry in children and adolescents. Thus, in addition to exercise being beneficial for a child's lungs and heart, it seems that aerobic exercise may also greatly improve on how their brain works.

AEROBIC EXERCISE AND COGNITION

Both cross-sectional and intervention studies have found aerobic exercise to influence a better performance on cognitive tasks in children and adolescents.

Some of the first reports of physical activity levels and cognition in children showed a positive relationship between activity levels and measurements of scholastic performance, such as mathematic and reading achievement (Sibley and Etnier, 2003; Castelli et al., 2007). Only within the past decade and a half has been an impetus to further examine how exercise impacts more on direct measures of cognition in children, with most studies focusing on executive measures of attention and cognitive control or inhibition (Sibley and Etnier, 2003; Hillman et al., 2005; Buck et al., 2008; Hillman et al., 2009; Stroth et al., 2009; Pontifex et al., 2010; Voss et al., 2011; Chaddock et al., 2012a).

As previously mentioned, aerobic exercise has been found to relate to improved performance on executive function tasks, including attention and inhibition (Chaddock et al., 2011a; Voss et al., 2011; Chaddock et al., 2012b), as well as better learning and memory in children (Chaddock et al., 2010a, 2011a) and adolescents (Herting and Nagel, 2012). Moreover, within the realm of learning and memory, it seems as if the influence of exercise might be especially relevant to hippocampal-dependent processes. In one study, Chaddock and colleagues (Chaddock et al., 2010a) examined memory performance for novel visual stimuli between higher- and lower-fit children. The novel visual stimuli were presented to participants using a relational (learning and recognizing visual triplets) or item-based paradigm (learning individual stimuli and recognizing them as either old or new). The results showed that lower-fit participants displayed a trend towards poorer performance on the material encoded relationally, though no differences were seen for item-based memory performance. A similar study was published by the same researchers, examining relational versus nonrelational encoding and recognition memory of face and house stimuli pairs (Chaddock et al., 2011a). Again, lower-fit individuals performed worse for recognition memory of house and face pairs encoded relationally, whereas no group differences were seen in performance on the nonrelational memory condition. Similarly, spatial associative memory, but not verbal memory, was found to relate to aerobic exercise in male adolescents (Herting and Nagel, 2012). These findings suggest that aerobic exercise may be especially important for specific processes within learning and remembering information.

REMAINING QUESTIONS AND FUTURE DIRECTIONS

While the initial findings from these studies seem promising, more research is needed in order to know what exercise and physical activity recommendations should be given to children and adolescents with respect to optimizing the influence of exercise on brain development.

First, these are the basic studies to examine how aerobic exercise influences the child and adolescent brain and behavior. As such, some of the findings are limited due to the cross-sectional nature of the data. To address this issue, the FITKids (through the University of Illinois–Urbana) and Active Brains Project (University of Toronto) are the two clinical exercise intervention studies that have been created to try and to show the effects (rather than just the associations) of aerobic exercise on brain and behavior in children. Initial findings from the FITKids study show that this is indeed a promising avenue for this line of investigation and that some of the cross-sectional brain activation findings do change with exercise. However, additional longitudinal experimental intervention studies are needed to determine more direct causal effects of aerobic exercise on brain structure and function.

Second, more research is needed to determine the dose–response relationships between aerobic fitness (e.g., frequency, duration) and brain structure and function. That is, additional longitudinal intervention studies are needed to concretely answer how often and for how long children and adolescents should exercise to benefit their brains. Moreover, although most of the studies to date have really focused on the aerobic component of exercise, more recently it has been found that nonaerobic benefits of exercise may also help to explain the relationships seen between exercise and brain structure and function. That is, changes occur to muscle, agility, and balance with both aerobic and nonaerobic exercise. These nonaerobic physiological processes may exert their own influences on the brain and behavior. In fact, resistance training and endurance factors have recently been shown to have similar benefits on spatial memory and neurogenesis as aerobic exercise in rodents, but are thought to do so through distinct physiological pathways (Kobilo et al., 2011; Cassilhas et al., 2012). Thus, studies are needed to determine how both aerobic and nonaerobic aspects of exercise may benefit the brain in youths.

Third, the cross-sectional child and adolescent studies have both found some similarities and differences in the effects of exercise. Beyond different samples and methods, these differences could also be due to exercises having different effects based on what brain processes are undergoing development at the time in which exercise occurs.

For example, a metaanalysis has shown age to moderate the effect sizes seen between aerobic exercise and cognition, with larger effect sizes for high school- and college-aged samples compared to studies in children and the elderly (Etnier et al., 1997). If future research supports these findings that suggest exercise has a larger effect during adolescence as compared to childhood, it will be important to disentangle the possible additive effects of exercise that may arise from childhood, as well as those solely related to aerobic exercise training during adolescence. This idea has yet to be fully examined, but preliminary research has found that aerobic fitness level and larger hippocampal volumes in 9–10-year-old predict spatial short-term memory performance (3s delayed match-to-sample) 1 year later (Chaddock et al., 2011b). These findings lend support for the idea that aerobic fitness could have lasting effects on the brain and behavior. If this is true, exercises performed during childhood may contribute to the positive relationships seen in adolescents, as well as later on during adulthood and even aging. Thus, future research is needed to directly test aerobic exercise effects on the brain and cognition using intervention studies during each developmental period, as well as longitudinal studies to capture if these effects endure across the lifespan.

Lastly, while there is strong evidence suggesting that exercise benefits the brain health in individuals of many ages, more research is needed to determine how exercise programs may benefit children and adolescents with cognitive or learning deficits. For example, attention deficit hyperactivity disorder (ADHD) is a widespread developmental disorder that is characterized by deficits in executive functioning processes, and can impede a child's development in social and scholastic settings (Barkley, 1997). However, a recent study examined brain waves using electroencephalogram (EEG) in preadolescent children with ADHD after exposure to an aerobic exercise intervention program (Huang et al., 2014). Children in the exercise intervention group did 40 min of aerobic exercise (achieving 50–60% maximal heart rate) and then 40 min of perceptual-motor exercises twice a week for 8 weeks. The control group abstained from aerobic exercise. Children in the exercise condition had changes in their brain waves from frontal and central regions relative to the control group. While the literature on aerobic interventions with behavioral outcome measures is varied and limited, these recent EEG findings suggest additional studies are needed to understand how aerobic exercise may influence the neural pathways that underlie the cognitive difficulties associated with ADHD.

SUMMARY

In conclusion, exercise during childhood and adolescents may have important consequences on the development of the brain and cognition. A few studies suggest that there is much to be gained by pursuing how exercise may benefit the brain of today's youth. As such, these findings may especially be important to consider by the education system and policymakers who strive to improve the way children learn, as it seems exercise through physical education and/or extracurricular avenues may be vital in helping maximize the development of each individual's cognitive capabilities and future success.

References

Armstrong, N., van Mechelen, W., 2008. Paediatric Exercise Science and Medicine. Oxford University Press Inc., New York.

Barkley, R.A., 1997. Behavioral inhibition, sustained attention, and executive functions: constructing a unifying theory of ADHD. Psychological Bulletin 121 (1), 65–94.

Basser, P.J., 1995. Inferring microstructural features and the physiological state of tissues from diffusion-weighted images. NMR in Biomedicine 8 (7–8), 333–344.

Black, J.E., Isaacs, K.R., Anderson, B.J., Alcantara, A.A., Greenough, W.T., 1990. Learning causes synaptogenesis, whereas motor activity causes angiogenesis, in cerebellar cortex of adult rats. Proceedings of the National Academy of Sciences of the United States of America 87 (14), 5568–5572.

Buck, S.M., Hillman, C.H., Castelli, D.M., 2008. The relation of aerobic fitness to stroop task performance in preadolescent children. Medicine & Science in Sports & Exercise 40 (1), 166–172.

Casey, B.J., Giedd, J.N., Thomas, K.M., 2000. Structural and functional brain development and its relation to cognitive development. Biological Psychology 54 (1–3), 241–257.

Cassilhas, R.C., Lee, K.S., Fernandes, J., Oliveira, M.G., Tufik, S., Meeusen, R., de Mello, M.T., 2012. Spatial memory is improved by aerobic and resistance exercise through divergent molecular mechanisms. Neuroscience 202, 309–317.

Castelli, D.M., Hillman, C.H., Buck, S.M., Erwin, H.E., 2007. Physical fitness and academic achievement in third- and fifth-grade students. Journal of Sport and Exercise Psychology 29 (2), 239–252.

Chaddock, L., Erickson, K.I., Prakash, R.S., Kim, J.S., Voss, M.W., Vanpatter, M., Pontifex, M.B., Raine, L.B., Konkel, A., Hillman, C.H., Cohen, N.J., Kramer, A.F., 2010a. A neuroimaging investigation of the association between aerobic fitness, hippocampal volume, and memory performance in preadolescent children. Brain Research 1358, 172–183.

Chaddock, L., Erickson, K.I., Prakash, R.S., VanPatter, M., Voss, M.W., Pontifex, M.B., Raine, L.B., Hillman, C.H., Kramer, A.F., 2010b. Basal ganglia volume is associated with aerobic fitness in preadolescent children. Developmental Neuroscience 32 (3), 249–256.

Chaddock, L., Erickson, K.I., Prakash, R.S., Voss, M.W., VanPatter, M., Pontifex, M.B., Hillman, C.H., Kramer, A.F., 2012a. A functional MRI investigation of the association between childhood aerobic fitness and neurocognitive control. Biological Psychology 89 (1), 260–268.

Chaddock, L., Hillman, C.H., Buck, S.M., Cohen, N.J., 2011a. Aerobic fitness and executive control of relational memory in preadolescent children. Medicine & Science in Sports & Exercise 43 (2), 344–349.

Chaddock, L., Hillman, C.H., Pontifex, M.B., Johnson, C.R., Raine, L.B., Kramer, A.F., 2012b. Childhood aerobic fitness predicts cognitive performance one year later. Journal of Sports Science and Medicine 30 (5), 421–430.

Chaddock, L., Pontifex, M.B., Hillman, C.H., Kramer, A.F., 2011b. A review of the relation of aerobic fitness and physical activity to brain structure and function in children. Journal of the International Neuropsychological Society 17 (6), 975–985.

Chaddock-Heyman, L., Erickson, K.I., Holtrop, J.L., Voss, M.W., Pontifex, M.B., Raine, L.B., Hillman, C.H., Kramer, A.F., 2014. Aerobic fitness is associated with greater white matter integrity in children. Frontiers in Human Neuroscience 8, 584.

Colcombe, S.J., Erickson, K.I., Scalf, P.E., Kim, J.S., Prakash, R., McAuley, E., Elavsky, S., Marquez, D.X., Hu, L., Kramer, A.F., 2006. Aerobic exercise training increases brain volume in aging humans. The Journals of Gerontology. Series A 61 (11), 1166–1170.

Dale, A.M., 1999. Optimal experimental design for event-related fMRI. Human Brain Mapping 8 (2–3), 109–114.

Davis, C.L., Tomporowski, P.D., McDowell, J.E., Austin, B.P., Miller, P.H., Yanasak, N.E., Allison, J.D., Naglieri, J.A., 2011. Exercise improves executive function and achievement and alters brain activation in overweight children: a randomized, controlled trial. Health Psychology 30 (1), 91–98.

Etnier, J.L., Salazar, W., Landers, D.M., Petruzzello, S.J., Han, M., Nowell, P., 1997. The influence of physical fitness and exercise upon cognitive functioning: a meta-analysis. Journal of Sport and Exercise Psychology 19, 249–277.

Fischl, B., Salat, D.H., Busa, E., Albert, M., Dieterich, M., Haselgrove, C., van der Kouwe, A., Killiany, R., Kennedy, D., Klaveness, S., Montillo, A., Makris, N., Rosen, B., Dale, A.M., 2002. Whole brain segmentation: automated labeling of neuroanatomical structures in the human brain. Neuron 33 (3), 341–355.

Fischl, B., van der Kouwe, A., Destrieux, C., Halgren, E., Segonne, F., Salat, D.H., Busa, E., Seidman, L.J., Goldstein, J., Kennedy, D., Caviness, V., Makris, N., Rosen, B., Dale, A.M., 2004. Automatically parcellating the human cerebral cortex. Cerebral Cortex 14 (1), 11–22.

Giedd, J.N., 2004. Structural magnetic resonance imaging of the adolescent brain. Annals of New York Academy of Sciences 1021, 77–85.

Giedd, J.N., Blumenthal, J., Jeffries, N.O., Castellanos, F.X., Liu, H., Zijdenbos, A., Paus, T., Evans, A.C., Rapoport, J.L., 1999. Brain development during childhood and adolescence: a longitudinal MRI study. Nature Neuroscience 2 (10), 861–863.

Giedd, J.N., Vaituzis, A.C., Hamburger, S.D., Lange, N., Rajapakse, J.C., Kaysen, D., Vauss, Y.C., Rapoport, J.L., 1996. Quantitative MRI of the temporal lobe, amygdala, and hippocampus in normal human development: ages 4–18 years. Journal of Comparitive Neurology 366 (2), 223–230.

Herting, M.M., Colby, J.B., Sowell, E.R., Nagel, B.J., 2014. White matter connectivity and aerobic fitness in male adolescents. Developmental Cognitive Neuroscience 7, 65–75.

Herting, M.M., Nagel, B.J., 2012. Aerobic fitness relates to learning on a virtual Morris Water Task and hippocampal volume in adolescents. Behavioural Brain Research 233 (2), 517–525.

Herting, M.M., Nagel, B.J., 2013. Differences in brain activity during a verbal associative memory encoding task in high- and low-fit adolescents. Journal of Cognitive Neuroscience 25 (4), 595–612.

Hillman, C.H., Buck, S.M., Themanson, J.R., Pontifex, M.B., Castelli, D.M., 2009. Aerobic fitness and cognitive development: event-related brain potential and task performance indices of executive control in preadolescent children. Developmental Psychology 45 (1), 114–129.

Hillman, C.H., Castelli, D.M., Buck, S.M., 2005. Aerobic fitness and neurocognitive function in healthy preadolescent children. Medicine & Science in Sports & Exercise 37 (11), 1967–1974.

Hillman, C.H., Pontifex, M.B., Castelli, D.M., Khan, N.A., Raine, L.B., Scudder, M.R., Drollette, E.S., Moore, R.D., Wu, C.T., Kamijo, K., 2014. Effects of the FITKids randomized controlled trial on executive control and brain function. Pediatrics 134 (4), e1063–e1071.

Huang, C.J., Huang, C.W., Tsai, Y.J., Tsai, C.L., Chang, Y.K., Hung, T.M., 2014. A preliminary examination of aerobic exercise effects on resting EEG in children with ADHD. Journal of Attention Disorders, 1–6.

Huettel, S.A., Song, A.W., McCarthy, G., 2009. Functional Magnetic Resonance Imaging. Sinauer Associates, Inc., Sunderland, MA.

Kim, H., 2011. Neural activity that predicts subsequent memory and forgetting: a meta-analysis of 74 fMRI studies. NeuroImage 54 (3), 2446–2461.

Kobilo, T., Yuan, C., van Praag, H., 2011. Endurance factors improve hippocampal neurogenesis and spatial memory in mice. Learning & Memory 18 (2), 103–107.

Krafft, C.E., Schwarz, N.F., Chi, L., Weinberger, A.L., Schaeffer, D.J., Pierce, J.E., Rodrigue, A.L., Yanasak, N.E., Miller, P.H., Tomporowski, P.D., Davis, C.L., McDowell, J.E., 2014. An 8-month randomized controlled exercise trial alters brain activation during cognitive tasks in overweight children. Obesity (Silver Spring) 22 (1), 232–242.

Morrow, J., Freedson, P., 1994. Relationships between habitual physical activity and aerobic fitness in adolescents. Pediatric Exercise Science 6 (4), 315–329.

Pontifex, M.B., Raine, L.B., Johnson, C.R., Chaddock, L., Voss, M.W., Cohen, N.J., Kramer, A.F., Hillman, C.H., 2010. Cardiorespiratory fitness and the flexible modulation of cognitive control in preadolescent children. Journal of Cognitive Neuroscience 23 (6), 1332–1345.

Raznahan, A., Shaw, P., Lalonde, F., Stockman, M., Wallace, G.L., Greenstein, D., Clasen, L., Gogtay, N., Giedd, J.N., 2011. How does your cortex grow? The Journal of Neuroscience: the Official Journal of the Society for Neuroscience 31 (19), 7174–7177.

Schaeffer, D.J., Krafft, C.E., Schwarz, N.F., Chi, L., Rodrigue, A.L., Pierce, J.E., Allison, J.D., Yanasak, N.E., Liu, T., Davis, C.L., McDowell, J.E., 2014. An 8-month exercise intervention alters frontotemporal white matter integrity in overweight children. Psychophysiology 51 (8), 728–733.

Sibley, B.A., Etnier, J.L., 2003. The relationship between physical activity and cognition in children: a meta-analysis. Pediatric Exercise Science 15, 243–256.

Sowell, E.R., Thompson, P.M., Leonard, C.M., Welcome, S.E., Kan, E., Toga, A.W., 2004. Longitudinal mapping of cortical thickness and brain growth in normal children. Journal of Neuroscience 24 (38), 8223–8231.

Stroth, S., Kubesch, S., Dieterle, K., Ruchsow, M., Heim, R., Kiefer, M., 2009. Physical fitness, but not acute exercise modulates event-related potential indices for executive control in healthy adolescents. Brain Research 1269, 114–124.

Uysal, N., Tugyan, K., Kayatekin, B.M., Acikgoz, O., Bagriyanik, H.A., Gonenc, S., Ozdemir, D., Aksu, I., Topcu, A., Semin, I., 2005. The effects of regular aerobic exercise in adolescent period on hippocampal neuron density, apoptosis and spatial memory. Neuroscience Letters 383 (3), 241–245.

Voss, M.W., Chaddock, L., Kim, J.S., Vanpatter, M., Pontifex, M.B., Raine, L.B., Cohen, N.J., Hillman, C.H., Kramer, A.F., 2011. Aerobic fitness is associated with greater efficiency of the network underlying cognitive control in preadolescent children. Neuroscience 199, 166–176.

3

Differential Expression of the Brain Proteome in Physical Training

T. Ravikiran[1], R. Vani[2], S. Anand[1]

[1]Bangalore University, Bengaluru, India; [2]Jain University, Bengaluru, India

Abstract

Proteomics is an emerging field of research facilitated by numerous advancements over the past few decades in protein separation. Two-dimensional gel electrophoresis followed by mass spectrometrical identification is a common approach to identify proteins. Studies on protein expression related to physical activity are limited. Exercise has beneficial effects on brain function, including the promotion of plasticity and the enhancement of learning and memory performance. Proteins involved in energy metabolism, synaptic plasticity, and signaling and stress response were upregulated in cerebral cortex and hippocampus of swim-trained rats. Thus our studies suggest that exercise elicits a significant differential protein expression pattern in cortical and hippocampal function. These proteins may be involved with neuronal recovery in terms of neurite formation and remodeling of synaptic connections. These findings form the basis for better understanding of protein alterations in the brain in response to physical activity.

INTRODUCTION

Proteomics is an emerging field of research facilitated by numerous advancements over the past few decades in protein separation, mass spectrometry (MS), genome sequencing/annotation, and protein search algorithms. The term "proteome" was first used by Wilkins et al. (1996) to describe the protein complement to the genome. Proteomics describes the protein population of a cell, characterized in terms of localization, posttranslational modification, interactions, and turnover, at any given time (Minton and Stone, 2010). It reveals different protein expression patterns under different dynamic situations. Many factors may influence the expression pattern of the proteins, such as stress, alterations in temperature, different growth conditions, and the effects of various treatments. The analysis of malfunctioning cellular processes would allow the identification of biomarkers useful for designing target specific drugs under disease conditions.

The standard tool for protein separation and visualization is still 2-DE (two-dimensional polyacrylamide gel electrophoresis), first described by O'Farrell (1975) and Klose (1975) and known as a classic gel-based proteomic tool. During the current genomic research era, gel-based methods have improved, and other protein separation and identification techniques, such as MS, have been developed, leading to substantial progress in molecular research (Fenn et al., 1989; Shevchenko et al., 1996). Based on molecular ionization and with the resulting ability to identify unknown proteins by molecular characterization, MS can be used almost in any protein identification research (Aebersold and Mann, 2003). The limitations of gel-based methods have addressed the development of novel gel-free techniques based on protein labeling, peptide fragmentation, and high throughput MS instruments to improve proteome data acquirement (Warren et al., 2010).

Physical exercise is widely suggested to benefit overall health and cognitive functions in both humans and animals (Fordyce and Wehner, 1993; Kramer et al., 1999; Laurin et al., 2001). Voluntary exercise (VE) was found to ameliorate some of the deleterious morphological and behavioral consequences of aging, increased levels of brain-derived neurotrophic factor and other growth factors, stimulate neurogenesis, increase resistance to brain insult, and improve learning and mental performance (Chen et al., 2007). Although some individual proteins have been described to be involved in exercise associated neuronal mechanisms, no systematic investigations have been performed to identify major candidates for exercise-related neuronal variations. Proteomics enables us to evaluate protein complexes, signaling pathways, and protein changes to further understand the protein interactions involved in the cellular machinery of exercise (Grant and Blackstock, 2001; Phizicky et al., 2003; Tyers and Mann, 2003). Knowledge about the intracellular protein machinery underlying the effects of exercise on different regions of the brain is limited.

In this chapter, we discuss the differential expression of proteins in cerebral cortex (CC) and hippocampus (HC) regions of the rat brain in response to physical exercise using proteomics approach.

METHODOLOGY

Exercise Training Regimens

Animal experiments are designed to test the impact of exercise on physiology and brain health, as animals are genetically homogenous, and their environment can be easily controlled allowing for more interventions than in clinical cases. Rats and mice are the most widely used models for exercise studies. There are different types of exercise paradigms such as swimming, treadmill, and voluntary wheel running. The modulatory role of exercise depends on the type of physical exercise, intensity, duration of exercise, and age. The detailed exercise protocols are discussed in the following sections.

Swimming Exercise

Swimming, as model for exercise performance, appears to be a natural behavior of rodents (Kramer et al., 2006). It is known that swimming training has been used as a suitable method of endurance training because of several benefits derived out of it over treadmill running. A few of these include the possible differences in the sympathoadrenal function between swimming and running, less mechanical stress and injury during swimming due to buoyancy and reduced effects of gravity, as well as better redistribution of blood flow among tissues without significant variations in cardiac output and heart rate that in turn minimizes the magnitude of injury caused due to the generation of free radicals.

In our studies, swimming exercise was done according to our earlier protocols (Devi and Kiran, 2004). Briefly, rats were made to swim in a rectangular glass tank ($77\,cm \times 38\,cm \times 39\,cm$) filled with water to a height depending on the age group, at $32 \pm 1°C$ for 5 days/week for 30 days with a load of 3% of their body weight tied to tails. Initially, they were made to exercise for 5 min/day with a progressive increase of 30 min/day, for a total training period of 4 weeks with 5 days/week. Sedentary controls were restricted to cage activity.

Treadmill Running

Treadmill running has a distinct advantage over other exercise forms, as the amount of external work done can be easily calculated and intensity and duration of exercise can be controlled. However, this regimen is considered as a stressor to rodents (Huang et al., 2006). Studies by Chen et al. (2008) and Kirchner et al. (2008) have adapted treadmill running as a model of exercise, wherein rats were forced to run on a treadmill for 2×20 min for 5 days/week with the horizontal floor moving at a speed of 20 m/min.

Voluntary Wheel Running

VE model mimics characteristics of human behavior by allowing animals to select how much to run and does not require aversive stimuli like electric shocks to motivate the rats to run in the wheels. Ding et al. (2006) used voluntary wheel running as a method of exercise performance. Briefly, the rats were given access to a wheel (diameter 31.8 cm, width 10 cm) that freely rotated against a resistance of 100 g and was connected to a computer system to monitor their revolutions.

SAMPLE PREPARATION

Rat brain was used in our study. After the completion of exercise regimen, the whole brains were rapidly removed from male rats. The CC and HC regions of the brain were separated by following the method of Glowinski and Iversen (1966). CC and HC regions were chosen, as they are involved in higher brain functions such as learning, memory, and perception. Therefore, we investigated the expression profile in the CC and HC regions of the brain in response to swimming training.

The tissues were homogenized or powdered in liquid nitrogen in lysis buffer containing 7M urea, 2M thiourea, 4% w/v CHAPS, 0.8% biolytes, 100mM dithiothreitol (DTT) and protease inhibitor cocktail. After centrifugation of the homogenate at 3000 × g for 10min the supernatant was collected and the total protein was estimated by Bradford method (Bradford, 1976) using bovine serum albumin as standard. The protein sample was precipitated using 10% TCA in acetone containing 20mM DTT and placed at −20°C for 45min. This was followed by centrifugation at 3000 × g for 10min. The resulting pellet was washed twice with acetone containing 20mM DTT and solubilized in rehydration buffer containing 7M urea, 2M thiourea, 50mM DTT, 4% CHAPS, 0.2% carrier ampholytes, and 0.0002% bromophenol blue.

TWO-DIMENSIONAL POLYACRYLAMIDE GEL ELECTROPHORESIS (2D-PAGE)

2D-PAGE is a sensitive technique that separates the proteins based on two physicochemical properties. In the first dimension, it separates the proteins based on their isoelectric points and in the second based on their relative mobility. Briefly, IPG strips were rehydrated for 12h at room temperature and isoelectric focusing was carried out for a total of 14,000VHr in a gradient mode. Following IEF, the strips were equilibrated and were applied on to 12.5% vertical slab gels for second dimension run. The protein gel maps of sedentary and trained animals were compared in terms of differential expression using a computer assisted software program like Image Master 2-D analysis software, PDQuest etc. (Fig. 3.1). The normalized volume (vol%) of each spot was automatically calculated by the software as a ratio of the volume of a particular spot to the total volume of all the spots present on the colloidal commassie/SYPRO Ruby/silver stained gels.

Mass Spectrometry

Statistically significant ($p < .05$) upregulated protein spots were excised and subjected to in-gel digestion with trypsin followed by matrix-assisted laser desorption/ionization time of flight mass spectrometric analysis according to the method described by Shevchenko et al. (1996). The excised spots were destained with 100 µL of 50% acetonitrile (ACN) in 25mM ammonium bicarbonate (NH_4HCO_3) for five times. Thereafter, the gel pieces were treated with 10mM DTT in 25mM NH_4HCO_3 and incubated at 56°C for 1h. This is followed by treatment with 55mM iodoacetamide in 25mM NH_4HCO_3 for 45min at room temperature (25 ± 2°C), washed with 25mM NH_4HCO_3 and ACN, dried in speed vac and rehydrated in 20 µL of 25mM NH_4HCO_3 solution containing 12.5ng/µL trypsin. The above mixture was incubated on ice for 10min and kept overnight for digestion at 37°C. After digestion, a short spin for 10min was given and the supernatant was collected in a fresh eppendorf tube. The gel pieces were re-extracted with 50µL of 1% trifluoroacetic acid (TFA) and ACN (1:1) for 15min with frequent vortexing. The supernatants were pooled together and dried using speed vac and were reconstituted in 5µL of 1:1 ACN and 1% TFA. Two microlitre of the above sample was mixed with 2µL of freshly prepared α-cyano-4-hydroxycinnamic acid matrix in 50% ACN and 1% TFA (1:1) and 1µL was spotted on target plate.

Protein Identification

Peptide mass fingerprints are characteristic of a particular protein and facilitate the identification of a particular protein using a suitable database (Table 3.1) that compares the experimental masses with that of the theoretical masses of trypsin-generated protein sequences. In our study, the protein identification was performed by database searches (PMF and MS/MS) using MASCOT program employing Biotools software. The similarity search for mass values was done with existing digests and sequence information from NCBInr and SwissProt database. The other search parameters were: fixed modification of carbamidomethyl (C), variable modification of oxidation (M), enzyme trypsin, peptide charge of 1+, and monoisotropic. According to the MASCOT probability analysis ($p < .05$), only significant hits were accepted for protein identification.

Differential Proteomic Analysis of CC and HC Regions of the Brain in Physically Trained Rats

Studies have shown that regular exercise improves brain function by modulating antioxidant status (Anand et al., 2014; Devi and Kiran, 2004; Somani et al., 1995). Exercise plays an important therapeutic role in preventing stroke, Alzheimer's and Parkinson's diseases (Mattson and Magnus, 2006; Mattson, 2005; Stummer et al., 1994). The effects

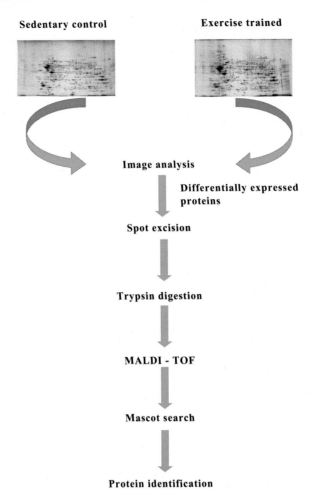

FIGURE 3.1   Schematic representation of the proteomics protocol.

TABLE 3.1   Peptide Mass Fingerprinting Search Engines for Protein Identification

Search Engines	URL
MOWSE	http://www.hgmp.mrc.ac.uk/Bioinformatics/Webapp/mowse
Mascot	http://www.matrixscience.com
MS-fit	http://prospector.ucsf.edu/ucsfhtml14.0/msfit.html
Peptident	http://ca.expasy.org/tools/peptident.html
ProFound	http://prowl.rockefeller.edu/profound_bin/webProfound.exe
SEQUEST	http://fields.scripps.edu/sequest
ExPASy	http://www.expasy.ch/tools

of exercise appears to be very complex and could include neurogenesis, increased capillarization, decreased oxidative damage, and increased proteolytic degradation (Radak et al., 2008). The molecular mechanisms behind these beneficial effects are not clearly understood. Using proteomic approach, we investigated the differential expression of proteins in CC and HC regions of the brain in response to swimming exercise. Most of the studies have focused on the modulation of hippocampus proteome in treadmill, voluntary, and wheel running rats (Kirchner et al., 2008; Ding et al., 2006; Chen et al., 2008). However, no studies are reported on the differential expression of CC proteome with exercise. To the best of our knowledge, this is the first study to investigate the comparative expression profile of CC and HC regions of the rat brain with swimming training. A number of candidate protein spots were identified that differed in expression levels and were classified into different functional classes (Table 3.2).

TABLE 3.2   Proteomic Identification of Upregulated Proteins in the CC and HC of Swim-Trained Rats

Functional Class	Protein Name
Energy-related enzymes	Glyceraldehyde-3-phosphate dehydrogenase, F-ATPase, glutamine synthetase etc.
Cytoskeletal proteins	Tubulin alpha, tubulin beta, actin etc.
Signaling proteins	Guanine nucleotide binding protein beta, annexin A3 etc.
Chaperones	78 kDa glucose-regulated protein and protein disulphide isomerase
Miscellaneous proteins	14-3-3 zeta/delta, albumin etc.

Proteins Involved in Energy Metabolism

Glycolysis plays an important role in maintaining normal synaptic function (Sultana et al., 2006; Ikemoto et al., 2003). We found glyceraldehyde-3-phosphate dehydrogenase (GAPDH), F-ATPase (Anand et al., 2014), and other metabolic enzymes involved in glutamate turnover, fatty acid metabolism, energy transduction, citric acid cycle in the CC and HC regions of swim-trained rats. A significant increase in the expression of metabolic enzymes was observed in the CC of aged animals compared to young ones. The increased expression of these enzymes may lead to improved glycolytic function, increased ATP production, and possible neuronal recovery from energy depletion. Ding et al. (2006) have also reported the upregulation of these metabolic enzymes in the HC of adult male rats subjected to VE.

Proteins Involved in Synaptic Plasticity

Cytoskeletal proteins form the structural integrity necessary for synaptic plasticity. Studies have shown that exercise induces neurogenesis in the adult brain (Ji et al., 2014; E et al., 2014). Our proteomic studies have revealed that swimming exercise can increase a diverse set of proteins related to cytoskeletal function. There was an upregulation of actin and tubulin in the CC of adult rat brain, whereas in HC region different subunits of tubulins were significantly expressed (Anand et al., 2014). These proteins function as scaffolding structures and have a vital role in transporting to various organelles and vesicular components. The expression of these two proteins are also observed in the HC of rats subjected to wheel running exercise (Ding et al., 2006). Ferreira et al. (2010) also showed modulation of cytoskeletal proteins in motor regions of the rat brain. Swimming exercise modulates the expression of cytoskeletal proteins in the CC and HC, which may play an important role in the exercise-dependent neuronal plasticity.

Proteins Involved in Signal Transduction

Signaling proteins play a vital role in functioning of the brain. Guanine nucleotide binding protein beta (GNB1) and annexin A3 (ANXA3) are modulated with exercise and may improve learning and memory performances. GNB1, a modulator in various transmembrane signaling pathways is required for GTPase activity. GNB1 was expressed in the CC of swim-trained rats, which may improve Ca^{2+} homeostasis, second messengers, cell cycle, and neurotransmission.

Annexin A3 belong to the lipocortin/annexin family that binds to phospholipids and membranes in a calcium-dependent manner. Studies by Weitzdorfer et al. (2008) reported that ANXA3 is related to brain development. Our studies showed an enhanced expression of ANXA3 in the CC and HC of adult rats. Chen et al. (2007) reported an enhanced expression of these signaling proteins in the HC of voluntary and treadmill exercise rats.

Chaperones

Chaperones are a category of proteins involved in protein import, folding, and assembly that help to cope with oxidative stress (Latchman, 2004). GRP78 (a constitutively expressed glucose-regulated protein) and PDIA3 (protein disulphide isomerase) are some of the important chaperones. GRP78 acts as a molecular chaperone by binding transiently to proteins crossing through the ER and helping their folding, assembly, and transport. GRP78 is the main constituent involved in the unfolded protein response (Pyrko et al., 2007). PDIA3 is a protein-thiol oxido-reductase chaperone from the thioredoxin superfamily that catalyzes the oxidation, reduction, and isomerization of protein disulfides. In the endoplasmic reticulum, PDIA3 catalyzes both the oxidation and isomerization of disulfides on nascent polypeptides (Laurindo et al., 2012; Noiva, 1999). These proteins were found to be enhanced in the HC region of exercised rats (Chen et al., 2008; Ding et al., 2006). In contrast, we have observed increased expression of these proteins in the CC region of swim-trained rats. Enhanced expression of GRP78 and PDIA3 in the trained rats may inhibit the accumulation of misfolded proteins and helps in maintaining the redox cell signaling and homeostasis.

Miscellaneous Proteins

Other proteins such as 14-3-3 zeta/delta and albumin were also upregulated with training. 14-3-3 zeta/delta, are small, cytosolic, and evolutionarily conserved protein expressed abundantly in the nervous system in humans and rodents as well. Our studies have demonstrated increase in their expression in the CC of trained rats (Anand et al., 2014). The protein also has an important role in the development and function of the nervous system besides learning and memory processes. An upregulation of albumin in the CC (Anand et al., 2014) and HC of trained animals suggests a higher intake of water and ions such as Ca^{2+}, Na^+, and K^+ to maintain the osmotic balance in the blood–brain barrier. Chen et al. (2007) have shown an over expression of these proteins in the hippocampal region of rats subjected to voluntary and treadmill exercise.

Our proteomics studies demonstrates the modulatory role of exercise in terms of significant expression of proteins related to key regulatory functions like energy metabolism, synaptic plasticity, signal transduction, and stress response in the CC and HC regions of rat brain. These findings have to be explored by future research and have to be complemented with data as to how exercise could modulate energy metabolism to interact with synaptic plasticity to affect brain function.

CONCLUSION

Although proteomics study has limitations, it offers many possibilities and approaches towards qualitative and quantitative analysis of proteins. Proteomics is still in its infancy in the areas of physical activity and brain as most of the proteomic studies have focused on neurological diseases. Our proteomic study lays foundation for further research on protein expression profile on other regions of the brain under different conditions of exercise. Proteomics research may help in better understanding of protein interactions at functional level, thereby leading to a new level of physiological understanding and therapeutics.

Acknowledgments

We acknowledge University Grants Commission (UGC), New Delhi, India (F. No. 34-267) for the financial assistance and University of Hyderabad, Hyderabad, India for proteomic analysis. We also thank Department of Microbiology and Biotechnology, Bangalore University, Bengaluru, India for providing necessary infrastructure facilities.

References

Aebersold, R., Mann, M., 2003. Mass spectrometry-based proteomics. Nature 422, 198–207.

Anand, S., Devi, S.A., Ravikiran, T., 2014. Differential expression of the cerebral cortex proteome in physically trained adult rats. Brain Research Bulletin 104, 88–91.

Bradford, M.M., 1976. A rapid and sensitive method for the quantitation of microgram quantities of protein utilizing the principle of protein-dye binding. Analytical Biochemistry 72, 248–254.

Chen, W.Q., Diao, W.F., Viidik, A., Skalicky, M., Hoger, H., Lubeg, G., 2008. Modulation of the hippocampal protein machinery in voluntary and treadmill exercising rats. Biochimica et Biophysica Acta 1784, 555–562.

Chen, W.Q., Viidik, A., Skalicky, M., Hoger, H., Lubec, G., 2007. Hippocampal signaling cascades are modulated in voluntary and treadmill exercise rats. Electrophoresis 28, 4392–4400.

Devi, S.A., Kiran, R.T., 2004. Regional responses of antioxidant system in exercise training and dietary vitamin E in aging rat brain. Neurobiology of Aging 25, 501–508.

Ding, Q., Vaynman, S., Souda, P., Whitelegge, J.P., Gomez-pinalla, F., 2006. Exercise effects energy metabolism and neural plasticity related proteins in the hippocampus as revealed by proteomic analysis. European Journal of Neuroscience 24, 1265–1276.

E, L., Burns, J.M., Swerdlow, R.H., 2014. Effect of high-intensity exercise on aged mouse brain mitochondria, neurogenesis, and inflammation. Neurobiology of Aging 35, 2574–2583.

Fenn, J.B., Mann, M., Meng, C.K., Wong, S.F., Whitehouse, C.M., 1989. Electrospray ionization for mass spectrometry of large biomolecules. Science 246, 64–71.

Ferreira, A.F.B., Real, C.C., Rodrigues, A.C., Alves, A.S., Britto, L.R.G., 2010. Moderate exercise changes synaptic and cytoskeletal proteins in motor regions of the rat brain. Brain Research 1361, 31–42.

Fordyce, D.E., Wehner, J.M., 1993. Physical activity enhances spatial learning performance with an associated alteration in hippocampal protein kinase C activity in C57BL/6 and DBA/2 mice. Brain Research 619, 111–119.

Glowinski, J., Iversen, L.L., 1966. Regional studies of catecholamines in the rat brain-I. Journal of Neurochemistry 13, 655–669.

Grant, S.G.N., Blackstock, W.P., 2001. Proteomics in neuroscience: from protein to network. Journal of Neuroscience 21, 8315–8318.

Huang, Q., Timofeeva, E., Richard, D., 2006. Regulation of corticotropin-releasing factor and its types 1 and 2 receptors by leptin in rats subjected to treadmill running-induced stress. Journal of Endocrinology 191, 179–188.

Ikemoto, A., Bole, D.G., Ueda, T., 2003. Glycolysis and glutamate accumulation into synaptic vesicles. Journal of Biological Chemistry 278, 5929–5940.

Ji, J.F., Ji, S.J., Sun, R., Li, K., Zhang, Y., Zhang, L.Y., Tian, Y., 2014. Forced running exercise attenuates hippocampal neurogenesis impairment and the neurocognitive deficits induced by whole-brain irradiation via the BDNF-mediated pathway. Biochemical and Biophysical Research Communications 443, 646–651.

Kirchner, L., Chen, W.Q., Afjehi-Sadat, L., Viidik, A., Skalicky, M., Hoger, H., Lubeg, G., 2008. Hippocampal metabolic proteins are modulated in voluntary and treadmill exercise rats. Experimental Neurology 212, 145–151.

Klose, J., 1975. Protein mapping by combined isoelectric focusing and electrophoresis of mouse tissues. A novel approach to testing for induced point mutations in mammals. Human-genetik 26, 231–243.

Kramer, A.F., Erickson, K.I., Colcombe, S.J., 2006. Exercise, cognition, and the aging brain. Journal of Applied Physiology 101, 1237–1242.

Kramer, A.F., Hahn, S., Cohen, N.J., Banich, M.T., McAuley, E., Harrison, C.R., Chason, J., Vakil, E., Bardell, L., Boileau, R.A., Colcombe, A., 1999. Ageing, fitness and neurocognitive function. Nature 400, 418–419.

Latchman, D.S., 2004. Protective effect of heat shock proteins in the nervous system. Current Neurovascular Research 1, 21–27.

Laurin, D., Verreault, R., Lindsay, J., MacPherson, K., Rockwood, K., 2001. Physical activity and risk of cognitive impairment and dementia in elderly persons. Archives of Neurology 58, 498–504.

Laurindo, F.R., Pescatore, L.A., Fernandes, D.C., 2012. Protein disulfide isomerase in redox cell signaling and homeostasis. Free Radical Biology and Medicine 52, 1954–1969.

Mattson, M.P., 2005. Energy intake, meal frequency, and health: a neurobiological perspective. Annual Review of Nutrition 25, 237–260.

Mattson, M.P., Magnus, T., 2006. Ageing and neuronal vulnerability. Nature Reviews Neuroscience 7, 278–294.

Minton, O., Stone, P.C., 2010. Review: the use of proteomics as a research methodology for studying cancer-related fatigue: a review. Palliative Medicine 24, 310–316.

Noiva, R., 1999. Protein disulfide isomerase: the multifunctional redox chaperone of the endoplasmic reticulum. Seminars in Cell & Developmental Biology 10, 481–493.

O'Farrell, P.H., 1975. High resolution two-dimensional electrophoresis of proteins. Journal of Biological Chemistry 250, 4007–4021.

Phizicky, E., Bastiaens, P.I., Zhu, H., Snyder, M., Fields, S., 2003. Protein analysis on a proteomic scale. Nature 422, 208–215.

Pyrko, P., Schonthal, A.M., Hofman, F.M., Chen, T.C., Lee, A.S., 2007. The unfolded protein response regulator GRP78/BiP as a novel target for increasing chemosensitivity in malignant gliomas. Cancer Research 67, 9809–9816.

Radak, Z., Chung, H.Y., Goto, S., 2008. Systemic adaptation to oxidative challenge induced by regular exercise. Free Radical Biology and Medicine 44, 153–159.

Shevchenko, A., Wilm, A., Vorm, O., Mann, M., 1996. Mass spectrometric sequencing of protein from silver-stained polyacrylamide gels. Analytical Chemistry 68, 850–858.

Somani, S.M., Frank, S., Rybak, L.P., 1995. Responses of antioxidant system to acute and trained exercise in rat heart subcellular fractions. Pharmacology Biochemistry and Behavior 51, 627–634.

Stummer, W., Weber, K., Tranmer, B., Baethmann, A., Kempski, O., 1994. Reduced mortality and brain damage after locomotor activity in gerbil forebrain ischemia. Stroke 25, 1862–1869.

Sultana, R., Poon, H.F., Cai, J., Pierce, W.M., Merchant, M., Klein, J.B., Markesbery, W.R., Butterfield, D.A., 2006. Identification of nitrated proteins in Alzheimer's disease brain using a redox proteomics approach. Neurobiological Disorders 22, 76–87.

Tyers, M., Mann, M., 2003. From genomics to proteomics. Nature 422, 193–197.

Warren, C.M., Geenen, D.L., Helseth Jr., D.L., Xu, H., Solaro, R.J., 2010. Sub-proteomic fractionation, iTRAQ, and OFFGEL-LC-MS/MS approaches to cardiac proteomics. Journal of Proteomics 73, 1551–1561.

Weitzdorfer, R., Hoger, H., Shim, K.S., Cekici, L., Pollak, A., Lubec, G., 2008. Changes of hippocampal signaling protein levels during postnatal brain development in the rat. Hippocampus 18, 807–813.

Wilkins, M.R., Sanchez, J.C., Gooley, A.A., Appel, R.D., Humphrey-Smith, I., Hochstrasser, D.F., Williams, K.L., 1996. Progress with proteome projects: why all proteins expressed by a genome should be identified and how to do it. Biotechnology and Genetic Engineering Reviews 13, 19–50.

4

Physical Exercise-Induced Changes in Brain Temperature

A.C. Kunstetter, W.C. Damasceno, C.G. Fonseca, S.P. Wanner

Federal University of Minas Gerais, Belo Horizonte, MG, Brazil

Abstract

Evidence suggests that brain temperature (T_{BRAIN}) is a more sensitive index than the temperature of peripheral tissues for determining physical performance and thermoeffector activity. Because direct measurements of T_{BRAIN} in exercising humans are not currently possible, several studies have been performed in rats to investigate the extent to which T_{BRAIN} increases during exercise and whether selective brain cooling occurs in mammals that do not possess a carotid rete. These studies have reported that (1) T_{BRAIN} increases during exercise and can reach values above 40°C when physical exertion is performed in a hot environment or during prolonged exertion (duration longer than 1 h) in a temperate environment; (2) a dorsoventral temperature gradient exists between brain regions, with the ventrally-located structures being warmer than the dorsally-located structures; (3) the observation of selective brain cooling in rats seems to depend on the brain site where temperature is measured; and (4) the exercise-induced increase in T_{BRAIN} negatively affects physical performance at different exercise intensities and ambient temperatures.

INTRODUCTION

The core body temperature (T_{CORE}) or deep body temperature corresponds to any temperature measured in the "core" compartment of the body, which comprises the abdominal, thoracic, and cranial cavities (IUPS Thermal Commission, 2001). Homeothermic animals maintain their T_{CORE} within narrow limits despite great fluctuations in the ambient temperature. This ability to tightly control the T_{CORE} is important for the maintenance of body homeostasis, and large deviations from the narrow limits of the T_{CORE} suggest the existence of systemic inflammation (Romanovsky et al., 2005).

Physical exercise accelerates the rate of heat production and leads to a rapid increase in the T_{CORE} that depends on exercise intensity and the ambient temperature (Galloway and Maughan, 1997; Wanner et al., 2015). Over a wide range of exercise intensities and ambient temperatures, humans and other mammals can attain a new, elevated steady-state T_{CORE} value, without presenting exaggerated or even levels of hyperthermia (Lind, 1963; Nielsen, 1966; Tanaka et al., 1988). However, physical exertion under conditions of noncompensable heat stress leads to a progressive and marked increase in the T_{CORE}, which may reach values above 40°C (Kunstetter et al., 2014; Tanaka et al., 1988). Noncompensable heat stress conditions are usually observed when exercise is performed in a hot environment and/or at a fast rate of metabolic heat production that exceeds the body's ability to dissipate heat to the environment via evaporation, convection, conduction, and radiation.

Exercise-induced hyperthermia negatively affects the ability to sustain prolonged physical exertion. In fact, several studies have reported a negative association between the increase in the T_{CORE} and physical (aerobic) performance, especially when prolonged exercise is performed in hot environments (Fuller et al., 1998; Gonzalez-Alonso et al., 1999; Walters et al., 2000). Notably, although the temperatures measured in the body core compartments are largely independent of fluctuations in ambient temperature, they are not homogeneous and do not respond in a similar manner (especially regarding their time course) to several arousing stimuli (Kiyatkin et al., 2002). In particular, several authors have associated hyperthermia-induced fatigue with an exaggerated increase in brain temperature (T_{BRAIN}) (Nybo, 2008; Nybo and Nielsen, 2001a). Indeed, evidence suggests that the T_{BRAIN} is a more sensitive index than the temperature of peripheral tissues for determining physical performance (Caputa et al., 1986; Fonseca et al., 2014) and thermoeffector activity (Gisolfi and Mora, 2000). In exercising humans, it has been hypothesized that an increase in rectal or esophageal temperatures is accompanied by a parallel increase in T_{BRAIN}, which ultimately augments the rate of perceived exertion (Nybo and Nielsen, 2001b) and changes cerebral function (Ftaiti et al., 2010).

Consistent with the aforementioned hypothesis, hyperthermia induced by prolonged exercise in hot environments reduces voluntary force production by the exercised muscles (Nybo and Nielsen, 2001a) and decreases electroencephalogram activity in the frontal cortex (Ftaiti et al., 2010; Nybo and Nielsen, 2001b), suggesting that hyperthermia inhibits the cortical areas responsible for motor activation. In addition, fatigue induced by exercise heat stress is not accompanied by reduction in the blood flow directed to the contracting muscles (Nielsen et al., 1990) or by increase in plasmatic concentrations of metabolic by products such as K^+, H^+, and lactate (Drust et al., 2005), indicating that hyperthermia-induced fatigue is not associated with peripheral alterations that could impair the ability of skeletal muscles to produce force. Considering these findings, Nybo (2008) proposed that the exercise-induced increase in T_{BRAIN} is perceived by hypothalamic thermosensors, which stimulate inhibitory projections from temperature-sensitive areas of the hypothalamus to cortical areas involved in motor control, reducing the central drive for muscle contraction.

Despite the major role assigned to the T_{BRAIN} increase in determining exercise performance, unfortunately, the temperature of brain structures cannot be directly measured in exercising humans. In this context, rodent experiments are essential to increase our understanding of the exercise-induced alterations in the T_{BRAIN} that may regulate performance or explain the central impairments caused by hyperthermia. Therefore, this book chapter aims to briefly review the data provided by our and other research groups regarding the effects of exercise on the T_{BRAIN} of rats and to discuss the effects of ambient temperature, exercise intensity, and exercise protocol on the T_{BRAIN} response to physical exertion as well as the role of the T_{BRAIN} in determining performance. We will also discuss the differences in the temperature responses of distinct brain regions to exercise. Finally, data that estimate the T_{BRAIN} in exercising humans will be presented.

MEASURING BRAIN TEMPERATURE DURING EXERCISE

Changes in the T_{BRAIN} of exercising rodents can be measured directly by a thermistor or thermocouple inserted into a specific brain region. For this purpose, a rat can be subjected to surgical implantation of a brain guide cannula that allows the insertion of the thermistor or thermocouple into the brain (Damasceno et al., 2015; Fonseca et al., 2014; Fuller et al., 1998; Hasegawa et al., 2008; Kunstetter et al., 2014; Walters et al., 1998a,b, 2000) or to surgical implantation of the thermocouple into a specific brain site (Caputa et al., 1991). In the former case, on the experimental day, the thermistor or thermocouple is inserted into the brain through the guide cannula immediately before the rat is subjected to exercise, with some investigators performing this procedure while the animal is under light anesthesia (Fuller et al., 1998; Hasegawa et al., 2008). In the latter case, the thermocouple is implanted into the rat brain, and the wires from the thermocouple are welded to a socket that is fixed to the skull. On the experimental day, the socket is then connected to the recording system before exercise is initiated.

EFFECTS OF EXERCISE ON T_{BRAIN}

Several studies have measured the T_{BRAIN} of exercising rats, as listed in the Table 4.1. All of these studies have evaluated the changes in the T_{BRAIN} of rats subjected to treadmill running and have reported an increase in this temperature at a wide range of exercise intensities and ambient temperatures. The magnitude of the exercise-induced increase in the T_{BRAIN} is affected by several factors, including: (1) ambient temperature; (2) exercise intensity; (3) exercise protocol; and (4) the brain site where the T_{BRAIN} is measured. The modulatory role of each of these factors on the T_{BRAIN} response to exercise will be discussed in the following sections.

The T_{BRAIN} increase observed during exercise can also be affected by the occurrence of selective brain cooling (SBC), which is defined as the capacity of maintaining the T_{BRAIN} at lower levels than the temperature of peripheral tissues (abdominal or rectal temperature), particularly during hyperthermic situations (Baker, 1982; Caputa et al., 1991). Some animal species such as the artiodactyls and felids have, in the base of their cranium, a specialized complex of medium-sized arteries (called the carotid rete) that lie in a pool of venous blood and increase the heat exchange between cooled venous blood and the arterial blood destined for the brain, allowing considerable cooling of this arterial blood and, consequently, the selective cooling of the brain (Baker, 1982). However, humans and rats do

TABLE 4.1 Studies That Have Evaluated the Effects of Physical Exercise on the Brain Temperature of Rats

	Methods					Results		
Author	Site of T_{BRAIN} Measurement	Other T_{CORE} Index Measured	Exercise Intensity	Ambient Temperature	Exercise Duration	T_{BRAIN} at the End of Exercise	Other T_{CORE} Index at the End of Exercise	T_{BRAIN}-T_{CORE} Temperature Differential
Caputa et al. (1991)	Hypothalamus	Rectal	25 m/min	31°C	30 min	41.0°C	41.2°C	−0.2°C
Fuller et al. (1998)	Hypothalamus	Abdominal	15 m/min 10% inclination	33°C and 38°C	25 min (33°C)[a] 22 min (38°C)[a]	40.1°C (33–38°C)	39.9°C (33–38°C)	+0.2°C
Walters et al. (1998a)	Hypothalamus	Rectal	13–21 m/min 8% inclination	24°C and 34°C	60 min	~39.6°C (24°C) ~41.0°C (34°C)	~40.2°C (24°C) ~41.4°C (34°C)	−0.6°C −0.4°C
Walters et al. (1998b)	Hypothalamus and cortex	Rectal	17 m/min 8% inclination	35°C	42.8 min[a]	~41.2°C (hypothalamus) ~40.4°C (cortex)	~41°C	+0.2°C −0.6°C
Walters et al. (2000)	Hypothalamus	Rectal	18 m/min 8% inclination	35°C	~38 min[a]	42.2°C	42.5°C	−0.2°C
Hasegawa et al. (2008)	Frontal cortex	Abdominal	26 m/min	18°C and 30°C	144 min (18°C)[a] 66 min (30°C)[a]	39.1°C (18°C) 40.5°C (30°C)	39.6°C (18°C) 41°C (30°C)	−0.5°C −0.5°C
Fonseca et al. (2014)	Hypothalamus	Abdominal	20 m/min 5% inclination	25°C and 12°C	31.5 min (25°C)[a] 67.1 min (12°C)[a]	39.2°C (25°C) 37.7°C (12°C)	38.9°C (25°C) 37.4°C (12°C)	+0.3°C +0.3°C
Kunstetter et al. (2014)	Frontal cortex	NM	18, 21 and 24 m/min; 5% inclination	25°C	201 min (S18)[a] 149 min (S21)[a] 62 min (S24)[a]	40.5°C (S18) 40.3°C (S21) 40.1°C (S24)	NM	NM
Damasceno et al. (2015)	Thalamus	Abdominal	21 m/min 5% inclination	24°C	113 min[a]	39.7°C	39.5°C	+0.2°C

NM, not measured or not evaluated.
[a]Exercise until fatigue. S18: 18 m/min; S21: 21 m/min; S24: 24 m/min.

I. OVERVIEW OF EXERCISE AND NEUROLOGICAL CHANGES

not possess a carotid rete, and therefore, the occurrence of SBC is still controversial in these species. Some investigators who have measured the T_{BRAIN} in exercising rats have observed the occurrence of SBC during exercise (Caputa et al., 1991; Hasegawa et al., 2008; Walters et al., 1998b), while others have not (Damasceno et al., 2015; Fonseca et al., 2014; Fuller et al., 1998). Moreover, recent studies performed by our group suggest that the observation of SBC is dependent on the site where the T_{BRAIN} is measured (Wanner et al., 2015). Therefore, in this chapter, the occurrence of SBC in running rats will also be discussed along with the description of the temperature response of the different brain sites to exercise.

Effects of Ambient Temperature

As observed for the abdominal and rectal temperatures (Rodrigues et al., 2003; Tanaka et al., 1988), the T_{BRAIN} increase in running rats is affected by the ambient temperature at which exercise is performed. Four studies have evaluated the effect of changing the ambient temperature on the T_{BRAIN} response to exercise (Fonseca et al., 2014; Fuller et al., 1998; Hasegawa et al., 2008; Walters et al., 1998b), and the results are summarized in Table 4.1. In these studies, higher ambient temperatures were associated with exaggerated brain hyperthermia relative to the lower ambient temperatures. Walters et al. (1998b) observed an approximately 1.5°C greater increase in hypothalamic temperature when rats exercised in a hot environment (34°C) compared to the experimental trial in a temperate environment (24°C). Similar results were reported by Hasegawa et al. (2008), who observed that the right frontal cortex temperature at the end of exercise was 1.4°C higher when the exercise was performed in a hot environment (30°C) compared to the trial in which rats exercised in a cool environment (18°C).

Not only the hot environments, but also cold environments influence the T_{BRAIN} of running rats. Fonseca et al. (2014) observed lower hypothalamic temperatures during exercise performed in a cold environment (12°C) compared to exercise performed in a temperate environment (25°C). Notably, the hypothalamic temperature remained unchanged when moderate-intensity exercise (20m/min) was performed at 12°C, as previously described for abdominal temperature (Guimaraes et al., 2013). The methods conducted in the latter experiments represent an important methodological approach for studying the effects of exercise on cerebral function while excluding the influence of the exercise-induced increase in T_{BRAIN}. Only one of the four studies mentioned above did not find any effect of the ambient temperature on the T_{BRAIN} increase induced by treadmill running. However, in this study, both experimental trials were performed in hot environments (33°C and 38°C) that likely represented noncompensable heat stress conditions to the exercising rats, as evidenced by the fact that their T_{BRAIN} increased sharply and progressively during the fatiguing treadmill running, without reaching a plateau (Fuller et al., 1998).

Another interesting factor regarding the effects of ambient temperature on exercise-induced increase in T_{BRAIN} is the level of hyperthermia attained at the interruption of exertion. When exercise is performed in a temperate or in a cool environment, the T_{BRAIN} reaches values close to 39°C at the end of the exercise and will rarely surpass 40°C. However, during exercise in hot environments (ambient temperatures higher than 30°C), the rats exhibit T_{BRAIN} values above 40°C upon the interruption of the exercise. These elevated T_{BRAIN} values may change brain function and, therefore, reduce exercise performance (as discussed later) or damage the blood–brain barrier and neuronal cells. In fact, when rats were passively warmed until reaching T_{BRAIN} values of 38°C, 39°C, 40°C, and 41°C, only those that attained T_{BRAIN} values above 40°C exhibited increased blood–brain barrier permeability, brain edema, and structural abnormalities in brain cells (Kiyatkin and Sharma, 2009). Moreover, Watson et al. (2005) provided evidence that exercise in hot environments may also affect the integrity of the blood–brain barrier in humans.

Effects of Exercise Intensity and Protocol

A recent study investigated the effects of the exercise intensity and protocol on the T_{BRAIN} increase induced by treadmill running (Kunstetter et al., 2014). In this study, the effect of exercise intensity was evaluated during constant-speed exercises performed at three different treadmill speeds: 18, 21, and 24m/min. In addition, the effect of the exercise protocol was evaluated by comparing the T_{BRAIN} responses between constant-speed exercises and an incremental-speed exercise (initial speed of 10m/min, with 1m/min increments every 3min).

During the initial phase of the constant-speed exercises (until the 8th min), rats exhibited the highest rates of T_{BRAIN} increase, which were independent of exercise intensity (Kunstetter et al., 2014). This marked and unspecific T_{BRAIN} increase was likely caused by animal handling, which is a stressful procedure required to insert the thermistor and to place the rat on the treadmill. Afterward, the T_{BRAIN} continued to increase at a slower rate, and exercise-induced hyperthermia became dependent on running speed. Higher values of T_{BRAIN} were observed for the highest exercise intensity (24m/min) relative to the other two intensities (18 and 21m/min) from the 23rd to the 31th min of exercise.

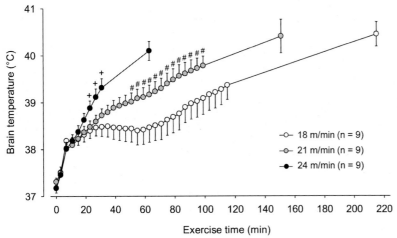

FIGURE 4.1 Cortical brain temperature of rats subjected to constant-speed exercise sessions on a treadmill at three different speeds (18, 21, and 24 m/min) until volitional fatigue. Data are reported as means ± SEM. +$P < 0.05$ compared to 18 and 21 m/min; #$P < 0.05$ compared to 18 m/min. *The graph was reprinted from Kunstetter, A.C., Wanner, S.P., Madeira, L.G., Wilke, C.F., Rodrigues, L.O., Lima, N.R., 2014. Association between the increase in brain temperature and physical performance at different exercise intensities and protocols in a temperate environment. Brazilian Journal of Medical and Biological Research 47, 679–688. Open-access manuscript.*

Moreover, the T_{BRAIN} was higher during exercise at 21 m/min than for a speed of 18 m/min from the 50th to the 100th min of exercise. A temperature plateau was not observed at 21 and 24 m/min, most likely because these intensities provoked elevated rates of heat production that had overcome the rat's ability to dissipate heat, which caused the T_{BRAIN} to increase constantly during exercise.

Despite the differences mentioned previously, no differences were observed in the average T_{BRAIN} between the three exercise intensities when the animals voluntarily terminated their effort (Fig. 4.1). Moreover, the rats subjected to the constant exercises fatigued with average T_{BRAIN} values above 40°C, irrespective of the treadmill speed (Kunstetter et al., 2014). Similar T_{BRAIN} values were previously observed in rats at the end of a fatiguing treadmill run in hot environments (see previous section), indicating that the hyperthermia-mediated changes in brain function may also play a role in determining exercise performance when prolonged constant-speed exercise is performed in a temperate environment. It is also likely that prolonged (more than 1 h), moderate-intensity exercise may affect the integrity of the blood–brain barrier and the structure of neural cells even when exertion is not associated with environmental thermal stress. Therefore, future studies should investigate the effects of T_{BRAIN} increase induced by prolonged exercise in a temperate environment on neuronal function related to exercise performance, blood–brain barrier integrity, and the morphology of neural cells.

Kunstetter et al. (2014) also observed that the running protocol affected the magnitude of exercise-induced brain hyperthermia. Although the incremental exercise increased the T_{BRAIN}, this increase was lower than that observed during constant exercises at 24 (Fig. 4.2) and at 21 m/min. The influence of the running protocol on the T_{BRAIN} increase may result from differences in the evolution of exercise intensity, which is an inherent characteristic of each running protocol. During the initial stages of the incremental exercise protocol, the power output by the animals and, consequently, the rate of heat production were low (e.g., 42 min were required for rats to begin running at 24 m/min). Moreover, at volitional fatigue, the average T_{BRAIN} was lower during the incremental exercise (39.3°C) than in the three constant exercise sessions (18 m/min: 40.45°C, 21 m/min: 40.31°C, 24 m/min: 40.10°C). These findings suggest that nonthermal factors, most likely metabolic factors, are more important for regulating fatigue than thermoregulation during an incremental exercise. In addition, these results suggest that incremental exercise in a temperate environment may not be the most adequate protocol for investigating the mechanisms by which high T_{BRAIN} values regulate prolonged performance.

Effects of the Brain Site Where T_{BRAIN} Is Measured

Most of the studies that have recorded the T_{BRAIN} in exercising rats have measured the temperature of the hypothalamus or the brain cortex. The selection of the hypothalamus as the site for temperature measurement seems obvious in considering that the hypothalamus is the brain center that modulates the recruitment of autonomic thermoeffectors (Romanovsky, 2007). Interestingly, the placement of a thermistor unilaterally in the hypothalamus does not affect the physical performance and the exercise-induced changes in the abdominal temperature, suggesting that unilateral hypothalamic lesions caused by the procedure for T_{BRAIN} measurement do not affect the rats' abilities to exercise and thermoregulate (Fonseca et al., 2014). The selection of the brain cortex for measuring the T_{BRAIN} is explained by the fact that the cortex is a more dorsally-located structure, and therefore, its temperature might be affected by the temperature of the cranial or sinus blood (Caputa et al., 1996). Again, the lesions caused by the

FIGURE 4.2 Cortical brain temperatures of rats subjected to a constant-speed exercise at 24 m/min or an incremental-speed exercise. Both exercises were performed on a treadmill until volitional fatigue. The data are expressed as means ± SEM. *$P < 0.05$ compared to constant-speed exercise at 24 m/min. *The graph was reprinted from Kunstetter, A.C., Wanner, S.P., Madeira, L.G., Wilke, C.F., Rodrigues, L.O., Lima, N.R., 2014. Association between the increase in brain temperature and physical performance at different exercise intensities and protocols in a temperate environment. Brazilian Journal of Medical and Biological Research 47, 679–688. Open-access manuscript.*

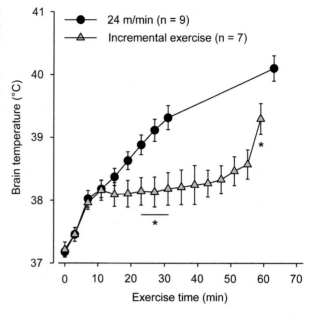

chronic placement of the guide cannula in the brain cortex do not change the physical performance of the rats (Kunstetter et al., 2014). Aside from measuring hypothalamic and cortical temperatures, a study conducted in our laboratory (Damasceno et al., 2015) measured the thalamic temperature of exercising rats because the thalamus is a brain structure involved in motor behavior control and is highly activated during locomotor activity (Holschneider and Maarek, 2008).

The temperature inside the brain is not homogenous: a dorsoventral gradient has been reported in resting (Kiyatkin, 2007; Kiyatkin et al., 2002; Walters et al., 1998a) and in exercising rats (Walters et al., 1998a), with more dorsally-located structures such as the cortex and striatum exhibiting lower temperatures than the ventral structures, including the hypothalamus and nucleus accumbens. Despite this dorsoventral temperature gradient, the temperatures of both the dorsal and ventral brain structures respond quite similarly to arousing stimuli (Kiyatkin et al., 2002) and exercise (Walters et al., 1998a). Indeed, Walters et al. (1998a) observed that a hypothalamic-cortex temperature gradient of 0.7°C in resting rats was constant throughout the exercise, even at volitional fatigue, indicating that hypothalamic and cortex temperatures have a similar rate of increase during exercise. However, two different groups of rats were used to evaluate the cortical brain and hypothalamic temperatures in the latter study. None of the studies that measured the T_{BRAIN} in exercising rats performed the measurement simultaneously at multiple brain sites in the same exercising rat, and therefore, future studies on this topic are warranted.

Considering the dorsoventral gradient in the T_{BRAIN} observed in resting and exercising animals, comparisons between the T_{BRAIN} and the temperature of the peripheral tissues (abdominal or rectal temperature) may lead to different qualitative results depending on the brain site where temperature is measured. In a series of studies performed in our laboratory, the T_{BRAIN} was measured in the thalamus (Damasceno et al., 2015), hypothalamus (Fonseca et al., 2014), and the cortex (Drummond LR and Wanner SP, unpublished data) simultaneously along with abdominal temperature during constant-speed exercises performed until volitional fatigue. As shown in Fig. 4.3, both the thalamic and hypothalamic temperatures increased more rapidly than abdominal temperature during the initial minutes of exercise. Then, the thalamic and hypothalamic temperatures reached a plateau, exhibiting an attenuated increase relative to the abdominal temperature (Fig. 4.3A and C). Therefore, the initial thalamic-abdominal temperature gradient (0.7°C) increased at the beginning of the exercise, reached its highest value (1.1°C) at the 6th min, and then decreased, approaching 0 after 30 min of treadmill running (Fig. 4.3B). Similarly, the initial hypothalamic-abdominal temperature gradient (0.2°C) increased during the initial minutes of running, reached a peak (0.8°C) at the 6th min, and then decreased toward preexercise values (Fig. 4.3D). The cortical–abdominal temperature differential also increased in response to exercise initiation and then decreased as exercise continued (Drummond LR and Wanner SP, unpublished data).

Aside from the similarities observed in the temperature response of the different brain regions to exercise, the brain–abdominal temperature gradient varied according to the site where the T_{BRAIN} was measured. While the thalamic and hypothalamic temperatures were always higher than the abdominal temperature throughout fatiguing exercises (Damasceno et al., 2015; Fonseca et al., 2014), the cortex temperature was lower than the abdominal temperature during the final moments of exercise, including the moment when the rats fatigued (Drummond LR and Wanner SP, unpublished data).

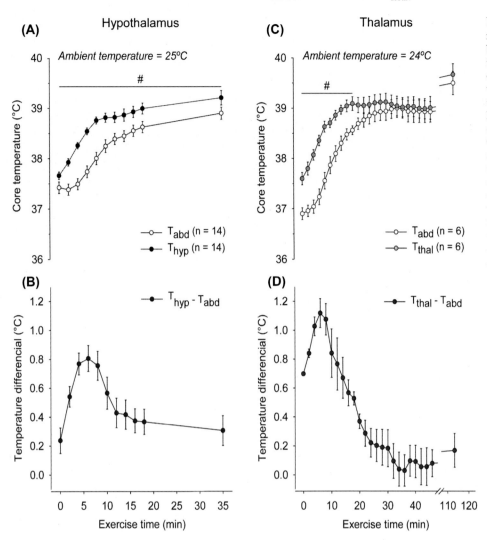

(A) Hypothalamus

(B)

(C) Thalamus

(D)

FIGURE 4.3 Brain and abdominal temperatures (panels A and C) and brain–abdominal temperature differentials (panels B and D) of rats subjected to constant-speed treadmill running until volitional fatigue. Panels A and B show the hypothalamic temperature and the hypothalamic-abdominal temperature differential, respectively, whereas, panels C and D show the thalamic temperature and the thalamic-abdominal temperature differential, respectively. The data are expressed as means±SEM. #$P < 0.05$ compared to the abdominal temperature. *The data were obtained from experiments reported in the following manuscripts: (A and B) hypothalamus—Fonseca, C.G., Pires, W., Lima, M.R., Guimarães, J.B., Lima, N.R., Wanner, S.P., 2014. Hypothalamic temperature of rats subjected to treadmill running in a cold environment. PLoS One 9, e111501. Open-access manuscript; (C and D) thalamus—Damasceno, W.C., Pires, W., Lima, M.R., Lima, N.R., Wanner, S.P., 2015. The dynamics of physical exercise-induced increases in thalamic and abdominal temperatures are modified by central cholinergic stimulation. Neuroscience Letters 590, 193–198.* Copyright © 2015 Elsevier. Used with permission.

These results are consistent with previous studies that observed higher hypothalamic temperatures (Fuller et al., 1998; Walters et al., 1998a, 2000) and lower cortical temperatures (Hasegawa et al., 2008; Walters et al., 1998a) than abdominal temperatures at volitional fatigue. Therefore, studies that have measured the cortical temperature have often reported the occurrence of SBC, while studies that have measured the temperature in subcortical regions (e.g., the thalamus and hypothalamus) have not observed SBC. Collectively, these results indicate that SBC might occur only in specific brain regions, most likely at dorsally-located regions. Again, future studies designed to compare the changes in T_{BRAIN} measured at different sites with changes in abdominal temperature in the same exercising rat are required to improve our knowledge of the occurrence of SBC during exercise, at least in this species.

This topic is of particular interest when discussing the role of T_{BRAIN} in determining exercise performance because SBC could improve exercise performance by attenuating brain hyperthermia. In vitro studies have indicated that neuronal cells are the most heat-sensitive cells of the body and are characterized by a low upper-temperature limit tolerated in hyperthermic conditions (Dewhirst et al., 2003). Therefore, SBC would improve the tolerance to physical exertion by maintaining the T_{BRAIN} at lower values and by protecting the brain against thermal damage.

The Association Between T_{BRAIN} Increases and Exercise Performance

The treadmill run is a forced exercise in which animals are often encouraged to run by light electrical stimulation provided by a grid located at the end of the treadmill belt. During this type of exercise, when animals become fatigued, their only option is to expose themselves to the electrical stimuli. In our studies, exercise is terminated when exposure lasts 10 s. Therefore, physical performance is usually determined by the running time or distance traveled until fatigue. Nevertheless, some investigators do not use electrical stimulation to force the rats to run on the treadmill and determine fatigue using different criteria (for a detailed discussion about fatigue definitions and criteria used for determining fatigue, please see Wanner et al., 2015).

As discussed in the previous sections, the T_{BRAIN} seems to be a more sensitive index for determining physical performance than the temperature of the peripheral tissues. The first evidence for this hypothesis was provided by Caputa et al. (1986), who reported that a lower increase in T_{BRAIN} (42.6°C) relative to the magnitude of the increase in the temperature of the abdominal aorta (43.5°C) was sufficient to promote feelings of fatigue, accelerating the termination of exercise in goats. In this context, other four studies have investigated the association between brain hyperthermia and exercise performance (Fonseca et al., 2014; Fuller et al., 1998; Kunstetter et al., 2014; Walters et al., 2000), and all have suggested that higher T_{BRAIN} values or higher rates of increase in T_{BRAIN} are associated with reduced total exercise time during constant-speed treadmill running. Fuller et al. (1998) and Walters et al. (2000) observed that the elevation of T_{BRAIN} prior to exercise initiation was a limiting factor for the attainment of the expected physical performance during treadmill running in hot environments. In fact, Walters et al. (2000) reported a negative correlation between high preexercise hypothalamic temperatures and total exercise time. Aside from these studies that have evaluated fatigue during exercise in hot environments, two studies performed in our laboratory indicate that the increase in T_{BRAIN} is also associated with a reduction in physical performance in a temperate environment (Fonseca et al., 2014; Kunstetter et al., 2014). During constant-speed exercises, Kunstetter et al. (2014) observed negative correlations between the rate of increase in T_{BRAIN} and total exercise time for each of the three treadmill speeds that were studied (Fig. 4.4). Interestingly, Fonseca et al. (2014) reported a significant and negative correlation between the increase in T_{BRAIN} and exercise performance at 25°C, while increases in abdominal temperature were not significantly correlated with the total exercise time. Collectively, these five studies support the hypothesis proposed by Nybo (2012), which states that exercise-induced increases in T_{BRAIN} play an important role in determining exercise performance. However, no study has described the physiological mechanism by which the increase in T_{BRAIN} decreases voluntary activation, inducing fatigue.

Brain Temperature in Exercising Humans

Direct measurements of the T_{BRAIN} cannot be performed in exercising humans. However, a seminal study performed by Nybo et al. (2002) proposed a methodological approach to indirectly evaluate the T_{BRAIN} in humans by measuring the temperatures of the jugular vein and arterial blood. The authors assumed that the temperature of the blood perfusing the brain equilibrates with that of the neuronal tissue, and therefore, the venous blood drained from the brain, flowing through the jugular vein, would represent the mean temperature of the cerebral tissue. These authors also proposed that the venous–arterial blood temperature gradient indicates the difference between the mean temperature of the neural tissue and the temperature of the blood supplying the brain. Because the metabolic

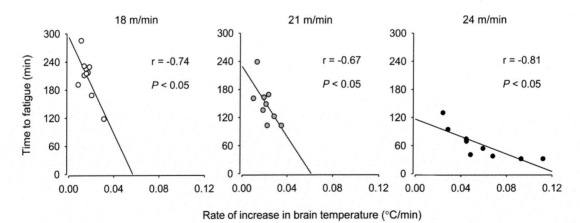

FIGURE 4.4   Correlations between time to fatigue and the rate of increase in cortical brain temperature calculated from the beginning until the end of constant exercises at three speeds: 18, 21, and 24 m/min. Data are reported as individual values. *The graph was reprinted from Kunstetter, A.C., Wanner, S.P., Madeira, L.G., Wilke, C.F., Rodrigues, L.O., Lima, N.R., 2014. Association between the increase in brain temperature and physical performance at different exercise intensities and protocols in a temperate environment. Brazilian Journal of Medical and Biological Research 47, 679–688. Open-access manuscript.*

heat produced by neuronal cells is dissipated primarily by cerebral blood flow, a larger venous–arterial blood temperature gradient is associated with increased heat drainage from the brain.

Nybo et al. (2002) observed that the jugular venous blood temperature increased progressively and in parallel with the increase in esophageal temperature during exercise performed in hot environments. In addition, the jugular venous blood temperature was always higher than the arterial blood and the esophageal temperature, indicating that the temperature of cerebral tissue is maintained at higher levels than the temperature of other "core" body compartments throughout the exercise period. During the initial minutes of exercise, the arterial temperature increased at a faster rate than the venous temperature, and the temperature differential was therefore narrowed relative to the differential at rest. This finding indicates that the increase in the human T_{BRAIN} during the initial minutes of exercise does not result from intra-brain heat production, and it may indicate a reduction in heat released from the brain, particularly during exertion in a hot environment. The authors also concluded that humans likely cannot selectively cool their brain during exercise, and therefore, the T_{BRAIN} will increase in parallel with the increase in the temperature of peripheral tissues. In contrast, the rat T_{BRAIN} increases more rapidly than the abdominal temperature in response to exercise, irrespective of where the T_{BRAIN} is measured. This early difference in the rate of increase in the T_{CORE} indexes likely results from intra-brain heat production. Notably, these inter-species comparisons should be interpreted cautiously because human data represent changes in the whole brain function, whereas the data collected in rats represent changes in the function of specific brain areas.

FINAL REMARKS

Because direct measurements of the T_{BRAIN} in exercising humans are not currently possible, several studies have been performed in rats to investigate the extent to which the T_{BRAIN} increases during exercise and whether SBC occurs in mammals that do not possess a carotid rete. These studies have reported that (1) the T_{BRAIN} increases during exercise and can reach values above 40°C when physical exertion is performed in a hot environment or during prolonged exertion (duration longer than 1 h) in a temperate environment; (2) a dorsoventral temperature gradient exists between brain regions, with the ventrally-located structures being warmer than the dorsally-located structures; (3) the observation of SBC in rats seems to depend on the brain site where temperature is measured; and (4) the exercise-induced increase in T_{BRAIN} negatively affects physical performance at different exercise intensities and ambient temperatures. Future studies are required to further understand how the temperature of different brain sites changes in response to physical exercise and to confirm the occurrence of SBC in specific brain structures of mammals that do not possess a carotid rete.

References

Baker, M.A., 1982. Brain cooling in endotherms in heat and exercise. Annual Review of Physiology 44, 85–96. http://dx.doi.org/10.1146/annurev.ph.44.030182.000505.

Caputa, M., Demick, A., Doklandy, K., Kurowicka, B., 1996. Anatomical and physiological evidence for efficacious selective brain cooling in rats. Journal of Thermal Biology 21 (1), 21–28. http://dx.doi.org/10.1016/0306-4565(95)00016-X.

Caputa, M., Feistkorn, G., Jessen, C., 1986. Effects of brain and trunk temperatures on exercise performance in goats. Pflügers Archiv 406 (2), 184–189. http://dx.doi.org/10.1007/BF00586681.

Caputa, M., Kamari, A., Wachulec, M., 1991. Selective brain cooling in rats resting in heat and during exercise. Journal of Thermal Biology 16 (1), 19–24. http://dx.doi.org/10.1016/0306-4565(91)90046-5.

Damasceno, W.C., Pires, W., Lima, M.R., Lima, N.R., Wanner, S.P., 2015. The dynamics of physical exercise-induced increases in thalamic and abdominal temperatures are modified by central cholinergic stimulation. Neuroscience Letters 590, 193–198. http://dx.doi.org/10.1016/j.neulet.2015.01.082.

Dewhirst, M.W., Viglianti, B.L., Lora-Michiels, M., Hanson, M., Hoopes, P.J., 2003. Basic principles of thermal dosimetry and thermal thresholds for tissue damage from hyperthermia. International Journal of Hyperthermia 19 (3), 267–294. http://dx.doi.org/10.1080/0265673031000119006.

Drust, B., Rasmussen, P., Mohr, M., Nielsen, B., Nybo, L., 2005. Elevations in core and muscle temperature impairs repeated sprint performance. Acta Physiologica Scandinavica 183 (2), 181–190. http://dx.doi.org/10.1111/j.1365-201X.2004.01390.x.

Fonseca, C.G., Pires, W., Lima, M.R., Guimaraes, J.B., Lima, N.R., Wanner, S.P., 2014. Hypothalamic temperature of rats subjected to treadmill running in a cold environment. PLoS One 9 (11), e111501. http://dx.doi.org/10.1371/journal.pone.0111501.

Ftaiti, F., Kacem, A., Jaidane, N., Tabka, Z., Dogui, M., 2010. Changes in EEG activity before and after exhaustive exercise in sedentary women in neutral and hot environments. Applied Ergonomics 41 (6), 806–811. http://dx.doi.org/10.1016/j.apergo.2010.01.008.

Fuller, A., Carter, R.N., Mitchell, D., 1998. Brain and abdominal temperatures at fatigue in rats exercising in the heat. Journal of Applied Physiology 84 (3), 877–883.

Galloway, S.D., Maughan, R.J., 1997. Effects of ambient temperature on the capacity to perform prolonged cycle exercise in man. Medicine & Science in Sports & Exercise 29 (9), 1240–1249.

Gisolfi, C.V., Mora, F., 2000. The Hot Brain: Survival, Temperature, and the Human Body. The Massachusetts Institute of Technology, Cambridge, MA.

Gonzalez-Alonso, J., Teller, C., Andersen, S.L., Jensen, F.B., Hyldig, T., Nielsen, B., 1999. Influence of body temperature on the development of fatigue during prolonged exercise in the heat. Journal of Applied Physiology 86 (3), 1032–1039.

Guimaraes, J.B., Wanner, S.P., Machado, S.C., Lima, M.R., Cordeiro, L.M., Pires, W., La Guardia, R.B., Silami-Garcia, E., Rodrigues, L.O., Lima, N.R., 2013. Fatigue is mediated by cholinoceptors within the ventromedial hypothalamus independent of changes in core temperature. Scandinavian Journal of Medicine & Science in Sports 23 (1), 46–56. http://dx.doi.org/10.1111/j.1600-0838.2011.01350.x.

Hasegawa, H., Piacentini, M.F., Sarre, S., Michotte, Y., Ishiwata, T., Meeusen, R., 2008. Influence of brain catecholamines on the development of fatigue in exercising rats in the heat. Journal of Physiology 586 (1), 141–149. http://dx.doi.org/10.1113/jphysiol.2007.142190.

Holschneider, D.P., Maarek, J.M., 2008. Brain maps on the go: functional imaging during motor challenge in animals. Methods 45 (4), 255–261. http://dx.doi.org/10.1016/j.ymeth.2008.04.006.

Kiyatkin, E.A., 2007. Brain temperature fluctuations during physiological and pathological conditions. European Journal of Applied Physiology 101 (1), 3–17. http://dx.doi.org/10.1007/s00421-007-0450-7.

Kiyatkin, E.A., Brown, P.L., Wise, R.A., 2002. Brain temperature fluctuation: a reflection of functional neural activation. European Journal of Neuroscience 16 (1), 164–168. http://dx.doi.org/10.1046/j.1460-9568.2002.02066.x.

Kiyatkin, E.A., Sharma, H.S., 2009. Permeability of the blood–brain barrier depends on brain temperature. Neuroscience 161 (3), 926–939. http://dx.doi.org/10.1016/j.neuroscience.2009.04.004.

Kunstetter, A.C., Wanner, S.P., Madeira, L.G., Wilke, C.F., Rodrigues, L.O., Lima, N.R., 2014. Association between the increase in brain temperature and physical performance at different exercise intensities and protocols in a temperate environment. Brazilian Journal of Medical and Biological Research 47 (8), 679–688. http://dx.doi.org/10.1590/1414-431X20143561.

Lind, A.R., 1963. A physiological criterion for setting thermal environmental limits for everyday work. Journal of Applied Physiology 18, 51–56.

Nielsen, B., 1966. Regulation of body temperature and heat dissipation at different levels of energy- and heat production in man. Acta Physiologica Scandinavica 68, 215–227.

Nielsen, B., Savard, G., Richter, E.A., Hargreaves, M., Saltin, B., 1990. Muscle blood flow and muscle metabolism during exercise and heat stress. Journal of Applied Physiology 69 (3), 1040–1046.

Nybo, L., 2008. Hyperthermia and fatigue. Journal of Applied Physiology 104 (3), 871–878. http://dx.doi.org/10.1152/japplphysiol.00910.2007.

Nybo, L., 2012. Brain temperature and exercise performance. Experimental Physiology 97 (3), 333–339. http://dx.doi.org/10.1113/expphysiol.2011.062273.

Nybo, L., Nielsen, B., 2001a. Hyperthermia and central fatigue during prolonged exercise in humans. Journal of Applied Physiology 91 (3), 1055–1060.

Nybo, L., Nielsen, B., 2001b. Perceived exertion is associated with an altered brain activity during exercise with progressive hyperthermia. Journal of Applied Physiology 91 (5), 2017–2023.

Nybo, L., Secher, N.H., Nielsen, B., 2002. Inadequate heat release from the human brain during prolonged exercise with hyperthermia. Journal of Physiology 545 (Pt 2), 697–704. http://dx.doi.org/10.1113/jphysiol.2002.030023.

Rodrigues, L.O., Oliveira, A., Lima, N.R., Machado-Moreira, C.A., 2003. Heat storage rate and acute fatigue in rats. Brazilian Journal of Medical and Biological Research 36 (1), 131–135. http://dx.doi.org/10.1590/S0100-879X2003000100018.

Romanovsky, A.A., 2007. Thermoregulation: some concepts have changed. Functional architecture of the thermoregulatory system. American Journal of Physiology - Regulatory, Integrative and Comparative Physiology 292 (1), R37–R46. http://dx.doi.org/10.1152/ajpregu.00668.2006.

Romanovsky, A.A., Almeida, M.C., Aronoff, D.M., Ivanov, A.I., Konsman, J.P., Steiner, A.A., Turek, V.F., 2005. Fever and hypothermia in systemic inflammation: recent discoveries and revisions. Frontiers in Bioscience 10, 2193–2216. http://dx.doi.org/10.2741/1690.

Tanaka, H., Yanase, M., Nakayama, T., 1988. Body temperature regulation in rats during exercise of various intensities at different ambient temperatures. The Japanese Journal of Physiology 38 (2), 167–177.

The Commission for Thermal Physiology of the International Union of Physiological Sciences (IUPS Thermal Commission), 2001. Glossary of terms for thermal physiology: third edition. The Japanese Journal of Physiology 51 (2), i–xxxvi.

Walters, T.J., Ryan, K.L., Belcher, J.C., Doyle, J.M., Tehrany, M.R., Mason, P.A., 1998a. Regional brain heating during microwave exposure (2.06 GHz), warm-water immersion, environmental heating and exercise. Bioelectromagnetics 19 (6), 341–353. http://dx.doi.org/10.1002/(SICI)1521-186X(1998)19:6<341::AID-BEM2>3.0.CO;2-1.

Walters, T.J., Ryan, K.L., Tate, L.M., Mason, P.A., 2000. Exercise in the heat is limited by a critical internal temperature. Journal of Applied Physiology 89 (2), 799–806.

Walters, T.J., Ryan, K.L., Tehrany, M.R., Jones, M.B., Paulus, L.A., Mason, P.A., 1998b. HSP70 expression in the CNS in response to exercise and heat stress in rats. Journal of Applied Physiology 84 (4), 1269–1277.

Wanner, S.P., Prímola-Gomes, T.N., Pires, W., Guimaraes, J.B., Hudson, A.S.R., Kunstetter, A.C., Fonseca, C.G., Drummond, L.R., Damasceno, W.C., Coelho, F.T., 2015. Thermoregulatory responses in exercising rats: methodological aspects and relevance to human physiology. Temperature 1, 1–19. http://dx.doi.org/10.1080/23328940.2015.1119615.

Watson, P., Shirreffs, S.M., Maughan, R.J., 2005. Blood–brain barrier integrity may be threatened by exercise in a warm environment. American Journal of Physiology - Regulatory, Integrative and Comparative Physiology 288 (6), R1689–R1694. http://dx.doi.org/10.1152/ajpregu.00676.2004.

DRUGS OF ABUSE WITH EXERCISE TO MODIFY NEUROLOGICAL STRUCTURE AND FUNCTION

5

Physical Activity as a Therapeutic Intervention for Addictive Disorders: Interactions With Methamphetamine

S.S. Somkuwar, M.J. Fannon-Pavlich, C.D. Mandyam

Committee on the Neurobiology of Addictive Disorders, La Jolla, CA, United States

Abstract

There is an increasing need for effective treatments to reduce propensity for relapse to the illicit psychostimulant methamphetamine in addicted individuals. Cognitive behavioral therapies are currently used with limited success and therefore pharmacotherapies could assist, yet no FDA approved medications are available. Preclinical studies demonstrate that this is partially attributed to the complex and dynamic neurobiology underlying methamphetamine addiction-like behavior. Therefore, therapeutic strategies to treat methamphetamine addiction, particularly the relapse stage of addiction, could revolutionize addiction treatment. In this context, preclinical studies demonstrate that voluntary exercise (sustained physical activity) may be beneficial. This chapter discusses the neurobiology of methamphetamine addiction and sustained physical activity deciphered using animal models and highlights the emerging mechanisms of wheel running in attenuating intake and in preventing relapse to methamphetamine seeking behavior in preclinical models of compulsive-like methamphetamine intake.

INTRODUCTION

Addiction or substance dependence is a mental disorder that involves the loss of behavioral control over drug taking and drug seeking, and involves impulsivity and compulsivity. The limited (often recreational) use of illicit drugs is distinct from the pattern of compulsive (escalated, unregulated) drug use and these uncontrolled behaviors materialize a chronic drug-dependent state which is a hallmark of addiction (Koob and Le Moal, 1997). The "cycle of addiction" can be divided into three stages: (1) binge/prolonged intoxication, (2) withdrawal/negative affect, and (3) preoccupation/anticipation (craving). The last stage of the addiction cycle helps define addiction in humans as a chronic relapsing disorder (Koob and Volkow, 2010).

Methamphetamine is a powerful psychostimulant and an illicit drug with high abuse potential, and subjects that are addicted to methamphetamine eventually become dependent on the drug and cannot abstain from it. For example, in the United States, 8% of all drug/alcohol treatment admissions involve methamphetamine and frequent relapses are common among those that are trying to abstain (SAMHSA, 2008). Furthermore, methamphetamine addiction takes emotional and financial tolls on society, cutting across ages, races, ethnicities, and genders and is a serious public health issue. According to the recent reports from the National Institutes on Drug Abuse (NIDA) there are no FDA approved medications for psychostimulant dependency in a primary care setting and only a few partially effective cognitive behavioral therapy options are available for methamphetamine addiction (Gonzales et al., 2010; McHugh et al., 2010; NIDA, 2011). Therefore, the need for effective treatment to reduce dependency to methamphetamine and reduce propensity for methamphetamine relapse is increasing. Notably, promising evidence from preclinical studies demonstrates that voluntary physical activity reduces methamphetamine consumption in animals that exhibit compulsive-like intake when physical activity is performed concurrently with the act of self-administering methamphetamine. Furthermore, physical activity during abstinence reduces reinstatement of methamphetamine seeking in rats that demonstrate higher propensity for relapse (Engelmann et al., 2014; Sobieraj et al., 2014). These studies demonstrate that physical activity could be a novel therapeutic approach to combat or reduce relapse in methamphetamine addicted individuals.

With respect to physical activity, its importance on the overall quality of life of an individual has piqued the interest of philosophers for centuries. The idea that mental stress adversely affects physical health is well accepted, and conversely, it is suggested that a healthy body will espouse a healthy mind (Phillips et al., 2014). In recent years, the benefits of exercise (physical activity via cardiovascular or aerobic exercise) on health and wellness have become increasingly well-known. Perhaps more relevant to this discourse, exercise offers relief from the symptoms of depression and anxiety, and improves mood (Blumenthal et al., 1999; DiLorenzo et al., 1999; Peluso and Guerra de Andrade, 2005). It is these properties that make exercise a valuable tool in disrupting the vicious feed-forward loop between mental illness and substance abuse (Jones et al., 2003; Koob, 2013; Polter and Kauer, 2014). Thus, the mechanisms by which voluntary exercise (sustained physical activity) affects the mammalian brain, particularly cognitive function, are of interest and the focus of several lines of scientific inquiry. The therapeutic effects of exercise extend into many different aspects of human life including the realm of substance use disorders. For example, recent reviews from clinical and preclinical studies have elaborated the potential of exercise or physical activity as a therapeutic intervention during the various stages of drug addiction, particularly, addiction to methamphetamine (Lynch et al., 2013; Somkuwar et al., 2015). While this chapter discusses the benefits of physical activity in the context of drug abuse, it should be noted that the reinforcing property of exercise is a double-edged sword; on one hand these properties make physical activity an effective treatment for addiction and on the other hand, it makes exercise itself potentially addictive (Kanarek et al, 2009). Nevertheless, preclinical research in the past few decades has conferred some clarity into circumstances where the benefits of physical activity may outweigh the risk in its use as a therapeutic strategy, particularly in the context of reward substitution with other reinforcing illicit drugs (Smith and Lynch, 2011). The following sections of the chapter will review animal models of drug reward and reinforcement and voluntary physical activity and will discuss the convergence of these behaviors in the context of neurobiology, neurotoxicity, and reward substitution.

ANIMAL MODELS OF DRUG REINFORCEMENT AND REWARD TO ILLICIT DRUGS

Drug-taking behavior has been demonstrated in rodent models of intravenous drug self-administration, in which rodents are trained to self-administer drugs by pressing a lever for an intravenous drug infusion in an operant conditioning chamber (Robbins and Everitt, 2002). Valid animal models of addiction should highlight dependence-like behaviors, such as escalation of drug intake over time and withdrawal symptoms when the drug is withheld (Ahmed and Koob, 1998). In that regard, intravenous drug self-administration with intermittent (1 h biweekly), limited (1 h daily), or long (extended >4 h daily) access have significant clinical relevance by illustrating a range of different drug seeking behaviors (Mandyam et al., 2007). An increase in drug availability or a history of drug intake has been shown to accelerate the development of dependence in humans (Gawin and Ellinwood, 1989; Kramer et al., 1967). In rats, extended access to drugs of abuse, including cocaine, methamphetamine, nicotine, heroin, and alcohol, produce an escalation of drug self-administration, suggesting compulsive-like drug intake and reflecting dependence-like behavior. Therefore, the extended access model may be particularly suitable for testing the hypothesis that alterations in adult brain plasticity induced by methamphetamine are partially responsible for the addictive behavior (Ahmed and Koob, 1998).

Reinstatement of drug-seeking behavior in rats is widely used as a model of craving to mimic the relapse stage of addiction often observed in the clinic (Shaham et al., 2003). This model is studied extensively to uncover the key brain regions, brain circuitry, neurotransmitters, and neuromodulators associated with reinstatement behavior. The paradigm extinguishes learned self-administration behavior by explicitly not rewarding (e.g., withholding intravenous drug infusion) the animal after the correct response is emitted (e.g., a correct lever response) and tests the ability of a priming stimulus to reinstate drug-seeking response (Shalev et al., 2002). The priming stimuli can be visual or auditory cues previously paired with drug self-administration (cue priming), acute noncontingent exposure to the drug (experimenter delivered, i.e., drug priming) or context (spatial location) where the drug was self-administered. Using the self-administration model of drug taking and reinstatement model of drug seeking, studies have shown that animals with compulsive-like methamphetamine intake also exhibit a higher propensity for relapse after a period of withdrawal or abstinence, thereby encompassing both addictive traits in a single subpopulation (Kitamura et al., 2006; Recinto et al., 2012). These findings demonstrate that these are powerful models for identifying neurobiological factors involved in determining risk for relapse and will improve our understanding of addiction-like behavior with regard to its translational value to the human population.

An alternative approach for assessing drug reward in animal models involves conditioned place preference (CPP), which determines the Pavlovian associations between rewarding effects of a drug and a contiguously presented stimulus, i.e., the context in which the rewarding effects of the drug are experienced (Bardo and Bevins, 2000). This conditioning approach is different from operant behavior, as it does not involve the animal "working" for the drug reward (e.g., no lever responses), but rather, it examines the preference for the context following the development of the association (Advokat, 1985). Furthermore, in this model animals receive passive administration of the drug (i.e., experimenter delivered), and are tested (cue/context) in a drug-free state (Bardo and Bevins, 2000). Although the operant self-administration and CPP models have face validity, the operant model of drug reward and reinstatement is more advantageous. For example, while CPP behavior fails to demonstrate drug dose-dependency, the self-administration model is useful for eliciting distinct drug intake patterns (limited versus compulsive-like intake of the drug) to mimic recreational use versus dependent use, to measure repeated operant responding to mimic an addict's drug-response pattern, and to produce high rates of relapse. Thus, the intravenous self-administration model of drug exposure appears to be the best suited for studying the neural mechanisms of drug reward and relapse.

ANIMAL MODELS OF SUSTAINED PHYSICAL ACTIVITY

Various animal models of physical activity have been utilized which can be broadly classified as either voluntary or as forced exercise (Arida et al, 2011). Voluntary wheel running is the most widely used model of voluntary exercise. In this paradigm, a wheel is placed in the home cage of the animal and the animal has *ad libitum* access to the wheel. In contrast, forced wheel running isolates the animal with the wheel by partitioning off access to any other area; rotation of the wheel can be controlled remotely (using a computer or other mechanism) to ensure that the animal is forced to run while on the wheel (Arida et al., 2011). Another forced exercise model is treadmill running, where an animal is forced to run on a motor-driven treadmill for a controlled amount of time (Arida et al., 2011). Swimming has also been used as an exercise model which involves the animal being forced to swim in a tank with access to a platform for resting (optional) without leaving the water (Segat et al., 2014). Both voluntary and forced exercise paradigms have proven effective animal models; while voluntary exercise is typically chosen to simulate human choices, forced exercise is suggested to more closely resemble more vigorous human exercise regimens (Voss et al., 2013). Environmental enrichment is another technique that provides greater opportunity for physical activity compared to standard housing conditions (Arida et al., 2011), but is a more complex paradigm with social and cognitive stimulation involved; thus, environmental enrichment is not solely measuring physical activity, and therefore will not be discussed further.

Utilizing these models of voluntary physical activity, emerging evidence suggests that wheel running is a positive reinforcer and the behavioral outcomes can appear similar to addiction to illicit substances (Kanarek et al., 2009). For example, in voluntary wheel running paradigms escalation of running activity has been reported (Engelmann et al., 2014). Such behavioral outcomes indicate that sustained physical activity has reinforcing properties that can lead to increased use over time. In addition, using the CPP task, rats were reported to prefer wheel-paired chambers compared to the chamber without wheel-pairing history (Greenwood et al., 2011), suggesting that access to running wheel is rewarding. Interestingly, wheel running has been shown to activate the mesolimbic reward pathway as seen with illicit drugs, and like methamphetamine, can increase extracellular dopamine in the ventral striatum (Fig. 5.1), further identifying the neuronal mechanism underlying the rewarding and reinforcing properties of wheel running. Combined, this body of research suggests that wheel running has rewarding properties, and can tap into the reward pathway associated with several illicit drugs and therefore, could be used as a reward substitute to reduce addiction-like behavior to illicit drugs.

CONVERGENCE BETWEEN METHAMPHETAMINE SELF-ADMINISTRATION AND SUSTAINED PHYSICAL ACTIVITY IN ANIMAL MODELS

Developmental effects on methamphetamine self-administration and wheel running: Drug consumption and wheel running in rodents is known to decrease as a function of age when adult (2–5-month-old) animals were compared with aged (10–20-month-old) animals (Gulve et al., 1993; Marshall et al., 2003; McCullough et al., 2013). However, few studies have demonstrated that these behaviors vary during development (between 2 and 5 months of age) in adult animals (Staples et al., 2015). Recent observations show that differences in both these consummatory behaviors is evidenced much before the geriatric age (10–20-month-old), particularly, when the age-difference between young adult and mature adult rats is merely 2 months (Staples et al., 2015; Fig. 5.2). For example, following the development of stable

FIGURE 5.1 Overlap of neural circuit underlying reward in animals experiencing methamphetamine and physical activity in the adult rodent brain: A schematic for the overarching effects of methamphetamine and physical activity on the reward, reinforcement and motivational centers of the adult rodent brain, particularly the medial prefrontal cortex (highlighted in green), the hippocampus (highlighted in blue), and striatum (highlighted in pink). *Reprinted from Sucharita, S., Somkuwar, Miranda, C., Staples, McKenzie, J., Fannon, Atoosa, Ghofranian and Chitra, D., Mandyam. Evaluating Exercise as a Therapeutic Intervention for Methamphetamine Addiction-Like Behavior. Tracking Effects of Exercise on Neuronal Plasticity 1, 59–77. Copyright (2015), with permission from IOS Press.*

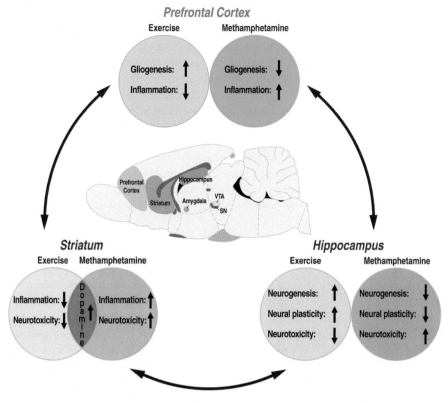

responding, young adult male rats (~3-month-old) self-administered 3-times more methamphetamine compared to mature adult counterparts (~5-month-old; Fig. 5.2A; unpublished observation). Effect of age on wheel running was also evaluated in male rats housed in special home cages with *ad libitum* wheel access. Young adult rats (2-month-old) showed greater running activity on the first day of wheel access compared to mature adult rats (4-month-old; Fig. 5.2B, modified from (Staples et al., 2015)). Further, young adult runners demonstrated an escalation in running output, an effect observed during the first 2 weeks; this behavior was not evident in the mature adult rats (Fig. 5.2C; modified from (Staples et al., 2015)). Given that the function of the reward circuitry dampens with age (Marschner et al., 2005), mature adults may not be as sensitive to the rewarding aspects of methamphetamine and wheel running as young adults. Taken together, these data further suggest that positive reinforcers (methamphetamine and wheel running) potentially affect common neurobiological factors, namely the reward circuit in the adult brain (Fig. 5.1).

Reward substitution between methamphetamine self-administration and wheel running: Data from preclinical research has repeatedly shown that wheel running reduces the amount of drug intake during self-administration sessions (for review see (Lynch et al., 2013)). With respect to methamphetamine in particular, access to running wheels during self-administration reduced self-administration during acquisition (Engelmann et al., 2014; Miller et al., 2012), and reduced and prevented compulsive-like intake (Engelmann et al., 2014). Furthermore, access to running wheels during protracted withdrawal from methamphetamine self-administration reduced responding during extinction (a behavioral inhibition paradigm where animals are tested for drug seeking behavior in the absence of the reinforcer) and reduced responding during context- and cue-induced reinstatement of methamphetamine seeking (Sobieraj et al., 2014). These results highlight that wheel running is preventing certain patterns of drug taking and seeking and provides protection against propensity for relapse. Additional findings demonstrate that withdrawal from access to running wheels was found to increase methamphetamine intake during acquisition compared to rats with continued access to wheels as well as compared to sedentary rats, suggesting a deprivation effect (Engelmann et al., 2014). Furthermore, escalation of methamphetamine intake did not differ between running wheel-withdrawn rats and sedentary rats (Engelmann et al., 2014), suggesting that the protective effect of wheel running in reducing methamphetamine taking may be contingent on continued availability (or contemporaneous availability) of the running wheel. This lends further credence to the hypothesis that the efficacy of physical activity (wheel running) depends on its ability to serve as a strong alternate rewarding and reinforcing agent. The subsequent sections will discuss the neurobiological mechanisms underlying the protective effects of wheel running in the context of drug (methamphetamine) addiction to elucidate the possibilities for future phamacotherapies that could assist with reducing drug taking and seeking behaviors.

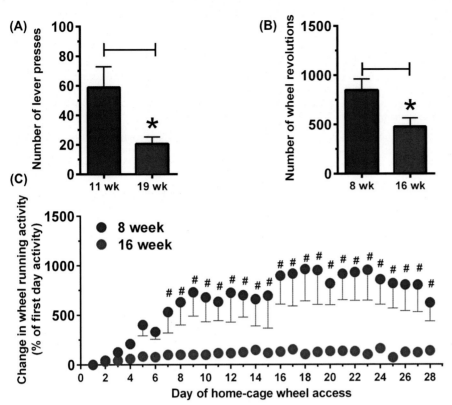

FIGURE 5.2   Methamphetamine self-administration (unpublished observation, (A)) and wheel running activity B–C in young adult (blue) and mature adult (red) rats. (A) Number of lever responses on active levers (reinforcing lever delivering 0.05 mg/kg methamphetamine per infusion intravenously) after 10 sessions of self-administration in young adult and mature adult rats. (B) Average of daily running activity measured as number of wheel revolutions per day for young adult and mature adult rats during the last week of 4-week running activity. (C) Percent change in running activity in young adult and mature adult rats from the first day of running to the last day of running. Asterisk in (A) denotes a significant decrease between young adult and mature adult animals self-administering methamphetamine and in (B) denotes a significant decrease in running activity (*$P \le .05$ versus young adult rats by unpaired t-test). Pound sign in (C) denotes significant increase (escalation) in running activity between young and mature runners over days of running (#$P < .05$ versus day one by repeated measures ANOVA). *Modified from Staples, M.C., Somkuwar, S.S., Mandyam, C.D., 2015. Developmental effects of wheel running on hippocampal glutamate receptor expression in young and mature adult rats. Neuroscience 305, 248–256.*

NEURAL MECHANISMS UNDERLYING REINFORCING EFFECTS OF METHAMPHETAMINE AND WHEEL RUNNING

Modulation of Neurotransmission in the Brain Reward Circuitry

Animal models of addiction have proved to be an immensely valuable tool for parsing out the neurobiological adaptations that contribute to the progression of addiction through the various stages of the addiction cycle (Koob and Volkow, 2010). For example, the key brain regions implicated in the reinstatement of drug seeking behavior include, but are not limited to, the medial prefrontal cortex, nucleus accumbens (ventral striatum), dorsal striatum, bed nucleus of the stria terminalis, central nucleus of the amygdala, basolateral amygdala, hippocampal regions, and ventral tegmental area (Crombag et al., 2008; Koob and Volkow, 2010; Robbins and Everitt, 2002; Shaham et al., 2003). Furthermore, the release of the neurotransmitters dopamine, glutamate, and corticotropin-releasing factor (CRF) in these key brain regions are considered essential for the rewarding effects of drug during the preoccupation/craving stage of addiction that contribute to relapse (Knackstedt and Kalivas, 2009; Koob, 1999). Finally, the overlapping effects of wheel running and drugs of abuse on these brain regions and neurotransmitters have been elegantly detailed in a recent review (Lynch et al., 2013) and is presented here from the perspectives of wheel running as a reward substitute for methamphetamine abuse (Table 5.1).

NEUROPROTECTION BY WHEEL RUNNING: SIGNIFICANT INTERACTIONS WITH METHAMPHETAMINE-INDUCED NEUROTOXICITY

Methamphetamine Affects Factors Associated With Neurotoxicity

Methamphetamine produces significant neurotoxicity. Briefly, methamphetamine reduces the function of dopamine transporters, vesicular monoamine transporters, tyrosine hydroxylase, and mitochondrial enzyme monoamine oxidase B, to produce excessive dopamine release in the dorsal and ventral striatum (Ares-Santos et al., 2013). The excess dopamine leads to striatal neurotoxicity via enhanced reactive oxygen species (ROS) and reactive nitrogen species, and via compromised mitochondrial function (Ares-Santos et al., 2013). Inflammation is another mechanism

TABLE 5.1   Wheel Running and Methamphetamine Alter Neurotransmission in the Reward and Reinforcement Centers of the Brain

Wheel Running	Methamphetamine	Interaction of Wheel Running and Methamphetamine
Acute running activity activates mesolimbic dopamine pathway (Greenwood et al., 2011).	Methamphetamine increases extracellular dopamine in the brain by increasing release and reducing uptake (Kish, 2008; Rothman and Baumann, 2003).	Wheel running blunts the dopaminergic response to initial methamphetamine experience (Chen et al., 2008; Marques et al., 2008).
Chronic running induces dopaminergic adaptations (Droste et al., 2006; Greenwood et al., 2011; Kolb et al., 2013; Sutoo and Akiyama, 1996). While some of these adaptations are beneficial, others may be detrimental and contribute to escalation of running activity, particularly when running wheel is withdrawn (Ferreira et al., 2006; Greenwood et al., 2011).	Chronic methamphetamine also leads to tolerance and hypofunctionality in the mesocorticolimbic dopamine system (O'Neil et al., 2006; Zhang et al., 2001). This contributes to compensatory escalation of methamphetamine intake, and may further enhance relapse vulnerability.	1. Chronic and continued access to running wheels attenuated escalation of and reinstatement of methamphetamine self-administration (Engelmann et al., 2014; Sobieraj et al., 2014). 2. Chronic wheel running cross-sensitized the reward system for other drugs, particularly when access to wheel is withdrawn (Engelmann et al., 2014; Ferreira et al., 2006).
Wheel running increased expression of group II metabotropic glutamate receptors (mGluR2/3) in striatum, and dampens glutamate release and signaling in the striatum and the hippocampus (Biedermann et al., 2012; Guezennec et al., 1998; Real et al., 2010).	Dysregulation of glutamatergic signaling and internalization-mediated decrease of mGluR2/3 in the prefrontal cortex, nucleus accumbens and dorsal striatum is evidenced in methamphetamine escalation (Crawford et al., 2013; Kufahl et al., 2013; Schwendt et al., 2012).	Activation of mGluR2/3 reduces methamphetamine seeking both before and after development of escalation (Crawford et al., 2013). This may be a mechanism underlying the protective effects of wheel running.
Molecular markers associated with the negative affect and dependence, like increased ΔFosB and dynorphin were also found to be upregulated by running activity (Nestler, 2001; Werme et al., 2002, 2000); withdrawal from running activity may result in the manifestation of negative affect (Kanarek et al., 2009; Kolb et al., 2013; Smith and Yancey, 2003).	Negative affect markers, ΔFosB and dynorphin, were upregulated by chronic methamphetamine (McDaid et al., 2006; Nestler, 2001; Wang and McGinty, 1995), all of which may increase relapse risk.	Wheel running mediated increase in ΔFosB and dynorphin, and manifestation of negative affect in wheel withdrawn subjects may be the neurochemical and behavioral bases, respectively, of cross-sensitization to methamphetamine.

This contributes to the value of exercise as a treatment for drug addiction.
For review, Foley, T.E., Fleshner, M., 2008. Neuroplasticity of dopamine circuits after exercise: implications for central fatigue. Neuromolecular Medicine 10 (2), 67–80.; Lynch, W.J., Peterson, A.B., Sanchez, V., Abel, J., Smith, M.A., 2013. Exercise as a novel treatment for drug addiction: a neurobiological and stage-dependent hypothesis. Neuroscience & Biobehavioral Reviews 37 (8), 1622–1644.

invoked in methamphetamine-induced neurotoxicity, and its effects are considerably potentiated by oxidative stress (Yamamoto and Bankson, 2005). Methamphetamine releases pro-inflammatory cytokines via activation of microglia and astroglia, which contribute to neuronal damage as well as cognitive deficits observed with chronic methamphetamine use (Clark et al., 2013). Therefore, it appears that the transition from recreational to compulsive-like methamphetamine use results from alterations in the reward circuitry in the brain which is assisted by neurotoxicity events such as oxidative stress and neuroinflammation (Everitt et al., 2008).

Wheel Running Modulates Factors Associated With Neurotoxicity

Emerging studies indicate that wheel running increases both antioxidant capacity and resistance against oxidative stress via regulating vasculature and blood flow (Mizuno et al., 2014; Toborek et al., 2013). Furthermore, physical activity, via modulation of oxidative pathways, as well as through independent mechanisms, has been shown to modulate trophic factor signaling in the brain to promote brain plasticity (for review see Phillips et al. (2014); Radak et al. (2014)). Specifically, wheel running increases brain-derived neurotrophic factor (BDNF) expression, activates its downstream signaling pathways, and increases cAMP response element binding protein, that subsequently upregulates other inducible transcription factors (Bechara et al., 2014; Ji et al., 2014; Perez-Gomez and Tasker, 2013). These molecular changes could manifest themselves as beneficial neuroplasticity changes (or reduced neurotoxicity effects) such as increasing cell survival (Novaes Gomes et al., 2014; Ploughman et al., 2014), formation of new synapses (synaptogenesis (Murphy and Segal, 1997)), and birth of new neurons (neurogenesis (van Praag et al., 2005)).

Furthermore, because ROS is known to dose-dependently modulate proliferation of neuronal progenitor cells in the hippocampus (Noble et al., 2005; Novaes Gomes et al., 2014), wheel running may modulate neurogenesis by regulating ROS in the hippocampus. Wheel running may also modulate the levels of trophic factors and ROS in brain regions rich in gliogenesis (generation of new glial cells, including astroglia and oligodendroglia) and contribute to glial homeostasis and affect neuronal function (Somkuwar et al., 2014). The medial prefrontal cortex, a brain region involved in executive function and impulse control (Balodis et al., 2013), is one region where this phenomena has been investigated (Mandyam et al., 2007). Specifically, voluntary wheel running in rats was shown to increase proliferation and survival of progenitor cells medial prefrontal cortex, and these new cells matured into new astroglia (~33%) and new oligodendroglia (~55%) (Mandyam et al., 2007). Thus, wheel running induced gliogenesis may be an antineurotoxic phenomena contributing to wheel running-induced improvement in cognition and executive function (Pinilla, 2006; Yu et al., 2006).

Overlap Between Methamphetamine and Wheel Running: Neurotoxicity Factors

The previous section demonstrates that the potential for overlap between methamphetamine and wheel running extends much deeper and is more complicated than simply modulating neurotransmission in the brain reward circuit (Fig. 5.1). For example, high levels of ROS is deleterious for brain function, and as observed in subjects exposed to high doses of methamphetamine, a high ROS load results in significant oxidative damage to lipids, proteins, and DNA, and contributes to neural cell death. Wheel running improves brain function via changes in redox homeostasis and contributes to increased resistance and tolerance to oxidative challenges, thereby promoting cell survival. Further, altered redox homeostasis establishes a conducive environment for increasing proliferation and survival of neurons and glia in several brain regions, including the hippocampus and the medial prefrontal cortex. However, very few studies have investigated these less conventional oxidative, trophic, and cell proliferation interactions between wheel running and methamphetamine. Notably, swimming (another form of physical activity) was found to attenuate amphetamine-reward and anxiety, which corresponded with wheel running-induced reduction in ROS and protein oxidation products in hippocampal homogenates (Segat et al., 2014). Studies conducted in animal models of methamphetamine addiction revealed that wheel running-induced attenuated acquisition and escalation of methamphetamine self-administration was associated with reduction of neuronal apoptosis and decreased expression of neuronal nitric oxide synthase (an enzyme critical for enhancing oxidative stress) in the ventral striatum (Engelmann et al., 2014). Other studies have supported that wheel running also attenuated methamphetamine-induced damage to dopamine and serotonin terminals in the dorsal and ventral striatum, potentially, by reducing methamphetamine-induced neurotoxicity (O'Dell and Marshall, 2014; O'Dell et al., 2012). Therefore, pro-neurotrophic and antineurotoxic mechanisms may mediate the beneficial effects of wheel running in reducing compulsive-like behavior in animals self-administering methamphetamine.

EXERCISE AS A THERAPEUTIC INTERVENTION FOR METHAMPHETAMINE ADDICTION

The previous sections have discussed that wheel running in rodents protects against propensity for reinstatement of drug seeking and that these behavioral outcomes are due to neural mechanisms and neuroprotection offered by wheel running. Therefore, given the complex and dynamic neurobiology underlying compulsive-like methamphetamine intake, and varied targets protected by wheel running, a single behavioral or pharmacological intervention for reducing drug relapse may not be sufficiently protective (Kalivas and Volkow, 2005; Koob and Volkow, 2010). Wheel running is reported to have negative relationships with the extent, duration, and frequency of drug use throughout the stages of initiation, prolonged intoxication, withdrawal, and relapse (Lynch et al., 2013), and thus, has been sought out as a potential noninvasive and nonpharmacological treatment in animal models. In humans, moderate exercise in methamphetamine dependent individuals significantly reduced depression symptom scores, with greater improvements observed in individuals with higher baseline depression (Haglund et al., 2014), suggesting that exercise could be a promising noninvasive nonpharmacological approach to reduce negative affect symptoms associated with chronic drug use. Importantly, since depression and poor mental health are risk factors for relapse to drug seeking (Koob, 2013), exercise could be propagated as a useful strategy for reducing relapse in methamphetamine dependent individuals. Most importantly, the low cost and easy-to-implement properties of exercise therapy make this all the more lucrative as a potential intervention.

In conclusion, the identification of the neuroplastic and neuromodulatory effects of wheel running in animal models over the past few decades has shed new light on the therapeutic and, more recently, the protective events that are associated with physical activity. While some information is available from animal models regarding the mechanisms underlying the interactions of wheel running with methamphetamine self-administration, several of the potential mechanisms have not been empirically evaluated. Future studies aimed at understanding the potential link between correlative decreases in methamphetamine intake and increase in running output in animal models will allow researchers to determine whether decrease in neurotoxicity by wheel running is behaviorally relevant to the reduced propensity for relapse. This may pave the way for future therapeutic possibilities for reducing relapse in addicted individuals.

Acknowledgments

The authors are supported by funds from the National Institute on Drug Abuse (DA034140) and National Institute on Alcohol Abuse and Alcoholism (AA020098 and AA006420).

References

Advokat, C., 1985. Evidence of place conditioning after chronic intrathecal morphine in rats. Pharmacology, Biochemistry, and Behavior 22 (2), 271–277. http://dx.doi.org/10.1016/0091-3057(85)90390-9.

Ahmed, S.H., Koob, G.F., 1998. Transition from moderate to excessive drug intake: change in hedonic set point. Science 282 (5387), 298–300. Retrieved from: http://www.ncbi.nlm.nih.gov/entrez/query.fcgi?cmd=Retrieve&db=PubMed&dopt=Citation&list_uids=9765157.

Ares-Santos, S., Granado, N., Moratalla, R., 2013. The role of dopamine receptors in the neurotoxicity of methamphetamine. Journal of Internal Medicine 273 (5), 437–453. http://dx.doi.org/10.1111/joim.12049.

Arida, R.M., Scorza, F.A., Gomes da Silva, S., Cysneiros, R.M., Cavalheiro, E.A., 2011. Exercise paradigms to study brain injury recovery in rodents. American Journal of Physical Medicine & Rehabilitation 90 (6), 452–465. http://dx.doi.org/10.1097/PHM.0b013e3182063a9c.

Balodis, I.M., Molina, N.D., Kober, H., Worhunsky, P.D., White, M.A., Rajita, S., Grilo, C.M., Potenza, M.N., 2013. Divergent neural substrates of inhibitory control in binge eating disorder relative to other manifestations of obesity. Obesity (Silver Spring) 21 (2), 367–377. http://dx.doi.org/10.1002/oby.20068.

Bardo, M.T., Bevins, R.A., 2000. Conditioned place preference: what does it add to our preclinical understanding of drug reward? Psychopharmacology 153 (1), 31–43.

Bechara, R.G., Lyne, R., Kelly, A.M., 2014. BDNF-stimulated intracellular signalling mechanisms underlie exercise-induced improvement in spatial memory in the male Wistar rat. Behavioural Brain Research 275, 297–306. http://dx.doi.org/10.1016/j.bbr.2013.11.015.

Biedermann, S., Fuss, J., Zheng, L., Sartorius, A., Falfan-Melgoza, C., Demirakca, T., Gass, P., Ende, G., Weber-Fahr, W., 2012. In vivo voxel based morphometry: detection of increased hippocampal volume and decreased glutamate levels in exercising mice. NeuroImage 61 (4), 1206–1212. http://dx.doi.org/10.1016/j.neuroimage.2012.04.010.

Blumenthal, J.A., Babyak, M.A., Moore, K.A., Craighead, W.E., Herman, S., Khatri, P., Waugh, R., Napolitano, M.A., Forman, L.M., Appelbaum, M., Doraiswamy, P.M., Krishnan, K.R., 1999. Effects of exercise training on older patients with major depression. Archives of Internal Medicine 159 (19), 2349–2356. Retrieved from: http://www.ncbi.nlm.nih.gov/pubmed/10547175.

Chen, H.I., Kuo, Y.M., Liao, C.H., Jen, C.J., Huang, A.M., Cherng, C.G., Su, S.W., Yu, L., 2008. Long-term compulsive exercise reduces the rewarding efficacy of 3,4-methylenedioxymethamphetamine. Behavioural Brain Research 187 (1), 185–189. http://dx.doi.org/10.1016/j.bbr.2007.09.014.

Clark, K.H., Wiley, C.A., Bradberry, C.W., 2013. Psychostimulant abuse and neuroinflammation: emerging evidence of their interconnection. Neurotoxicity Research 23 (2), 174–188. http://dx.doi.org/10.1007/s12640-012-9334-7.

Crawford, J.T., Roberts, D.C., Beveridge, T.J., 2013. The group II metabotropic glutamate receptor agonist, LY379268, decreases methamphetamine self-administration in rats. Drug and Alcohol Dependence 132 (3), 414–419. http://dx.doi.org/10.1016/j.drugalcdep.2013.07.024.

Crombag, H.S., Bossert, J.M., Koya, E., Shaham, Y., 2008. Review. Context-induced relapse to drug seeking: a review. Philosophical Transactions of the Royal Society London Series B, Biological Sciences 363 (1507), 3233–3243. http://dx.doi.org/10.1098/rstb.2008.0090 pii:R06784853K242644.

DiLorenzo, T.M., Bargman, E.P., Stucky-Ropp, R., Brassington, G.S., Frensch, P.A., LaFontaine, T., 1999. Long-term effects of aerobic exercise on psychological outcomes. Preventive Medicine 28 (1), 75–85. http://dx.doi.org/10.1006/pmed.1998.0385.

Droste, S.K., Schweizer, M.C., Ulbricht, S., Reul, J.M., 2006. Long-term voluntary exercise and the mouse hypothalamic-pituitary-adrenocortical axis: impact of concurrent treatment with the antidepressant drug tianeptine. Journal of Neuroendocrinology 18 (12), 915–925. http://dx.doi.org/10.1111/j.1365-2826.2006.01489.x pii:JNE1489.

Engelmann, A.J., Aparicio, M.B., Kim, A., Sobieraj, J.C., Yuan, C.J., Grant, Y., Mandyam, C.D., 2014. Chronic wheel running reduces maladaptive patterns of methamphetamine intake: regulation by attenuation of methamphetamine-induced neuronal nitric oxide synthase. Brain Structure & Function 219 (2), 657–672. http://dx.doi.org/10.1007/s00429-013-0525-7.

Everitt, B.J., Belin, D., Economidou, D., Pelloux, Y., Dalley, J.W., Robbins, T.W., 2008. Review. Neural mechanisms underlying the vulnerability to develop compulsive drug-seeking habits and addiction. Philosophical Transactions of the Royal Society of London Series B, Biological Sciences 363 (1507), 3125–3135. http://dx.doi.org/10.1098/rstb.2008.0089 pii:2G5556313GX38610.

Ferreira, A., Lamarque, S., Boyer, P., Perez-Diaz, F., Jouvent, R., Cohen-Salmon, C., 2006. Spontaneous appetence for wheel-running: a model of dependency on physical activity in rat. European Psychiatry 21 (8), 580–588. http://dx.doi.org/10.1016/j.eurpsy.2005.02.003. pii: S0924-9338(05)00049-0.

Foley, T.E., Fleshner, M., 2008. Neuroplasticity of dopamine circuits after exercise: implications for central fatigue. Neuromolecular Medicine 10 (2), 67–80. http://dx.doi.org/10.1007/s12017-008-8032-3.

Gawin, F.H., Ellinwood Jr., E.H., 1989. Cocaine dependence. Annual Review of Medicine 40, 149–161. Retrieved from: http://www.ncbi.nlm.nih.gov/entrez/query.fcgi?cmd=Retrieve&db=PubMed&dopt=Citation&list_uids=2658744.

Gonzales, R., Mooney, L., Rawson, R.A., 2010. The methamphetamine problem in the United States. Annual Review of Public Health 31, 385–398. http://dx.doi.org/10.1146/annurev.publhealth.012809.103600.

Greenwood, B.N., Foley, T.E., Le, T.V., Strong, P.V., Loughridge, A.B., Day, H.E., Fleshner, M., 2011. Long-term voluntary wheel running is rewarding and produces plasticity in the mesolimbic reward pathway. Behavioural Brain Research 217 (2), 354–362. http://dx.doi.org/10.1016/j.bbr.2010.11.005.

Guezennec, C.Y., Abdelmalki, A., Serrurier, B., Merino, D., Bigard, X., Berthelot, M., Peres, M., 1998. Effects of prolonged exercise on brain ammonia and amino acids. International Journal of Sports Medicine 19 (5), 323–327. http://dx.doi.org/10.1055/s-2007-971925.

Gulve, E.A., Rodnick, K.J., Henriksen, E.J., Holloszy, J.O., 1993. Effects of wheel running on glucose transporter (GLUT4) concentration in skeletal muscle of young adult and old rats. Mechanisms of Ageing and Devlopment 67 (1–2), 187–200.

Haglund, M., Ang, A., Mooney, L., Gonzales, R., Chudzynski, J., Cooper, C.B., Dolezal, B.A., Gitlin, M., Rawson, R.A., 2014. Predictors of depression outcomes among abstinent methamphetamine-dependent individuals exposed to an exercise intervention. The American Journal of Addiction. http://dx.doi.org/10.1111/j.1521-0391.2014.12175.x.

Ji, J.F., Ji, S.J., Sun, R., Li, K., Zhang, Y., Zhang, L.Y., Tian, Y., 2014. Forced running exercise attenuates hippocampal neurogenesis impairment and the neurocognitive deficits induced by whole-brain irradiation via the BDNF-mediated pathway. Biochemical and Biophysical Research Communications 443 (2), 646–651. http://dx.doi.org/10.1016/j.bbrc.2013.12.031.

Jones, E.M., Knutson, D., Haines, D., 2003. Common problems in patients recovering from chemical dependency. American Family Physician 68 (10), 1971–1978. Retrieved from: http://www.ncbi.nlm.nih.gov/pubmed/14655806.

Kalivas, P.W., Volkow, N.D., 2005. The neural basis of addiction: a pathology of motivation and choice. The American Journal of Psychiatry 162 (8), 1403–1413. http://dx.doi.org/10.1176/appi.ajp.162.8.1403 pii.

Kanarek, R.B., D'Anci, K.E., Jurdak, N., Mathes, W.F., 2009. Running and addiction: precipitated withdrawal in a rat model of activity-based anorexia. Behavioural Neuroscience 123 (4), 905–912. http://dx.doi.org/10.1037/a0015896 pii:2009-10928-024.

Kish, S.J., 2008. Pharmacologic mechanisms of crystal meth. CMAJ 178 (13), 1679–1682. http://dx.doi.org/10.1503/cmaj.071675.

Kitamura, O., Wee, S., Specio, S.E., Koob, G.F., Pulvirenti, L., 2006. Escalation of methamphetamine self-administration in rats: a dose-effect function. Psychopharmacology 186 (1), 48–53. Retrieved from: http://www.ncbi.nlm.nih.gov/entrez/query.fcgi?cmd=Retrieve&db=PubMed&dopt=Citation&list_uids=16552556.

Knackstedt, L.A., Kalivas, P.W., 2009. Glutamate and reinstatement. Current Opinion in Pharmacology 9 (1), 59–64. http://dx.doi.org/10.1016/j.coph.2008.12.003 pii:S1471-4892(08)00199-9.

Kolb, E.M., Rezende, E.L., Holness, L., Radtke, A., Lee, S.K., Obenaus, A., Garland Jr., T., 2013. Mice selectively bred for high voluntary wheel running have larger midbrains: support for the mosaic model of brain evolution. The Journal of Experimental Biology 216 (Pt. 3), 515–523. http://dx.doi.org/10.1242/jeb.076000.

Koob, G.F., 1999. Stress, corticotropin-releasing factor, and drug addiction. Annals of the New York Academy of Sciences 897, 27–45. Retrieved from: http://www.ncbi.nlm.nih.gov/entrez/query.fcgi?cmd=Retrieve&db=PubMed&dopt=Citation&list_uids=10676433.

Koob, G.F., 2013. Addiction is a reward deficit and stress surfeit disorder. Frontiers in Psychiatry 4, 72. http://dx.doi.org/10.3389/fpsyt.2013.00072.

Koob, G.F., Le Moal, M., 1997. Drug abuse: hedonic homeostatic dysregulation. Science 278 (5335), 52–58. Retrieved from: http://www.ncbi.nlm.nih.gov/entrez/query.fcgi?cmd=Retrieve&db=PubMed&dopt=Citation&list_uids=9311926.

Koob, G.F., Volkow, N.D., 2010. Neurocircuitry of addiction. Neuropsychopharmacology 35 (1), 217–238. http://dx.doi.org/10.1038/npp.2009.110 pii:npp2009110.

Kramer, J.C., Fischman, V.S., Littlefield, D.C., 1967. Amphetamine abuse. Pattern and effects of high doses taken intravenously. JAMA 201 (5), 305–309. Retrieved from: http://www.ncbi.nlm.nih.gov/entrez/query.fcgi?cmd=Retrieve&db=PubMed&dopt=Citation&list_uids=6071725.

Kufahl, P.R., Watterson, L.R., Nemirovsky, N.E., Hood, L.E., Villa, A., Halstengard, C., Zautra, N., Olive, M.F., 2013. Attenuation of methamphetamine seeking by the mGluR2/3 agonist LY379268 in rats with histories of restricted and escalated self-administration. Neuropharmacology 66, 290–301. http://dx.doi.org/10.1016/j.neuropharm.2012.05.037.

Lynch, W.J., Peterson, A.B., Sanchez, V., Abel, J., Smith, M.A., 2013. Exercise as a novel treatment for drug addiction: a neurobiological and stage-dependent hypothesis. Neuroscience & Biobehavioral Reviews 37 (8), 1622–1644. http://dx.doi.org/10.1016/j.neubiorev.2013.06.011 pii:S0149-7634(13)00166-8.

Mandyam, C.D., Wee, S., Eisch, A.J., Richardson, H.N., Koob, G.F., 2007. Methamphetamine self-administration and voluntary exercise have opposing effects on medial prefrontal cortex gliogenesis. The Journal of Neuroscience 27 (42), 11442–11450. http://dx.doi.org/10.1523/JNEUROSCI.2505–07.2007 pii:27/42/11442.

Marques, E., Vasconcelos, F., Rolo, M.R., Pereira, F.C., Silva, A.P., Macedo, T.R., Ribeiro, C.F., 2008. Influence of chronic exercise on the amphetamine-induced dopamine release and neurodegeneration in the striatum of the rat. Annals of the New York Academy of Sciences 1139, 222–231. http://dx.doi.org/10.1196/annals.1432.041.

Marschner, A., Mell, T., Wartenburger, I., Villringer, A., Reischies, F.M., Heekeren, H.R., 2005. Reward-based decision-making and aging. Brain Research Bulletin 67 (5), 382–390. http://dx.doi.org/10.1016/j.brainresbull.2005.06.010.

Marshall, C.E., Dadmarz, M., Hofford, J.M., Gottheil, E., Vogel, W.H., 2003. Self-administration of both ethanol and nicotine in rats. Pharmacology 67 (3), 143–149 doi:10/67801.

McCullough, M.J., Gyorkos, A.M., Spitsbergen, J.M., 2013. Short-term exercise increases GDNF protein levels in the spinal cord of young and old rats. Neuroscience 240, 258–268. http://dx.doi.org/10.1016/j.neuroscience.2013.02.063.

McDaid, J., Graham, M.P., Napier, T.C., 2006. Methamphetamine-induced sensitization differentially alters pCREB and DeltaFosB throughout the limbic circuit of the mammalian brain. Molecular Pharmacology 70 (6), 2064–2074. http://dx.doi.org/10.1124/mol.106.023051.

McHugh, R.K., Hearon, B.A., Otto, M.W., 2010. Cognitive behavioral therapy for substance use disorders. Psychiatric Clinics of North America 33 (3), 511–525. http://dx.doi.org/10.1016/j.psc.2010.04.012.

Miller, M.L., Vaillancourt, B.D., Wright Jr., M.J., Aarde, S.M., Vandewater, S.A., Creehan, K.M., Taffe, M.A., 2012. Reciprocal inhibitory effects of intravenous d-methamphetamine self-administration and wheel activity in rats. Drug and Alcohol Dependence 121 (1–2), 90–96. http://dx.doi.org/10.1016/j.drugalcdep.2011.08.013.

II. DRUGS OF ABUSE WITH EXERCISE TO MODIFY NEUROLOGICAL STRUCTURE AND FUNCTION

Mizuno, M., Iwamoto, G.A., Vongpatanasin, W., Mitchell, J.H., Smith, S.A., 2014. Exercise training improves functional sympatholysis in sponta-neously hypertensive rats through a nitric oxide-dependent mechanism. American Journal of Physiology Heart and Circulatory Physiology 307 (2), H242–H251. http://dx.doi.org/10.1152/ajpheart.00103.2014.

Murphy, D.D., Segal, M., 1997. Morphological plasticity of dendritic spines in central neurons is mediated by activation of cAMP response ele-ment binding protein. Proceedings of the National Academy of Sciences of the United States of America 94 (4), 1482–1487. Retrieved from: http://www.ncbi.nlm.nih.gov/pubmed/9037079.

Nestler, E.J., 2001. Molecular neurobiology of addiction. The American Journal on Addictions 10 (3), 201–217. Retrieved from: http://www.ncbi.nlm.nih.gov/entrez/query.fcgi?cmd=Retrieve&db=PubMed&dopt=Citation&list_uids=11579619.

NIDA, 2011. Topics in Brief: Methamphetamine Addiction: Progress, but Need to Remain Vigilant. The Science of Drug Abuse and Addiction.

Noble, M., Mayer-Proschel, M., Proschel, C., 2005. Redox regulation of precursor cell function: insights and paradoxes. Antioxidants & Redox Signaling 7 (11–12), 1456–1467. http://dx.doi.org/10.1089/ars.2005.7.1456.

Novaes Gomes, F.G., Fernandes, J., Vannucci Campos, D., Cassilhas, R.C., Viana, G.M., D'Almeida, V., de Moraes Rêgo, M.K., Buainain, P.I., Cavalheiro, E.A., Arida, R.M., 2014. The beneficial effects of strength exercise on hippocampal cell proliferation and apoptotic signaling is impaired by anabolic androgenic steroids. Psychoneuroendocrinology 50, 106–117. http://dx.doi.org/10.1016/j.psyneuen.2014.08.009.

O'Dell, S.J., Marshall, J.F., 2014. Running wheel exercise before a binge regimen of methamphetamine does not protect against striatal dopaminer-gic damage. Synapse 68 (9), 419–425. http://dx.doi.org/10.1002/syn.21754.

O'Dell, S.J., Galvez, B.A., Ball, A.J., Marshall, J.F., 2012. Running wheel exercise ameliorates methamphetamine-induced damage to dopamine and serotonin terminals. Synapse 66 (1), 71–80. http://dx.doi.org/10.1002/syn.20989.

O'Neil, M.L., Kuczenski, R., Segal, D.S., Cho, A.K., Lacan, G., Melega, W.P., 2006. Escalating dose pretreatment induces pharmacodynamic and not pharmacokinetic tolerance to a subsequent high-dose methamphetamine binge. Synapse 60 (6), 465–473. http://dx.doi.org/10.1002/syn.20320.

Peluso, M.A., Guerra de Andrade, L.H., 2005. Physical activity and mental health: the association between exercise and mood. Clinics (Sao Paulo) 60 (1), 61–70. http://dx.doi.org/10.1590/S1807-59322005000100012.

Perez-Gomez, A., Tasker, R.A., 2013. Transient domoic acid excitotoxicity increases BDNF expression and activates both MEK- and PKA-dependent neurogenesis in organotypic hippocampal slices. BMC Neuroscience 14, 72. http://dx.doi.org/10.1186/1471-2202-14-72 pii:1471-2202-14-72.

Phillips, C., Baktir, M.A., Srivatsan, M., Salehi, A., 2014. Neuroprotective effects of physical activity on the brain: a closer look at trophic factor signaling. Frontiers in Cell Neuroscience 8, 170. http://dx.doi.org/10.3389/fncel.2014.00170.

Pinilla, F.G., 2006. The impact of diet and exercise on brain plasticity and disease. Nutrition and Health 18 (3), 277–284. Retrieved from: http://www.ncbi.nlm.nih.gov/entrez/query.fcgi?cmd=Retrieve&db=PubMed&dopt=Citation&list_uids=17180873.

Ploughman, M., Austin, M.W., Glynn, L., Corbett, D., 2014. The effects of poststroke aerobic exercise on neuroplasticity: a systematic review of animal and clinical studies. Translational Stroke Research. http://dx.doi.org/10.1007/s12975-014-0357-7.

Polter, A.M., Kauer, J.A., 2014. Stress and VTA synapses: implications for addiction and depression. The European Journal of Neuroscience 39 (7), 1179–1188. http://dx.doi.org/10.1111/ejn.12490.

Radak, Z., Ihasz, F., Koltai, E., Goto, S., Taylor, A.W., Boldogh, I., 2014. The redox-associated adaptive response of brain to physical exercise. Free Radical Research 48 (1), 84–92. http://dx.doi.org/10.3109/10715762.2013.826352.

Real, C.C., Ferreira, A.F., Hernandes, M.S., Britto, L.R., Pires, R.S., 2010. Exercise-induced plasticity of AMPA-type glutamate receptor subunits in the rat brain. Brain Research 1363, 63–71. http://dx.doi.org/10.1016/j.brainres.2010.09.060.

Recinto, P., Samant, A.R., Chavez, G., Kim, A., Yuan, C.J., Soleiman, M., Grant, Y., Edwards, S., Wee, S., Koob, G.F., George, O., Mandyam, C.D., 2012. Levels of neural progenitors in the hippocampus predict memory impairment and relapse to drug seeking as a function of excessive meth-amphetamine self-administration. Neuropsychopharmacology 37 (5), 1275–1287. http://dx.doi.org/10.1038/npp.2011.315 pii:npp2011315.

Robbins, T.W., Everitt, B.J., 2002. Limbic-striatal memory systems and drug addiction. Neurobioliogy of Learning and Memory 78 (3), 625–636. http://dx.doi.org/10.1006/nlme.2002.4103.

Rothman, R.B., Baumann, M.H., 2003. Monoamine transporters and psychostimulant drugs. European Journal of Pharmacology 479 (1–3), 23–40.

SAMHSA, 2008. Results from the 2007 National Survey on Drug Use and Health: Detailed Tables. Substance Abuse and Mental Health Services Administration, Office of Applied Studies.

Schwendt, M., Reichel, C.M., See, R.E., 2012. Extinction-dependent alterations in corticostriatal mGluR2/3 and mGluR7 receptors following chronic methamphetamine self-administration in rats. PLoS One 7 (3), e34299. http://dx.doi.org/10.1371/journal.pone.0034299 pii:PONE-D-12-00743.

Segat, H.J., Kronbauer, M., Roversi, K., Schuster, A.J., Vey, L.T., Roversi, K., Pase, C.S., Antoniazzi, C.T., Burger, M.E., 2014. Exercise modifies amphet-amine relapse: behavioral and oxidative markers in rats. Behavioural Brain Research 262, 94–100. http://dx.doi.org/10.1016/j.bbr.2014.01.005.

Shaham, Y., Shalev, U., Lu, L., De Wit, H., Stewart, J., 2003. The reinstatement model of drug relapse: history, methodology and major findings. Psychopharmacology 168 (1–2), 3–20. http://dx.doi.org/10.1007/s00213-002-1224-x.

Shalev, U., Grimm, J.W., Shaham, Y., 2002. Neurobiology of relapse to heroin and cocaine seeking: a review. Pharmacological Reviews 54 (1), 1–42. Retrieved from: http://www.ncbi.nlm.nih.gov/entrez/query.fcgi?cmd=Retrieve&db=PubMed&dopt=Citation&list_uids=11870259.

Smith, M.A., Lynch, W.J., 2011. Exercise as a potential treatment for drug abuse: evidence from preclinical studies. Frontiers in Psychiatry 2, 82. http://dx.doi.org/10.3389/fpsyt.2011.00082.

Smith, M.A., Yancey, D.L., 2003. Sensitivity to the effects of opioids in rats with free access to exercise wheels: mu-opioid tolerance and physical dependence. Psychopharmacology 168 (4), 426–434. http://dx.doi.org/10.1007/s00213-003-1471-5.

Sobieraj, J.C., Kim, A., Fannon, M.J., Mandyam, C.D., 2014. Chronic wheel running-induced reduction of extinction and reinstatement of metham-phetamine seeking in methamphetamine dependent rats is associated with reduced number of periaqueductal gray dopamine neurons. Brain Structure & Function. http://dx.doi.org/10.1007/s00429-014-0905-7.

Somkuwar, S.S., Staples, M.C., Galinato, M.H., Fannon, M.J., Mandyam, C.D., 2014. Role of NG2 expressing cells in addiction: a new approach for an old problem. Frontiers in Pharmacology 5, 279. http://dx.doi.org/10.3389/fphar.2014.00279.

Somkuwar, S.S., Staples, M.C., Fannon, M.J., Ghofranian, A., Mandyam, C.D., 2015. Evaluating exercise as a therapeutic intervention for metham-phetamine addiction-like behavior. Brain Plasticity. http://dx.doi.org/10.3233/BPL-150007.

Staples, M.C., Somkuwar, S.S., Mandyam, C.D., 2015. Developmental effects of wheel running on hippocampal glutamate receptor expression in young and mature adult rats. Neuroscience 305, 248–256. http://dx.doi.org/10.1016/j.neuroscience.2015.07.058.

Sutoo, D.E., Akiyama, K., 1996. The mechanism by which exercise modifies brain function. Physiology & Behavior 60 (1), 177–181. Retrieved from: http://www.ncbi.nlm.nih.gov/pubmed/8804660.

Toborek, M., Seelbach, M.J., Rashid, C.S., Andras, I.E., Chen, L., Park, M., Esser, K.A., 2013. Voluntary exercise protects against methamphetamine-induced oxidative stress in brain microvasculature and disruption of the blood–brain barrier. Molecular Neurodegeneration 8, 22. http://dx.doi.org/10.1186/1750-1326-8-22.

van Praag, H., Shubert, T., Zhao, C., Gage, F.H., 2005. Exercise enhances learning and hippocampal neurogenesis in aged mice. The Journal of Neuroscience 25 (38), 8680–8685. http://dx.doi.org/10.1523/JNEUROSCI.1731-05.2005 pii:25/38/8680.

Voss, M.W., Vivar, C., Kramer, A.F., van Praag, H., 2013. Bridging animal and human models of exercise-induced brain plasticity. Trends in Cognitive Sciences 17 (10), 525–544. http://dx.doi.org/10.1016/j.tics.2013.08.001.

Wang, J.Q., McGinty, J.F., 1995. Dose-dependent alteration in zif/268 and preprodynorphin mRNA expression induced by amphetamine or methamphetamine in rat forebrain. The Journal of Pharmacology and Experimental Therapeutics 273 (2), 909–917. Retrieved from: http://www.ncbi.nlm.nih.gov/pubmed/7752096.

Werme, M., Thoren, P., Olson, L., Brene, S., 2000. Running and cocaine both upregulate dynorphin mRNA in medial caudate putamen. The European Journal of Neuroscience 12 (8), 2967–2974. http://dx.doi.org/10.1046/j.1460-9568.2000.00147 (pii).

Werme, M., Messer, C., Olson, L., Gilden, L., Thoren, P., Nestler, E.J., Brene, S., 2002. ΔFosB regulates wheel running. The Journal of Neuroscience 22 (18), 8133–8138 pii:22/18/8133.

Yamamoto, B.K., Bankson, M.G., 2005. Amphetamine neurotoxicity: cause and consequence of oxidative stress. Critical Reviews in Neurobiology 17 (2), 87–117 pii:04c698ea6529efba, 51741a1b2a4b5a60.

Yu, F., Kolanowski, A.M., Strumpf, N.E., Eslinger, P.J., 2006. Improving cognition and function through exercise intervention in Alzheimer's disease. Journal of Nursing Scholarship 38 (4), 358–365. Retrieved from: http://www.ncbi.nlm.nih.gov/entrez/query.fcgi?cmd=Retrieve&db=PubMed&dopt=Citation&list_uids=17181084.

Zhang, Y., Loonam, T.M., Noailles, P.A., Angulo, J.A., 2001. Comparison of cocaine- and methamphetamine-evoked dopamine and glutamate overflow in somatodendritic and terminal field regions of the rat brain during acute, chronic, and early withdrawal conditions. Annals of the New York Academy of Sciences 937, 93–120. Retrieved from: http://www.ncbi.nlm.nih.gov/pubmed/11458542.

Pharmacological Intervention of Brain Neurotransmission Affects Exercise Capacity

X. Zheng[1], H. Hasegawa[2]

[1]Shanghai University of Sport, Shanghai, China; [2]Hiroshima University, Higashihiroshima, Japan

Abstract

Neurotransmitters in the brain, especially monoamines, are modulated by exercise. Interplay between exercise and monoamines, was initially explained by the "central fatigue hypothesis," which increased brain serotonin release have been attributed to the onset of fatigue during prolonged exercise. However, because of the complexity of brain functions, it is unlikely that a single neurotransmitter system is responsible for central fatigue. Several other mechanisms are involved, and the evidence supports the role of brain dopamine (DA) and noradrenaline (NA). In recent decennia, Roelands and Meeusen (2010) suggested that brain serotonin, DA, and NA might play an important role in thermoregulation and hyperthermia-induced fatigue, specifically when exercising in the heat. It opened a window of opportunity for several research groups that tried to manipulate performance, and to delay or induce fatigue by different pharmacological interventions that affected brain monoamine release, at normal and high ambient temperatures.

INTRODUCTION

The nervous system can affect all forms of physiological activity. The central nervous system (CNS) is composed of the brain and the spinal cord. Exercise can benefit brain health and function. Brain neurotransmitters, especially monoamines, are modulated by exercise. Interplay between exercise and monoamines were initially derived from the "central fatigue hypothesis," in which increased brain serotonin (5-HT) release has been attributed to the onset of fatigue during prolonged exercise. However, because of the complexity of brain functions, it is unlikely that a single neurotransmitter system is responsible for central fatigue. Several other mechanisms are appeared to be involved, and evidence supports the role of the brain catecholamines (dopamine (DA), noradrenaline (NA)) in the causation of central fatigue. Davis and Bailey (1997) hypothesized that central fatigue is the result of changes in the ratio of 5-HT and DA. They suggested that a low 5-HT/DA ratio favored improved exercise performance, through increased arousal, motivation, and optimal muscular coordination, while increased 5-HT/DA ratio resulted in decreased performance. In recent decennia, Roelands and Meeusen (2010) suggested that central fatigue could be related to a change in the synthesis and metabolism of brain monoamines. Moreover, hyperthermia has been considered as causative factor for central fatigue, especially in the heat. Since 5-HT, DA, and NA can mediate thermoregulatory responses, it can be expected that alterations in these monoamine concentrations contribute to changes in thermoregulation, and consequently to the onset of fatigue, specifically when exercising in the heat. It opened a window of opportunity for several research groups that tried to manipulate performances, and to delay or induce fatigue, by different pharmacological interventions that affected brain monoamine release at normal and high ambient temperatures.

THE STRUCTURE AND FUNCTION OF THE NERVOUS SYSTEM

The basic unit of the nervous system is the neuron. A typical neuron is composed of the cell body, dendrites, and axon. The axon is the neuronal transmitter. Near its end, an axon splits into numerous branches. These are the axon terminals or the terminal fibrils. A nerve impulse (an electrical charge) is the signal that passes from one neuron to the next. Impulse transmissions from one neuron to another have to cross synapses. The neuron sending the impulse across the synapse is called the presynaptic neuron; therefore, axon terminals are called presynaptic terminals. The neuron receiving the impulse on the other side of the synapse is called as the postsynaptic neuron. There is a narrow gap between the presynaptic and postsynaptic membranes, which is called the synaptic cleft. When the impulse reaches the presynaptic terminal, the synaptic vesicles respond by releasing chemicals into the synaptic cleft. These neurotransmitters diffuse across the synaptic cleft and bind to the postsynaptic receptors. Once this binding happens, the impulse is transmitted, and the neurotransmitter is either destroyed by enzymes, or actively returned to the presynaptic neuron, via auto-receptors in the presynaptic membrane (Erlanger and Gasser, 1968).

Neurotransmitters are the chemicals that allow the transmission of signals from one neuron to the next across synapses. There are more than 40 identified neurotransmitters. These can be categorized into either small-molecule, rapid-acting neurotransmitters which are responsible for most neural transmissions; or into neuropeptide, slow-acting neurotransmitters. The small-molecule, rapid-acting neurotransmitters are divided into three types: acetylcholine, amines such as monoamine, and amino acids. Catecholamines and 5-HT are the major monoamine neurotransmitters that are believed to be modulated by exercise (Erlanger and Gasser, 1968).

PHYSIOLOGICAL PROPERTIES OF MONOAMINES

DA, NA, and 5-HT are the main players in the monoamine neurotransmitter family. All three monoaminergic neurons modulate a wide range of functions in the CNS. To learn more about DA, NA, and 5-HT, we will briefly discuss their biosynthesis and their central pathways.

The Serotoninergic System

5-HT-containing neurons are present in the mesencephalon, pons, and medulla oblongata. They are mainly located in the raphe nuclei. Effect fibers innervate the substrantia nigra, various thalamic centers, nucleus caudatus, putamen, nucleus accumbens, cortex, and hippocampus. Other serotoninergic cells innervate the ventral horn of the spinal cord and the medulla (Meeusen and De Meirleir, 1995; Fig. 6.1).

There are a number of receptor subtypes that mediate the central and peripheral actions of 5-HT (Table 6.1). There are seven types of receptors ($5-HT_{1-7}$) with further subtypes (A–D) of $5HT_1$ and $5HT_2$. $5-HT_1$ receptors occur mainly in the CNS, and in the case of $5-HT_{1D}$, in some blood vessels. The general actions of the $5-HT_1$ receptor group are neural inhibition and vasoconstriction. $5-HT_2$ and $5-HT_3$ receptors occur in greater numbers outside the CNS, and their effects are generally excitatory (Barnes and Sharp, 1999). The precise localization of 5-HT neurons in the brain has allowed their electrical activity to be studied in detail. In vertebrates, certain behavioral and physiological functions are related to 5-HT pathways. These include various behavioral responses, control of mood and emotions, sleep/wakefulness, sensory transmission, and body temperature (Rang et al., 1999).

The synthesis of 5-HT requires two enzymatic steps (Fig. 6.2). The dietary amino acid precursor tryptophan is first hydroxylated by tryptophan hydroxylase to L-5-hydroxytryptophan, and then decarboxylated to 5-HT. 5-HT is metabolized by two enzymes into 5-hydroxy-indoleacetic acid (Meeusen and De Meirleir, 1995).

FIGURE 6.1   Serotonin neurons and major pathways in the rat brain. *DRN*, dorsal raphe nucleus; *MRN*, median raphe nucleus; *NRM*, nucleus raphes magnus; *NRO*, nucleus raphe obscures; *NRPa*, nucleus raphe pallidus.

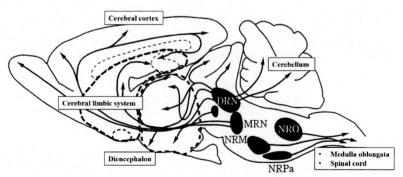

TABLE 6.1 Serotonin Receptor Subtypes and Their Main Effects

Receptor	Location	Main Effects
1A	Central nervous system	Neuronal inhibition
		Behavioral effects: Sleep, feeding, anxiety
1B	Central nervous system	Behavioral effects
1D	Central nervous system	Behavioral effects: locomotion
	Blood vessels	Cerebral vasoconstriction
2A	Central nervous system	Behavioral effects
	Peripheral nervous system	Platelet aggregation
	Smooth muscle	Smooth muscle contraction
	Platelets	Vasoconstriction/vasodilatation
2B	Gastric fundus	Contraction
2C	Central nervous system	Cerebrospinal fluid secretion
	Choroid plexus	
3	Peripheral nervous system	Emesis
	Central nervous system	Behavioral effects: anxiety

Modified from Barnes, N.M., Sharp, T., 1999. A review of central 5-HT receptors and their function. Neuropharmacology 38, 1083–1152.

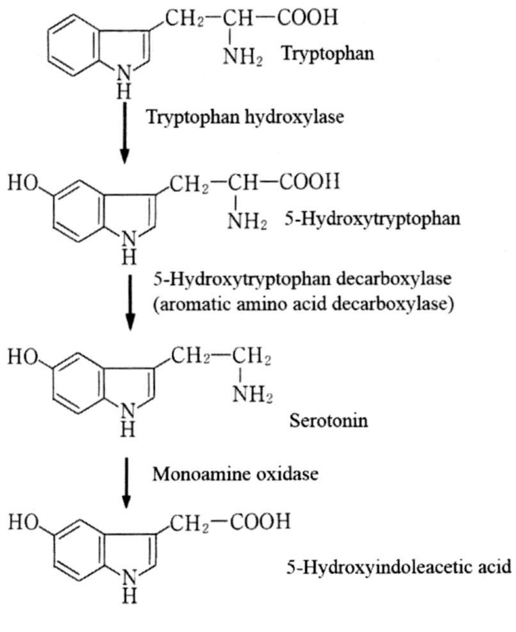

CH_2—CH—$COOH$
NH_2 Tryptophan

Tryptophan hydroxylase

HO CH_2—CH—$COOH$
NH_2 5-Hydroxytryptophan

5-Hydroxytryptophan decarboxylase
(aromatic amino acid decarboxylase)

HO CH_2—CH_2
NH_2 Serotonin

Monoamine oxidase

HO CH_2—$COOH$

5-Hydroxyindoleacetic acid

FIGURE 6.2 Biosynthesis and catabolism of the serotonin. *Modified by Meeusen, R., De Meirleir, K., 1995. Exercise and brain neurotransmission. Sports Medicine 20, 160–188.*

The Dopaminergic System

Dopaminergic, noradrenergic, and adrenergic cell groups form the primary catecholaminergic innervations of the CNS. The cells in each of these neurotransmitter systems arise from relatively small compact nuclei in vertebrates. Dahlstrom and Fuxe (1964) classified them into 14 groups and extensively described them. They categorized them from A1–14, caudally to rostrally (Oliff and Gallardo, 1999).

DA neurons form three main systems within the brain (Fig. 6.3). The nigrostriatal pathway has cell bodies in the substantia nigra, and its axons terminate in the corpus striatum. The mesolimbic/mesocortical pathway has cell bodies which occur in groups in the midbrain, and project to parts of the limbic system, nucleus accumbens, amygdaloid nucleus, and the cortex. Finally, the tuberohypophyseal system is a group of neurons with axons that run from the hypothalamus to the pituitary gland, and its secretions regulate prolactin (PRL; Bridge, 2002).

Two types of DA receptors (D_1 and D_2) were originally distinguished by pharmacological and biochemical techniques. Further subtypes (D_1–D_5) have been revealed by gene cloning. The distribution and function of these receptors are shown in Table 6.2. The receptors are grouped into two main families, D_1 and D_2, whose actions linked to stimulation and inhibition of adenylate cyclase, respectively. The functions of the DA pathways are divided broadly into three categories: motor control (nigrostriatal system), behavioral effects (mesolimbic and mesocortical systems), and endocrine control (tuberohypophyseal system; Bridge, 2002).

The rate-limiting step in the biosynthesis of DA is the hydroxylation of tyrosine to dihydroxypheylalanine (DOPA) by the enzyme tyrosine hydroxylase. The majority of tyrosine hydroxylase is located in the catecholamine nerve terminals. Tyrosine hydroxylase activity can be inhibited by catecholamines, suggesting a feedback inhibitory effect. DOPA is decarboxylated to DA by the enzyme dopa-decarboxylase (aromatic amino acid decarbosylase). The activity of this enzyme is not rate limiting in the synthesis of catecholamines, and is therefore not a regulatory factor in their formation. DA is first metabolized to 3,4-dihydroxyphenylacetic acid (DOPAC) by monoamine oxidase and aldehyde oxidase, under normal conditions. DOPAC is further metabolized into homovanillic acid (HVA) by catechol-O-methyltransferase (Fig. 6.4; Meeusen and De Meirleir, 1995).

FIGURE 6.3   Dopamine neurons and major pathways in the rat brain. *NAcc*, nucleus accumbens.

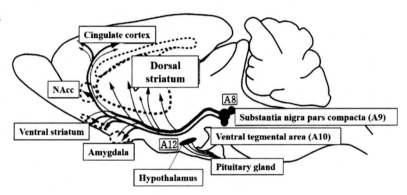

TABLE 6.2   Dopamine Receptor Subtypes and Their Main Effects

Receptor	Location	Main Effects
D1	Cortex	Arousal, mood
	Limbic system	Emotion, stereotypic behavior
	Basal ganglia	Motor control
	Hypothalamus	Autonomic and endocrine control
D2	Cortex	Arousal, mood
	Limbic system	Emotion, stereotypic behavior
	Basal ganglia	Motor control
	Pituitary gland	Endocrine control
D3	Limbic system	Emotion, stereotypic behavior
	Basal ganglia	Motor control
D4	Limbic system	Emotion, stereotypic behavior
	Basal ganglia	Motor control
D5	Basal ganglia	Motor control
	Hypothalamus	Autonomic and endocrine control

Modified from Rang, H.P., Dale, M.M., Ritter, J.M., 1999. Pharmacology. Churchill Livingstone, Edinburgh (Chapter 4).

II. DRUGS OF ABUSE WITH EXERCISE TO MODIFY NEUROLOGICAL STRUCTURE AND FUNCTION

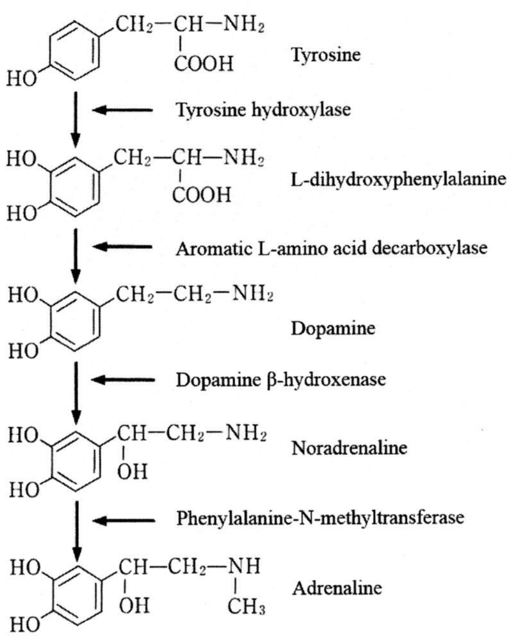

FIGURE 6.4 Biosynthesis and catabolism of the catecholamines. *Modified from Meeusen, R., De Meirleir, K., 1995. Exercise and brain neurotransmission. Sports Medicine 20, 160–188.*

The Noradrenergic System

Noradrenergic cells are found more caudally in the brainstem (Fig. 6.5). The noradrenergic cell group consists of the locus coeruleus (LC), and A6 cell group. It is one of the most well conserved cell groups in the brain, being preserved in all vertebrate species. Located in the rostral pons, it projects widely throughout the neuoaxis. Smaller collections of NA neurons are located in the lateral tegmental system and caudal pons. Recent anatomical studies suggest a greater degree of specificity and topographical organization of the LC/NA system that has been previously appreciated. The LC provides immense noradrenergic inputs to the neocortex, hippocampus, thalamus, septum, cerebellum, and brain stem. Interestingly, the striatum is nearly devoid of any NA innervations (Oliff and Gallardo, 1999).

Traditionally, noradrenergic receptors are divided into three types: α_1, α_2, and β. So far, three α_1 subtypes (α_{1a}, α_{1b}, α_{1d}), four α_2-receptor subtypes (α_{2A-D}), and three β subtypes (β_{1-3}) receptors have been identified. The α_1 and β receptors are present primarily at postsynaptic sites, whereas α_2-receptors exist at both the pre- and postsynaptic terminals. The distribution and functions of α_1, α_2, and β_1 receptors are shown in Table 6.3. Binding of NA to an α_1 receptor, activates phospholipase C, which in turn produces inositol 1,4,5-trisphosphate and diacylglycerol, regulates intracellular Ca^{2+} concentration, and activates protein kinase C. The main function of the α_2 receptor is to increase glycogenesis in neurons. β receptor can either activate cAMP-dependent protein kinase through activating adenylyl cyclase and cAMP, or cause apoptosis via the Src family tyrosine kinase dependent pathway. Activation of these receptors carries out a variety of tasks in the CNS (Lin and Kuo, 2013).

In noradrenergic neurons, DA is converted into NA through dopamine β-hydroxylase. The enzymes responsible for the catabolism of NA are monoamine oxidase and catechol-*O*-methyltransferase. The main metabolite of NA is 3-methosy-4-hydroxyphenyleneglycol (Meeusen and De Meirleir, 1995).

MONOAMINE AND EXERCISE

Monoamines have been shown to be modulated by exercise. Using different exercise protocols, measurement methods, and training levels, animal studies examined brain 5-HT, DA, NA, and their metabolite levels. They aimed to explore the effects of physiological stimuli on monoamine release in the entire brain and in specific regions.

Changes in Serotonin With Exercise

Numerous animal studies have examined the effects of acute exercise on the 5-HT system. Several studies have found that acute bouts of exercise increased 5-HT levels in the entire brain (Acworth et al., 1986; Barchas and Freedman, 1963; Romanwski and Grabiec, 1974). Using homogenates, Dey at al. (1992) studied 5-HT levels in

FIGURE 6.5   Noradrenaline neurons and major pathways in the rat brain.

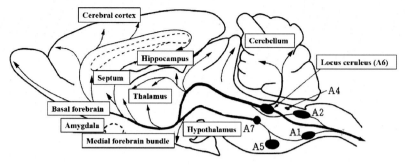

TABLE 6.3   Noradrenaline Receptor Subtypes and Their Main Effects

Receptor	Location	Main Effects
α_1	Smooth muscle	Vasoconstriction
	Hypothalamus	Elevated blood pressure
		Mydriasis
		Decreased ability to defecate and/or urinate
α_2	Nerve endings	Vasodilatation
	Stomach	Lowers blood pressure
	Hypothalamus	Constipation
β_1	Heart	Increased heart rate
	Fat cells	Increased cardiac output and force of contraction
	Kidneys	Increased conduction
	Posterior lobe of pituitary gland	Lipolysis
		Release of rennin
		Release of antidiuretic hormone

Modified from Lemke, D.M., 2007. Sympathetic storming after severe traumatic brain injury. Critical Care Nurse 27, 30–37.

different brain regions during acute exercise. They observed that acute exercise significantly increased the synthesis and metabolism of 5-HT in the brain stem and hypothalamus, and that there were no changes in the cerebral cortex and hippocampus. Measuring neurotransmitter levels in homogenates made no distinction between extracellular and intracellular levels and gave no indication of neurotransmitter release. Using the microdialysis method to explore neurotransmitter release during exercise in vivo, several studies showed that running on the treadmill increased the release of 5-HT in the hippocampus (Gomez-Merino et al., 2001a,b; Meeusen et al., 1996), ventral cortex (Gomez-Merino et al., 2001a), and ventral funiculus of the spinal cord (Gerin et al., 1995). However, Gerin and his coworkers reported no changes in the release of 5-HT, in the ventral horn and spinal cord during exercise (Gerin et al., 1994; Gerin and Privat, 1996, 1998). Hasegawa et al. observed that 5-HT release in the preoptic area and anterior hypothalamus (PO/AH) did not change while running at constant (Hasegawa et al., 2008; Takatsu et al., 2010; Zheng and Hasegawa, 2016) or incremental speeds on the treadmill (Hasegawa et al., 2011). Moreover, Wilson and Marsden (1996) observed that acute exercise only increased 5-HT release in the hippocampus of rats with good running ability. Altogether, there was no consensus on the effects of acute exercise on 5-HT system. The 5-HT levels following acute exercise was brain region dependent; was affected by training levels; the type of exercise performed such as wheel running, treadmill running, and swimming; the intensity of the exercise; and the method used for measurement. Therefore, the "central fatigue hypothesis," with increased release of brain 5-HT was challenged.

Changes in DA With Exercise

To clarify the effects of acute exercise on brain DA, some animal studies focused on DA synthesis and metabolism. Bliss and Aillion (1971) reported that both swimming and running increased the levels of HVA, a DA metabolite, in the entire brain. Chaouloff et al. (1986) found that similar changes in DA metabolism occurred following running, among trained rats. Sheldon et al. (1975) incorporated [14C] tyrosine into [14C] DA, to clarify the effect of exercise on DA synthesis and turnover in the entire brain, while being forced to run. However, he found no changes in the DA synthesis. Regional analyses indicated that DA metabolism was enhanced during exercise in the midbrain, hippocampus, striatum, and hypothalamus (Chaouloff et al., 1987; Heyes et al., 1988). Using the microdialysis method, Hasegawa et al. (2000) reported that the level of DOPAC, a DA metabolite, was increased in the rat hypothalamus during treadmill exercise. Moreover, Bailey et al. (1993) found elevated levels of brain DA and DOPAC, in rats after 1h of exercise. However, these levels decreased and returned to resting states with the onset of fatigue. From these studies, it could be hypothesized that acute exercise increased central dopaminergic activity, and DA might play an important role in mediating central fatigue.

Changes in Noradrenaline With Exercise

Acute bouts of exercise yielded conflicting results with respect to changes in the levels of NA in the whole brain. Several studies have reported that NA levels in the entire brain decreased, following swimming or running (Barchqas and Freedman, 1963; Cicardo et al., 1986; Moore and Larivière, 1964). In contrast, Acworth et al. (1986) reported that the brain NA level did not change following the running. Some studies showed that the brain NA level in trained rats increased following exercise (Acworth et al., 1986; De Castro and Duncan, 1985; Östman and Nybäck, 1976). Moreover, in one review, Meeusen and De Meirleir (1995) summarized studies that examined the effects of acute exercise on NA levels in specific brain regions. They showed that NA levels decreased due to acute exercise in the brain stem, hippocampus, pons-medulla, midbrain, and hypothalamus, while NA levels in the striatum, cortex, and preoptic area increased. Interestingly, using the microdialysis method, Meeusen et al. (1997a) reported that levels of NA and DA in the striatum increased during exercise in both trained and untrained rats. Thereafter, using the same method of measurement, other studies also showed that acute exercise increased NA and DA in the PO/AH, despite different exercise intensities (Hasegawa et al., 2008; Takatsu et al., 2010; Zheng et al., 2014). Recently, Hasegawa et al. (2011) found that increased extracellular NA and DA release in the PO/AH during incremental treadmill running was accompanied by increased exercise intensity. In summary, acute exercise stimulated the NA system in specific brain regions.

DRUGS MANIPULATING BRAIN MONOAMINE AND EXERCISE PERFORMANCE

Because of the known effects of 5-HT on sleep, lethargy, and loss of motivation, increased brain 5-HT release was first suggested to be associated with central fatigue. Bailey et al. (1993) suggested that 5-HT could influence fatigue through the inhibition of the DA system, during exercise. An increase in brain DA level could improve arousal, reward, motivation, and control all aspects of motor behavior, speed, and posture, DA could play an ergogenic effect on exercise. Moreover, increased release of NA might induce anxiety behavior (Sciolion and Holmes, 2012), and affect mood, motivation, and stress response. Therefore, stimulation of brain NA release by acute exercise might be one of the factors causing central fatigue. However, the precise role of brain monoamines in regulating fatigue and exercise performance remained elusive. To clarify the effects of monoamine on exercise performance, drug-induced alterations of brain monoamine levels have been conducted.

Selective Serotonin Reuptake Inhibitor (SSRI)

Three types of the SSRI drugs have been used to clarify the effects of 5-HT on central fatigue in human studies. Blockade of 5-HT reuptake by SSRIs increases synaptic 5-HT concentrations, and thereby stimulates the many behavioral and physiological adaptations mediated by the transmitter. Wilson and Maughan (1992) were the first to use the SSRI paroxetine at normal temperatures and reported a decrease in the time taken to develop fatigue. They attributed this to an increase in serotonergic activity. Thereafter, using the time taken to develop fatigue as the end point, Strüder et al. (1998) studied 10 male cyclists. The time taken to develop exhaustion was significantly reduced by the administration of 20mg of paroxetine. However, there was no difference in PRL release, an index of hypothalamic 5-HT activity, between the placebo and paroxetine. The single low dose used in both these studies might have had a 5-HT antagonist effect through the activation of inhibitory 5-HT_{1A} auto-receptors in the pathway (Artigas et al., 1996) controlling PRL release. Recently, Teixeira-Coelho et al. (2014) showed that performance in a time taken to develop exhaustion trial, decreased significantly after administration of paroxetine, in the group with higher aerobic capacity.

However, Strachan et al. (2004) examined the effects of acute paroxetine administration in the heat. While the drug induced a slight increase in core body temperature at rest and during exercise, the time taken to develop exhaustion, perceived exertion, and the hormonal response to exercise were not different between the groups. In addition, several studies used another SSRI, fluoxetine, at normal ambient temperature (Davis et al., 1993; Meeusen et al., 2001). Only Davis et al. (1993) observed that fluoxetine decreased the time taken to develop exhaustion. Moreover, using the SSRI citalopram, Roelands et al. (2009a) reported that exercise performance, physiological and subjective responses were not different between the two trials conducted at normal and high ambient temperatures. These conflicted results could have been caused by the use of different types of drugs and indicated that these results could also be "drug-specific."

Selective Serotonin Receptor Agonist

Buspirone can stimulate PRL release by activating postsynaptic hypothalamic 5-HT_{1A} receptors. The prolactino-trophic effects of buspirone are complicated by its DA D_2 receptor blocking action. Indeed, it was originally thought that the PRL releasing mechanism of buspirone was dopaminergic. Therefore, the PRL response to buspirone might be due to a combination of hypothalamic 5-HT_{1A} stimulation, and pituitary D_2 receptor blockade. Marvin et al. (1997) reported that the rating of perceived exertion and plasma PRL levels during exercise were increased after buspirone ingestion, whereas the time taken to develop fatigue was reduced under normal conditions. However, when buspirone was administered at high temperatures, despite the increased time taken to develop fatigue and high rectal temperature, the proportion of PRL response attributable to a nonserotonergic component (most likely dopaminergic) correlated with the exercise duration, rectal temperature at fatigue, and the rate of temperature rise (Bridge et al., 2003). These results suggested that higher activation of the hypothalamic dopaminergic pathways predicted exercise tolerance in the heat.

Selective Serotonin Receptor Antagonist

Several studies used selective 5-HT receptor antagonists to inhibit the brain serotoninergic system during exercise. Meeusen et al. (1997b) used the $5\text{-HT}_{2A/2C}$ receptor antagonist ritanserin during exercise, which was performed at 65% of the maximal aerobic power output. The authors gave 0.3 mg/kg of ritanserin or a placebo at 24 h and immediately before the test, but found no difference in the time taken to develop fatigue between the trials, which were held at 18°C. A 5-HT_{2C} receptor antagonist pizotifen increased rectal and skin temperatures during exercise, but did not affect performance in the 40-km time trials, which were held in the heat.

DA Reuptake Inhibitor

Methylphenidate (MPH), an amphetamine-like stimulant, is a well-known DA reuptake inhibitor. MPH occupies the DA transporter and has a fivefold-higher affinity for it, than for the NA transporter. Swart et al. (2009) reported that MPH improved performance under exhaustion at a fixed rate of perceived exertion under normal ambient temperatures. However, Roelands et al. (2008b) administered MPH to subjects and let them perform 60 min of constant intensity exercise, followed by a 30-min time trial at both normal and high ambient temperatures. They found that the cycling performance improved by only 16% in the heat, an outcome that coincided with an average maximal core temperature of 40°C, which was much higher than the placebo trial, in which an average maximal core temperature of 39.1°C was obtained. Similar results were not found at normal ambient temperatures. In addition, both the rating of perceived exertion and thermal sensation were not different between the two trials conducted in the heat. This indicated that the subjects did perceive producing more power and consequently more heat. The authors concluded that the "safety switch" or the mechanisms existing in the body to prevent harmful effects were overridden by drug administration. Taken together, these data indicated that increased brain DA levels played an important role in delaying central fatigue.

DA Receptor Agonist

At normal ambient temperatures, Heyes et al. (1985) administered the DA agonist apomorphine to rats that had 6-hydroxydopamine (which destroys DA nerve terminals) induced lesions of the central dopaminergic pathways to determine the influence of central dopaminergic activity on exercise. The rats with lesions and without apomorphine administration ran for a shorter time before exhaustion set in than the control rats. Administration of apomorphine resulted in the rats with lesions running significantly longer than the control rats. The authors suggested that increasing central dopaminergic activity delayed fatigue. In addition, Balthazar et al. (2009) injected DA intracerebroventricularly (ICV) into rats, 1 min before they were made to run on a treadmill, to activate central dopaminergic pathways during exercise. These rats ran until they were fatigued at normal ambient temperatures. DA delayed fatigue despite high-heat storage, and an elevated core temperature at the point of fatigue ($\geq 40°C$). These results suggested that central DA pathways were involved in the ability of CNS neurons to detect and prevent thermal damage to the brain even at normal ambient temperatures. In addition, they also found that the activation of DA pathways in the CNS increased the core temperature and the heat production response. ICV injection of DA increased the core temperature. This might result from the activation of DA pathways in the nigrostriatal and the mesocorticolimbic brain systems that stimulated heat production responses.

Selective DA Receptor Antagonist

DA receptor antagonists block dopaminergic pathway translation. Balthazar et al. (2010) reported that injection of DA D_1 receptor antagonist SCH23390, and D_2 receptors antagonist eticlopride into the brain stimulated exercise-induced fatigue under normal ambient temperatures. They hypothesized that the impaired exercise performance could be due to inhibition of a common reward circuit caused by the blockage of DA neurotransmission. This led to reduced motivation and voluntary locomotion that therefore increased perceived exertion. Another possible explanation was that the blockage of DA neurotransmission in the PO/AH inhibited heat loss responses and decreased heat tolerance. However, these studies did not measure brain DA levels and heat loss responses. Therefore, there is no evidence for these hypotheses.

Caffeine

Caffeine is an adenosine receptor antagonist that can cross the blood–brain barrier. Thus, it can block adenosine receptors, increase arousal, spontaneous behavioral activity, affect blood flow regulation, stimulate neuronal excitability and synaptic transmission in the brain, and increase neurotransmitter release, especially that of DA (Zheng and Hasegawa, 2015). It is well established that caffeine has effects on central DA release, in addition to blocking negative interactions between adenosine A_1/DA D_1 and adenosine A_{2a}/DA D_2 receptors, in striatal and limbic brain regions (Zheng and Hasegawa, 2015). Such effects strongly implicated the role of DA in caffeine improved exercise performance. Caffeine exerts ergogenic effects at normal ambient temperature. However, few studies have examined the effects of caffeine or adenosine receptor antagonism on exercise capacity, thermoregulation, and neurotransmitter release. Recently, we observed that caffeine could increase the run time to developing fatigue, core temperature, heat production, and heat loss responses (Zheng et al., 2014). Caffeine could also increase extracellular DA release in the PO/AH of exercising rats, with no effects on NA and 5-HT. In caffeine trials, rats continued exercising despite passing the critical core temperature level. In addition, a nonselective adenosine receptor agonist (5′-N-ethylcarboxamidoadenosine [NECA]) decreased the run time to fatigue, core temperature, heat production, heat loss, and extracellular DA release at rest and during exercise, but increased the body heat rate. The combinational injection of caffeine inhibited these NECA-induced alterations (Zheng and Hasegawa, 2016). These results indicated that caffeine-increased brain DA release, through blockage of adenosine receptors, and might be related to hyperthermic and ergogenic effects. Furthermore, increased DA release in the PO/AH caused by caffeine might stimulate heat loss responses, delay body heat rating, increase the development of heat resistance, and override the critical core temperature.

Moreover, acute caffeine ingestion by humans yielded conflicting results with respect to changes in thermoregulation while exercising in the heat. The effects of caffeine on performance and thermoregulation in hot environments needs to be studied further. In a preloaded time trial, Cheuvront et al. (2009) showed that a high dose of caffeine (9 mg/kg), increased the rectal temperature and induced no change in exercise performance. Roelands et al. (2011) reported that a moderate dose of caffeine (6 mg/kg), increased T_{core} during a time trial at 30°C and failed to improve exercise performance. Conversely, Ganio et al. (2011) observed that a low dose (3 mg/kg) produced no change in core temperature, but improved the time trial performance in the heat. Recently, Pitchford et al. (2014) found that 3 mg/kg of caffeine improved the time trial performance, inhibited the increased the rating of perceived exertion, and did not change physiological responses during exercise. According to these studies, caffeine supplementation at low doses resulted in a worthwhile improvement of cycling time trial performance and inhibited central fatigue in the heat.

Noradrenaline Reuptake Inhibitor

Reboxetine is widely prescribed as an antidepressant; it occupies the NA transporter, and thereby increases the concentration of NA in the synaptic cleft. In a recent review, Roelands et al. (2015) summarized all human reboxetine studies. Piacentini et al. (2002) investigated the effects of reboxetine on fatigue and hormonal parameters, on humans under normal ambient temperature. The authors failed to show any changes in performance in the self-pace test, although other studies reported decreased performances after reboxetine administration (Roelands et al., 2008a; Klass et al., 2012). Furthermore, using transcranial magnetic stimulation, Klass et al. (2012) reported that reboxetine administration reduced exercise performance at normal ambient temperature, with a significant decrease in voluntary activation. This suggested that NA contributed to the development of supraspinal fatigue during prolonged exercise. In the heat, subjects performed 20% worse after reboxetine administration when compared with placebo.

DA/Noradrenaline Reuptake Inhibitor

Bupropion is a DA/NA reuptake inhibitor. It possesses a pharmacological profile intermediate between that of tricyclic antidepressants and amphetamine-like stimulants. When compared with the tricyclics, bupropion inhibits DA uptake more effectively than NA, in animals. Watson et al. (2005) examined the effect of bupropion on exercise performance and thermoregulation, under normal and warm conditions. They found that subjects completed the time trial faster by 9% at 30°C when bupropion was administered, but not at 18°C. Bupropion appeared to enable the maintenance of an elevated power output and a higher core temperature, with the same perceived effort and thermal discomfort, as reported in the placebo trials. More specially, bupropion allowed core temperature to increase to ≥40°C at the end of exercise. These results suggested that bupropion acted on central DA and NA neurotransmission to maintain motivation and arousal, and enabled subjects to sustain a higher power output despite reaching the critical core temperature level.

Roelands et al. (2009a,b) reported that chronic bupropion administration did not influence TT performance at 30°C, and that subjects did not reach core temperature values as high as those observed during the acute bupropion administration. They proposed that bupropion was primarily under NA influence when administered chronically, and resulted in no effect on exercise performance, as was previously found by Piacentini et al. (2002) after acute administration of NA reuptake inhibitor under normal ambient temperatures. Furthermore, Roelands et al. (2008a) observed that NA reuptake inhibition induced a decrease in exercise performance, at both normal and high ambient temperatures. According to these studies, the acuteness of the DA pathways appeared to play a part in acute bupropion-induced increase in time trial performance and hyperthermia.

To clarify the precise mechanism behind the ergogenic effects of DA and NA in the heat, Hasegawa et al. (2008) examined the effects of bupropion on exercise performance, thermoregulation, and neurotransmitter release, in rats exercising at 30°C. They showed that an acute dose of bupropion significantly improved the time taken to develop fatigue, increased both core and brain temperatures during exercise, and overrode the critical core temperature. These changes in temperature were accompanied by an increase in extracellular DA and NA concentrations in the PO/AH during exercise. Animal studies suggested that bupropion mainly affected DA reuptake. Therefore, they suggested that protective mechanisms are dampened or overridden, when DA levels in the brain were manipulated. As bupropion has a higher potency for DA than NA among animals, DA in the PO/AH might play an important role in overriding critical core temperature levels.

SUMMARY

It has been suggested that the central fatigue caused by acute exercise is possibly related to changes in the synthesis and metabolism of brain monoamines. To clarify the mechanism, experiments using different drugs and exercise have been examined. Due to the different pharmacological tools used, experiments involving the 5-HT system did not demonstrate similar results. 5-HT might be involved in central fatigue, but probably in combination with other neurotransmitters. Increased DA has been shown to delay fatigue, especially at high temperatures. While central dopaminergic activity could limit or override inhibitory signals from the CNS for continued exercise, core temperature thresholds for exercise cessation could be bypassed by high levels of brain DA. However, since the "safety brake" in these individuals is eliminated, we suggest that there is a potential danger for development of harmful hyperthermia. In contrast, increased NA and DA have been shown to induce fatigue, at both normal and high ambient temperatures. Taken together, the interaction of DA and NA possibly extend the safe limits of hyperthermia. Nevertheless, the interaction of brain NA with DA-inhibited hyperthermic central fatigue, needs to be investigated further.

References

Acworth, I., Nicholass, J., Morgan, B., Newsholme, E.A., 1986. Effect of sustained exercise on concentrations of plasma aromatic and branched-chain amino acids and brain amines. Biochemical and Biophysical Research Communications 137, 149–153.

Artigas, F., Romero, L., De Montigny, C., Blier, P., 1996. Acceleration of the effect of selected antidepressant drugs in major depression by 5-HT1A antagonists. Trends in Neurosciences 19, 378–383.

Bailey, S.P., Davis, J.M., Ahlborn, E.N., 1993. Neuroendocrine and substrate responses to altered brain 5-HT activity during prolonged exercise to fatigue. Journal of Applied Physiology 74, 3006–3012.

Balthazar, C.H., Leite, L.H., Rodrigues, A.G., Coimbra, C.C., 2009. Performance-enhancing and thermoregulatory effects of intracerebroventricular dopamine in running rats. Pharmacology, Biochemistry and Behavior 93, 465–469.

Balthazar, C.H., Leite, L.H., Ribeiro, R.M., Soares, D.D., Coimbra, C.C., 2010. Effects of blockade of central dopamine D1 and D2 receptors on thermoregulation, metabolic rate and running performance. Pharmacological Reports 62, 54–61.

Barchas, J., Freedman, D., 1963. Brain amines: response to physiological stress. Biochemical Pharmacology 12, 1232–1235.

Barnes, N.M., Sharp, T., 1999. A review of central 5-HT receptors and their function. Neuropharmacology 38, 1083–1152.

Bliss, E., Aillion, J., 1971. Relationship of stress and activity on brain dopamine and homovanillic acid. Life Sciences 10, 1161–1169.

Bridge, W.M., 2002. Mechanisms of Fatigue during Prolonged Exercise in the Heat. The University of Birmingham Press, Birmingham.

Bridge, M.W., Weller, A.S., Rayson, M., Jones, D.A., 2003. Responses to exercise in the heat related to measures of hypothalamic serotonergic and dopaminergic function. European Journal of Applied Physiology 89, 451–459.

Chaouloff, F., Laude, D., Guezennec, Y., Elghozi, J.L., 1986. Motor activity increases tryptophan, 5-hydroxyindoleacetic acid, and homovanillic acid in ventricular cerebrospinal fluid of the conscious rat. Journal of Neurochemistry 46, 1313–1316.

Chaouloff, F., Laude, D., Merino, D., Serrurrier, B., Guezennec, Y., Elghozi, J., 1987. Amphetamine and alpha-methyl-p-tyrosine affect the exercise-induced imbalance between the availability of tryptophan and synthesis of serotonin in the brain of the rat. Neuropharmacology 26, 1099–1106.

Cheuvront, S.N., Ely, B.R., Kenefick, R.W., Michniak-Kohn, B.B., Rood, J.C., Sawka, M.N., 2009. No effect of nutritional adenosine receptor antagonists on exercise performance in the heat. American Journal of Physiology, Regulatory, Integrative and Comparative Physiology 296, 394–401.

Cicardo, V.H., Carbone, S.E., De Rondina, D.C., Mastronardi, I.O., 1986. Stress by forced swimming in the rat, effects of mianserin and moclobemide on GABAergic and monoaminergic systems in the brain. Comparative Biochemistry and Physiology Part C: Comparative Pharmacology 83, 133–135.

Dahlstrom, A.B., Fuxe, K., 1964. Evidence for the existence of monoamine-containing neurons in the central nervous system. I. Demonstration of monoamines in the cell bodies of the brainstem neurons. Acta Physiologica Scandinavica 62, 1–55.

Davis, J.M., Bailey, S.P., 1997. Possible mechanisms of central nervous system fatigue during exercise. Medicine and Science in Sports and Exercise 29, 45–57.

Davis, J.M., Bailey, S.P., Jackson, D.A., Strasner, A.B., Morehouse, S.L., 1993. Effects of a serotonin (5-HT) agonist during prolonged exercise to fatigue in humans. Medicine and Science in Sports and Exercise 25, S78.

De Castro, J., Duncan, G., 1985. Operantly conditioned running: effects on brain catecholamine concentrations and receptor densities in the rate. Pharmacology, Biochemistry and Behavior 23, 495–500.

Dey, S., Singh, R., Dey, P., 1992. Exercise training: significance of regional alterations in serotonin metabolism of rat brain in relation to antidepressant effect of exercise. Physiology and Behavior 52, 1095–1099.

Erlanger, J., Gasser, H.S., 1968. Electrical Signs of Nervous Activity. University of Pennsylvania Press, Pennsylvania.

Ganio, M.S., Johnson, E.C., Klau, J.F., Anderson, J.M., Casa, D.J., Maresh, C.M., Volek, J.S., Armstrong, L.E., 2011. Effect of ambient temperature on caffeine ergogenicity during endurance exercise. European Journal of Applied Physiology 111, 1135–1146.

Gerin, C., Becquet, D., Privat, A., 1995. Direct evidence for the link between monoaminergic descending pathways and motor activity: I. A study with microdialysis probes implanted in the ventral funiculus of the spinal cord. Brain Research 704, 191–201.

Gerin, C., Legrand, A., Privat, A., 1994. Study of 5-HT release with chronically implanted microdialysis probe in the ventral horn of the spinal cord of unrestrained rats during exercise on a treadmill. The Journal of Neuroscience Methods 52, 129–141.

Gerin, C., Privat, A., 1996. Evaluation of the function of microdialysis probes permanently implanted into the rat CNS and coupled to an on-line HPLC system of analysis. The Journal of Neuroscience Methods 66, 81–92.

Gerin, C., Privat, A., 1998. Direct evidence for the link between monoaminergic descending pathways and motor activity: II. A study with microdialysis probes implanted in the ventral horn of the spinal cord. Brain Research 794, 169–173.

Gomez-Merino, D., Béquet, F., Berthelot, M., Chennaoui, M., Guezennec, C.Y., 2001a. Site-dependent effects of an acute intensive exercise on extracellular 5-HT and 5-HIAA levels in rat brain. Neuroscience Letters 301, 143–146.

Gomez-Merino, D., Béquet, F., Berthelot, M., Riverain, S., Chennaoui, M., Guezennec, C.Y., 2001b. Evidence that the branched-chain amino acid L-valine prevents exercise-induced release of 5-HT in rat hippocampus. International Journal of Sports Medicine 22, 317–322.

Hasegawa, H., Yazawa, T., Yasumatsu, M., Otokawa, M., Aihara, Y., 2000. Alteration in dopamine metabolism in the thermoregulatory center of exercising rats. Neuroscience Letters 289, 161–164.

Hasegawa, H., Piacentini, M.F., Sarre, S., Michotte, Y., Ishiwata, T., Meeusen, R., 2008. Influence of brain catecholamines on the development of fatigue in exercising rats in the heat. The Journal of Physiology 586, 141–149.

Hasegawa, H., Takatsu, S., Ishiwata, T., Tanaka, H., Sarre, S., Meeusen, R., 2011. Continuous monitoring of hypothalamic neurotransmitters and the thermoregulatory responses in exercising rats. Journal of Neuroscience Methods 202, 119–123.

Heyes, M.P., Garnett, E.S., Coates, G., 1985. Central dopaminergic activity influences rat ability to exercise. Life Sciences 36, 671–677.

Heyes, M.P., Garnett, E.S., Coates, G., 1988. Nigrostriatal dopaminergic activity is increased during exhaustive exercise stress in rats. Life Sciences 42, 1537–1542.

Klass, M., Roelands, B., Levenez, M., Fontenelle, V., Pattyn, N., Meeusen, R., 2012. Effects of noradrenaline and dopamine on supraspinal fatigue in well-trained men. Medicine and Science in Sports and Exercise 44, 2299–2308.

Lemke, D.M., 2007. Sympathetic storming after severe traumatic brain injury. Critical Care Nurse 27, 30–37.

Lin, T.W., Kuo, Y.M., 2013. Exercise benefits brain function: the monoamine connection. Brain Science 11, 39–53.

Marvin, G., Sharma, A., Aston, W., Field, C., Kendall, M.J., Jones, D.A., 1997. The effects of buspirone on perceived exertion and time to fatigue in man. Experimental Physiology 82, 1057–1060.

Meeusen, R., De Meirleir, K., 1995. Exercise and brain neurotransmission. Sports Medicine 20, 160–188.

Meeusen, R., Piacentini, M.F., Van Den Eynde, S., Magnus, L., De Meirleir, K., 2001. Exercise performance is not influenced by a 5-HT reuptake inhibitor. International Journal of Sports Medicine 22, 329–336.

Meeusen, R., Smolders, I., Sarre, S., De Meirleir, K., Keizer, H., Serneels, M., Ebinger, G., Michotte, Y., 1997a. Endurance training effects on neurotransmitter release in rat striatum: an in vivo microdialysis study. Acta Physiologica Scandinavica 159, 335–341.

Meeusen, R., Roeykens, J., Magnus, L., Keizer, H., De Meirleir, K., 1997b. Endurance performance in humans: the effect of a dopamine precursor or a specific serotonin (5-HT2A/2C) antagonist. International Journal of Sports Medicine 17, 571–577.

Meeusen, R., Thorré, K., Chaouloff, F., Sarre, S., Meirleir, K., Ebinger, G., Michotte, T., 1996. Effects of tryptophan and/or acute running on extracellular 5-HT and 5-HIAA levels in the hippocampus of food-deprived rats. Brain Research 740, 245–252.

Moore, K.E., Larivière, E.W., 1964. Effects of stress and d-amphetamine on rat brain catecholamines. Biochemical Pharmacology 13, 1098–1100.

Oliff, H.S., Gallardo, K.A., 1999. The effect of nicotine on developing brain catecholamine systems. Frontiers in Bioscience 4, 883–897.

Östman, I., Nybäck, H., 1976. Adaptive changes in central and peripheral noradrenergic neurons in rats following chronic exercise. Neuroscience 1, 41–47.

Piacentini, M.F., Meeusen, R., Buyse, L., De Schutter, G., De Meirleir, K., 2002. No effect of a noradrenergic reuptake inhibitor on performance in trained cyclists. Medicine and Science in Sports and Exercise 34, 1189–1193.

Pitchford, N.W., Fell, J.W., Leveritt, M.D., Desbrow, B., Shing, C.M., 2014. Effect of caffeine on cycling time-trial performance in the heat. Journal of Science and Medicine in Sport 17, 445–449.

Rang, H.P., Dale, M.M., Ritter, J.M., 1999. Pharmacology. Churchill Livingstone, Edinburgh (Chapter 4).

Roelands, B., Buyse, L., Pauwels, F., Delbeke, F., Deventer, K., Meeusen, R., 2011. No effect of caffeine on exercise performance in high ambient temperature. European Journal of Applied Physiology 111, 3089–3095.

Roelands, B., Goekint, M., Heyman, E., Piacentini, M.F., Watson, P., Hasegawa, H., Buyse, L., Pauwels, F., De Schutter, G., Meeusen, R., 2008a. Acute norepinephrine reuptake inhibition decreases performance in normal and high ambient temperature. Journal of Applied Physiology 105, 206–212.

Roelands, B., Hasegawa, H., Watson, P., Piacentini, M.F., Buyse, L., De Schutter, G., Meeusen, R., 2008b. The effects of acute dopamine reuptake inhibition on performance. Medicine and Science in Sports and Exercise 89, 451–459.

Roelands, B., Goekint, M., Buyse, L., Pauwels, F., De Schutter, G., Piacentini, F., Hasegawa, H., Watson, P., Meeusen, R., 2009a. Time trial performance in normal and high ambient temperature: is there a role for 5-HT? European Journal of Applied Physiology 107, 119–126.

Roelands, B., Hasegawa, H., Watson, P., Piacentini, M.F., Buyse, L., De Schutter, G., Meeusen, R., 2009b. Performance and thermoregulatory effects of chronic bupropion administration in the heat. European Journal of Applied Physiology 105, 493–498.

Roelands, B., De Pauw, K., Meeusen, R., 2015. Neurophysiological effects of exercise in the heat. Scandinavian Journal of Medicine and Science in Sports (Suppl. 1), 65–78.

Roelands, B., Meeusen, R., 2010. Alterations in central fatigue by pharmacological manipulations of neurotransmitters in normal and high ambient temperature. Sports Medicine 40, 229–246.

Romanowski, W., Grabiec, S., 1974. The role of serotonin in the mechanism of central fatigue. Acta Physiologica Polonica 25, 127–134.

Sciolion, N.R., Holmes, P.V., 2012. Exercise offers anxiolytic potential: a role for stress and brain noradrenergic-galaninergic mechanisms. Neuroscience and Biobehavioral Reviews 36, 1965–1984.

Sheldon, M.I., Sprscjer, S., Smith, C.B., 1975. A comparison of the effects of morphine and forced running upon the incorporation of 14-C-tyrosine into 14-C-catecholamines in mouse brain, heart and spleen. The Journal of Pharmacology and Experimental Therapeutics 193, 564–575.

Strachan, A.T., Leiper, J.B., Maughan, R.J., 2004. Paroxetine administration to influence human exercise capacity, perceived effort or hormone responses during prolonged exercise in a warm environment. Experimental Physiology 89, 657–664.

Strüder, H.K., Hollmann, W., Platen, P., Donike, M., Gotzmann, A., Weber, K., 1998. Influence of paroxetine, branched-chain amino acids and tyrosine on neuroendocrine system responses and fatigue in humans. Hormone and Metabolic Research 30, 188–194.

Swart, J., Lamberts, R.P., Lambert, M.I., St Clair Gibson, A., Lambert, E.V., Skowno, J., Noakes, T.D., 2009. Exercising with reserve: evidence that the central nervous system regulates prolonged exercise performance. British Journal of Sports Medicine 43, 782–788

Teixeira-Coelho, F., Uendeles-Pinto, J.P., Serafim, A.C., Wanner, S.P., De Matos Coelho, M., Soares, D.D., 2014. The paroxetine effect on exercise performance depends on the aerobic capacity of exercising individuals. Journal of Sports Science and Medicine 13, 232–243.

Takatsu, S., Ishiwata, T., Meeusen, R., Sarre, S., Hasegawa, H., 2010. Serotonin release in the preoptic area and anterior hypothalamus is not involved in thermoregulation during low-intensity exercise in a warm environment. Neuroscience Letters 482, 7–11.

Watson, P., Hasegawa, H., Roelands, B., Piacentini, M.F., Looverie, R., Meeusen, R., 2005. Acute dopamine/noradrenaline reuptake inhibition enhances human exercise performance in warm, but not temperate conditions. The Journal of Physiology 565, 873–883.

Wilson, W., Marsden, C., 1996. In vivo measurement of extracellular serotonin in the ventral hippocampus during treadmill running. Behavioural Pharmacology 7, 101–104.

Wilson, W.M., Maughan, R.J., 1992. Evidence for a possible role of 5-hydroxytryptamine in the genesis of fatigue in man: administration of paroxetine, a 5-HT re-uptake inhibitor, reduces the capacity to perform prolonged exercise. Experimental Physiology 77, 921–924.

Zheng, X., Hasegawa, H., 2015. Central dopaminergic neurotransmission plays an important role in thermoregulation and performance during endurance exercise. European Journal of Sport Science 19, 1–11.

Zheng, X., Hasegawa, H., 2016. Administration of caffeine inhibited adenosine receptor agonist-induced decreases in motor performance, thermoregulation, and brain neurotransmitter release in exercising rats. Pharmacology, Biochemistry, and Behavior 140, 82–89.

Zheng, X., Takatsu, S., Wang, H., Hasegawa, H., 2014. Acute intraperitoneal injection of caffeine improves endurance exercise performance in association with increasing brain dopamine release during exercise. Pharmacology, Biochemistry, and Behavior 122, 136–143.

The Endocannabinoid System and Chronic Disease: Opportunity for Innovative Therapies

A. Yoder

University of Arizona, Tucson, AZ, United States

Abstract

Knowledge of the endocannabinoid system is relatively new and lacks depth. Regardless of the lack of knowledge about how the endocannabinoid system works, why it may be activated or inhibited, or what effects it may have, recent evidence suggests that an understanding of the endocannabinoid system could be extremely important in preventing, managing, or even treating certain chronic conditions. An inadequate understanding of many neurological disorders leads to poor health outcomes for many individuals due to a lack of effective therapies for treating disorders that are complex and poorly understood. As more knowledge is gained about the endocannabinoid system, more therapies that treat symptoms and may even reverse some conditions are developed, but many uses of the endocannabinoid system are only theories at this time. The opportunities for viable therapeutic treatments that focus on the endocannabinoid system provide strong justification for increasing research of the endocannabinoid system.

INTRODUCTION

The goal of the following chapter is to suggest physiological and psychological effects of the endocannabinoid system on health in a number of circumstances. This chapter outlines a number of different literature sources that have been published in the past 20 years dealing with chronic conditions, the endocannabinoid system, and other neurotransmitters. It provides evidence of the possible physiological and psychological systems by which humans promote the idea that the endocannabinoid system may be an important factor to consider ways in which we aim to treat and manage certain chronic conditions.

HISTORY OF THE RUNNER'S HIGH

Many distance runners, whether elites or amateurs, often associate marathon running with pain, adversity, and agony. Despite the commonality of suffering, the number of finishers have increased exceptionally. Runningusa.org reports an estimated 25,000 finishers in 1976 and, due to steady increases over the past 37 years, ~541,000 total finishers in 2013. Races like the New York City ING Marathon and the Bank of America Chicago Marathon have increased to nearly 50,000 finishers in a single race. Why would a race associated with excessive pain and hardship become increasingly popular?

Examining the history of the marathon may help promote the idea that there are other benefits to distance running which may explain why the marathon attracts so many runners. Today's marathon is named after the Greek town Marathon and the story of Phidippides. In 5th century BC, the Persian Empire began their conquest to expand into Greece by sailing into the bay of Marathon and engaging Athenian troops in the fields of Marathon (Christensen et al., 2009). During a 5-day pause from fighting, the Athenian general defending Marathon sent a herald named Phidippides, who was known for his running abilities, to Sparta for assistance fighting the Persian army (Christensen et al., 2009). Over 3 days, Phidippides ran an estimated 500 km to Sparta and then back to

Marathon to report that the Spartans would not send reinforcements to Marathon (Christensen et al., 2009). The Athenian's attacked and defeated the Persian army without the Spartans (Christensen et al., 2009). After driving the Persians from Marathon, Phidippides was sent 40 km to Athens to report their victory (Christensen et al., 2009). Upon delivering the news, it is believed that Phidippides collapsed and died (Christensen et al., 2009). The modern marathon was first introduced in the 1898 Olympics as a 40 km race on the same route Phidippides is thought to have taken to Athens (Christensen et al., 2009). Although there is a lack of strong historical evidence that the story of Phidippides is true, his story suggests that some psychological drive may produce absurd physiological capabilities.

EFFECTS OF ENDOCANNABINOID SYSTEM STIMULATION

As running and other physically taxing sports have increased in popularity, the desire to understand the psychological and physiological characteristics of physical activity has increased as well. The physiology of physical activity has been important in understanding health outcomes and experimental analysis of exercise has increased tremendously. Many recent studies have found acute physical activity to cause analgesia (Dietrich and McDaniel, 2004). Exercise-induced hypoalgesia and analgesia has been studied since the 1980s and many peer reviewed texts outline hypoalgesia in subjects shortly after a number of different exercises including cycling, running, and swimming (Sparling et al., 2003). However, the exact mechanisms which cause analgesia and hypoalgesia after physical activity are commonly debated (Dietrich and McDaniel, 2004). For many years, postexercise analgesia was thought to be caused by endorphins (Dietrich and McDaniel, 2004). However, other factors, like the endocannabinoid system, have been found to play a role in hypoalgesia and analgesia (Dietrich and McDaniel, 2004).

An anxiolytic effect is another psychological effect often observed in exercising individuals and more specifically in distance runners. The combination of anxiolytic and analgesic effects along with a feeling of euphoria during and after intense running has been labeled as the "runner's high" (Boecker et al., 2008). These specific effects are not always observed by distance runners, but there are many factors which may contribute to this lack of consistency (Dietrich and McDaniel, 2004). Until recently, the idea that endorphins control and produce anxiolysis, analgesia, and feelings of euphoria dominated most thoughts about the "runner's high" (Dietrich and McDaniel, 2004). Endorphins were predicted to increase opioid receptor activity in the central nervous system which lead to the observed effects of distance running (Dietrich and McDaniel, 2004). Many now discredit the theory that changes in endorphin levels are the source of the "runner's high" based on the lack of conclusive and specific evidence that details the effects of increased endorphin levels on endogenous opioid receptors (Boecker et al., 2008). Most studies outlined increased plasma endorphin levels, specifically beta-endorphin levels, in peripheral areas (Boecker et al., 2008). Evidence that increased peripheral endorphin levels lead to an increase of endorphins crossing the blood–brain barrier where endogenous opioid receptors could be affected was inconclusive (Boecker et al., 2008). As studies were unable to show the ability of endorphins to have a significant impact on opioid receptors in the brain, which was commonly understood as the mechanism for the feelings of the "runner's high," exercise scientists began to examine other possible mechanisms for exercise-induced analgesia, anxiolysis, and euphoria.

In 1988, cannabinoid ligands were first developed, allowing for the characterization of endocannabinoid receptors (Di Marzo et al., 1998). The discovery of cannabinoid ligands led to the distinction between cannabinoid receptor 1 (CB1) and cannabinoid receptor 2 (CB2) (Di Marzo et al., 1998). Albeit playing a major role in the effects of marijuana, CB1 and other cannabinoid receptors have shown to be activated by internal stimuli naturally found in the human body (Di Marzo et al., 1998). At the time of their discovery CB1 and CB2 were known to interact with $\Delta 9(-)$-tetrahydrocannabinol (THC), but there was no evidence of endocannabinoids which interacted with CB1 and CB2 (Di Marzo et al., 1998). The idea that the human body would have a specific receptor that could be activated by a substance found in the plant, THC the main psychoactive chemical in marijuana, but did not interact with any endogenous substances was puzzling, and studying CB1 receptors eventually led to the discovery of anandamide (AEA) (Di Marzo et al., 1998). AEA is a CB1 receptor agonist and when tested in mice, produced similar effects of THC including locomotor activity limitations and analgesia (Campos and Guimarães, 2009). Cross-tolerance between AEA and THC also showed the link between AEA and CB1 receptor stimulation (Campos and Guimarães, 2009). Along with AEA, other endocannabinoids, including 2-arachidonoylglycerol (2-AG), have been discovered and have been shown to be CB1 and CB2 receptor agonists (Di Marzo et al., 1998).

Although the physiological effects of increased endocannabinoid levels, specifically AEA and AG-2, are rather consistent, the mechanism for the observable effects is still undetermined. Increased amounts of AEA and AG-2 correlate to anxiolysis and analgesia, as observed in mice and in humans (Di Marzo et al., 1998). However, endocannabinoids have different and sometimes contradicting effects depending on location (Di Marzo et al., 1998). For example, in the CB1 receptor agonists in the basal ganglia cause inhibition of reuptake of GABA which limits GABA-mediated neurotransmission, but in the globus pallidus, CB1 receptor agonists enhance GABA-mediated neurotransmission (Di Marzo et al., 1998). Although the endocannabinoid system can have multiple physiological effects and the exact mechanism of action is not clearly defined, endocannabinoid stimulation is correlated with decrease in anxiety behaviors and increase in pain threshold that correspond to the symptoms described as the "runner's high."

Understanding the neurological changes that occur during and after running could be of major importance when attempting to explain the rewarding feelings that may cause runners to engage in extremely demanding exercise like marathons or ultra-marathons. Prior to discovering neurological changes caused by exercise, it might be assumed that the sense of accomplishment may drive people to take on challenging and painful tasks. However, we now know that Phidippides may have been able to complete his exhaustive run to Athens because of other factors than his motivation to complete his duties as a herald. The increased pain threshold due to the stimulation of the endocannabinoid system may have hidden his perception of bodily functions and played a role in Phidippides's decision to run himself to death on his mission.

An animal study published by the National Academy of Sciences of the United States of America helps to outline endocannabinoid behavior during acute exercise using a mouse running wheel model (Fuss et al., 2015). The goal of their study was to link increased levels of AEA and AG-2 acting as CB1 and CB2 receptor agonists proceeding running to anxiolysis and analgesia (Fuss et al., 2015). Mice were separated into two groups, a run group and a control group. To allow mice to become accustomed to a running wheel, both groups were allowed to run on a running wheel for 3 days and averaged a distance of 5.4 km per day (Fuss et al., 2015). After 3 days of unrestricted access, both groups were inhibited from running on the wheel for 2 days (Fuss et al., 2015). On the 6th day, the run group was again given unrestricted access to the running wheel and mice in the run group ran an average of 6.5 km while the control group was again restricted from running. After the 6th day, plasma concentrations of AEA and AG-2 were measured in both groups (Fuss et al., 2015). The run group was shown to have significantly higher plasma concentrations of AEA and AG-2. Anxiety-like behaviors (using a dark–light box) and thermal pain sensitivity (using a hotplate) were also measured immediately following the 6th day of running (Fuss et al., 2015). Mice that were a part of the run group showed decreased anxiety by spending significantly more time in the anxiety contributing lit compartment than the control group (Fuss et al., 2015). Pain threshold also increased in mice that were given access to the running wheel on the 6th day (Fuss et al., 2015). This showed that running reduced anxiety-like behavior, increased pain threshold, and increased plasma concentrations of endocannabinoids AEA and AG-2, but did not directly link endocannabinoids to the observed behaviors.

To show that behavioral changes were connected to CB1 receptors, the experiment was repeated, but the run group was treated with CB1 and CB2 antagonists (AM251 and AM630, respectively) (Fuss et al., 2015). To show that endorphins, which also increased in plasma concentrations in the run group, did not cause the observed behavioral changes, mice were treated with naloxone, a known inhibitor of endorphin signaling (Fuss et al., 2015). Mice in the run group that were treated with naloxone showed the same changes in anxiety-like behaviors and thermal pain sensitivity as untreated mice in the run group in the first experiment (Fuss et al., 2015). Mice in the run group that were treated with the CB2 antagonist AM630 showed the same behavioral changes as untreated and naloxone treated mice in the run group (Fuss et al., 2015). However, mice in the run group that were treated with the CB1 antagonist AM251 showed no significant behavioral changes compared to the control group which did not run (Fuss et al., 2015). This displayed the connection between CB1 receptors primarily activated by AEA and reduced anxiety-like behavior and decreased pain sensitivity (Fuss et al., 2015).

The mechanism for reduced anxiety-like behavior of CB1 receptors was further outlined based on predictions that CB1 receptors located on GABAergic neurons played a role in producing emotional benefits when running (Fuss et al., 2015). Previously, this was noted by removing CB1 receptors on GABAergic neurons and measuring the time that mice accessed a running wheel (Fuss et al., 2015). Mice without CB1 receptors on GABAergic neurons used the running wheel significantly less than the normal mice with CB1 receptors present on GABAergic neurons (Fuss et al., 2015). To evaluate the role of GABAergic neurons in anxiety-like behavior, CB1 receptors were removed from one group of the mice and the same running procedures were used (Fuss et al., 2015). After running on the 6th day, the dark-box anxiety test was used to determine anxiety-like behavior in mice with and without CB1 receptors present on GABAergic neurons (Fuss et al., 2015). The control group, which did no running on the 6th day, with CB1 receptors showed significantly more anxiety behavior than the run group with CB1 receptors (Fuss et al., 2015). However, anxiety behavior in mice without CB1 receptors on GABAergic neurons increased significantly, even when compared to the control group with CB1 receptors, and the control group and the run group without CB1 receptors were almost identical (Fuss et al., 2015). This showed that even without increased endocannabinoid stimulation, CB1 receptors on GABAergic neurons decrease anxiety-like behavior, linking GABAergic neurons with decreased anxiety (Fuss et al., 2015).

When data about the effects of endocannabinoids was originally found in mice it was extrapolated to humans, but since then many studies have shown that the endocannabinoid system also plays a similar role in anxiolysis and analgesia in humans. A study conducted at the School of Applied Physiology at the Georgia Institute of Technology aimed to show that the endocannabinoid system was stimulated by acute moderate exercise (Sparling et al., 2003). Participants in the study were assigned to either running, cycling, or sedentary group and each participant in their group either did moderate running or cycling or remained seated for 45 min (Sparling et al., 2003). Moderate exercise was defined as 70–80% of maximum heart rate. Blood sampling was used to measure plasma concentrations of AEA and AG-2 pre- and postexercise in all three groups (Sparling et al., 2003). In the two exercising groups, both AEA and AG-2 plasma concentrations increased significantly while the sedentary group showed little change in AEA and AG-2 plasma concentrations (Sparling et al., 2003).

A human study has also displayed exercise induced hypoalgesia controlled by the endocannabinoid system (Koltyn, 2000). The study also displayed that opioid antagonists, like endorphins, are most likely not the underlying cause of exercise induced hypoalgesia (Koltyn, 2000). Participants underwent thermal and pressure pain tests before and after exercise (Koltyn, 2000). Participants were also divided into two groups and one group received the opioid-antagonist naloxone while the other group received a placebo (Koltyn, 2000). There was a significant increase in pain threshold and decreased levels of pain perception after exercise in both groups (Koltyn, 2000). The placebo group and the naloxone group both had increased pain thresholds, but there was no significant difference between the pain thresholds of the placebo and naloxone groups (Koltyn, 2000). Both groups also showed a significant decrease in pressure pain ratings after running and again there was no significant difference between the placebo and naloxone groups (Koltyn, 2000). The data revealed that exercise did induce analgesia, but opioid antagonists had little effect on levels of analgesia during exercise, suggesting the possibility of nonopioid antagonists inducing analgesia (Koltyn, 2000). Pre- and postplasma concentrations of endocannabinoids, both AEA and AG-2, were measured for all participants and postmeasurements were shown to be significantly higher for both AG-2 and AEA, along with a number of other endocannabinoids (Koltyn, 2000). Although the exact effects of endocannabinoids were not tested in this study, it showed that nonopioid antagonists are a more likely cause for exercise-induced hypoalgesia and endocannabinoids may produce those effects (Koltyn, 2000).

Later studies have concluded that the endocannabinoid system does play a major role in producing analgesic and anxiolytic effects in humans, although the mechanisms of endocannabinoids are still uncertain, endocannabinoids play a role in neurotransmitter activity resulting in analgesia and anxiolysis (Dietrich and McDaniel, 2004). Effects of endocannabinoids are most often attributed to inhibition of glutamate transmission, inhibition of dopamine reuptake, and inhibition of GABA reuptake (Dietrich and McDaniel, 2004). As more of the central and peripheral effects of endocannabinoids are found and understood, manipulating the endocannabinoid system as a therapy for various chronic diseases becomes increasingly feasible.

POSSIBILITIES OF THERAPEUTIC USES OF THE ENDOCANNABINOID SYSTEM IN CHRONIC CONDITIONS

The physical health benefits of running are frequently observed and most Americans are at least aware that running produces cardiovascular benefits that have a positive effect on overall health. However, the psychological and neurological benefits have become clearer in recent years. Running is most often seen as a mode of prevention of chronic diseases like obesity and heart disease due to physical health benefits, but what if the psychological effects of running could be used to prevent chronic conditions and help manage symptoms of conditions like anxiety disorders and depression as well?

BRAIN DERIVED NEUROTROPIC FACTOR AND DEPRESSION

There is no single mechanism that has proven to be the cause of depression, but decreased brain-derived neurotropic factor (BDNF) has been shown to cause some forms of depression (Heyman et al., 2012). Decreased levels of BDNF often occur due to hippocampal atrophy that has been found in some cases of depression (Heyman et al., 2012). In a study of cyclists who underwent 60 min of intense cycling and blood concentrations of AEA, AG-2, and

BDNF were taken before and after exercise (Heyman et al., 2012). Increased plasma concentrations of AEA correlated with increased levels of BDNF, both due to acute exercise (Heyman et al., 2012). This study describes how exercise may be a possible alternative to antidepressant drugs that stimulate the release of BDNF (Heyman et al., 2012). Using exercise to stimulate the endocannabinoid system and also to increase BDNF may be a valuable treatment for depression due to hippocampal atrophy, but further research is necessary to prove endocannabinoid stimulation effective before it can be thought of as a way of treating depression (Bugg and Head, 2011).

CHRONIC PAIN

Hundreds of billions of dollars are spent every year to treat chronic pain in America. This cost measures only the cost of medications and does not measure the negative effects of using analgesic medications consistently over a long period of time (Gaskin and Richard, 2011). When used appropriately, exercise can significantly improve symptoms of chronic pain and can be a beneficial alternative or addition to pharmacological treatments used for pain reduction (Kaufmann et al., 2009). Many chronological pain disorders, like chronic regional pain syndrome and fibromyalgia, are incurable and have a poor long-term prognosis (Kaufmann et al., 2009). Along with chronic pain sensations, depression and anxiety are often associated with chronic pain. Exercise has occasionally been used to treat symptoms of chronic pain long before the discovery of the endocannabinoid system, but exercise may be proven more effective in treating chronic pain as the benefits of the endocannabinoid system are further studied (Kaufmann et al., 2009). AEA and AG-2 have already shown to be positively correlated with analgesia and anxiolysis (Jayamanne et al., 2006). If stimulating the endocannabinoid system through exercise can be proven to be an effective treatment for depression, exercise could be shown to treat three different symptoms of chronic pain which are extremely detrimental to the quality of life in many disorders (Taylor et al., 2015). Opioids are a common treatment for acute pain, for example, morphine prescribed after surgery, but opioids have proven to be mostly ineffective in treating chronic pain (Naugle et al., 2012). However, the endocannabinoid system works through nonopioid antagonists, again suggesting that the endocannabinoid system can be used to treat symptoms of chronic pain (Naugle et al., 2012).

There are many adverse side effects of pharmacological pain treatment and physiological and psychological dependence are common. There are side effects to endocannabinoid stimulation as well, but most side effects are thought to be beneficial when increased endocannabinoids are a result of physical activity (Koltyn, 2000). A short list of the side effects of physical activity includes cardiovascular and psychological benefits along with decreased risk of type 2 diabetes and some types of cancers. Replacing the adverse side effects of pharmacological pain treatments with the beneficial effects of exercise make exercise an even more favorable treatment of chronic pain. Many studies have outlined the effects of physical activity on treating depression and anxiety in patients with chronic pain disorders and have proven that physical activity can help with pain management and improve mood (Naugle et al., 2012). Even though the mechanisms for elevated mood are still unsure, nonrelated studies have suggested that elevated mood in response to exercise is correlated with the endocannabinoid system (Sparling et al., 2003). Linking the endocannabinoid system to elevated mood in individuals with chronic pain could be crucial in developing a more effective nonpharmacological treatment for pain (Micale et al., 2013). At this point, a plethora of different modes of physical activity (like yoga, Tai Chi, and running) are used to treat chronic pain, but if the exact mechanism by which symptoms are improved is determined, a more efficient manner of improving common symptoms can be developed (Bushnell et al., 2013).

EPILEPSY

The fact that the endocannabinoid acts through modifying specific neuronal signaling implies that it may be used as an effective way of treating and managing certain neurological disorders. Recent discoveries have linked the endocannabinoid system to certain neurotransmitters and as the neurological effects of endocannabinoids are better understood, their application seems more plausible (Koltyn, 2000). Since 1990, the correlation between the abundance of CB1 receptors and levels of glutamate and GABA neurotransmitters has been known (Katona and Freund, 2008). Activation of CB1 receptors consistently results in the depletion of neurotransmitters and inhibits transmission across the synaptic cleft (Katona and Freund, 2008). CB1 receptors are predominantly found on presynaptic neurons and may be useful in controlling neurotransmission when an excess of neurotransmitters causes functional disabilities (Katona and Freund, 2008). Deleting CB1 receptors on glutamatergic neurons in mice caused reduced seizure threshold and often resulted in death; showing CB1 receptors play a clear role in controlling glutamate activity

(Katona and Freund, 2008). The role of CB1 receptors on glutamatergic neurons may prove significantly important in managing epilepsy and reducing seizures that are a result of increased glutamate neurotransmission. Patients with intractable temporal lobe epilepsy have been shown to have a large decrease in CB1 receptors, specifically in areas that have been found to play a major role in epileptogenesis (Katona and Freund, 2008). There is significant evidence that shows that 2-AG signaling is increased during excess neuronal activity (Katona and Freund, 2008).

Head trauma has been found to increase endocannabinoid levels and decreased brain edema has been noted in instances when trauma increases the presence of 2-AG (Nagayama et al., 1999). Neuronal death is also common in head trauma and CB1 agonists have been shown to decrease neuronal death by up to 50% in animal studies (Nagayama et al., 1999). In these studies, CB1 activation was caused by exogenous cannabinoids, but these external stimuli have shown to have the same impact on CB1 receptors as endocannabinoids (Nagayama et al., 1999). Therefore, endocannabinoids can be considered to serve as a protective factor for neurological damage due to head trauma. Brain damage can also occur from excitotoxicity due to overstimulation by many neurotransmitters (Nagayama et al., 1999). In another mouse study, kainic acid was used to overstimulate glutamate transmission which leads to seizures and neuronal cell death (Marsicano et al., 2003). In some mice, CB1 receptors were actively removed and epileptic threshold and neuronal cell death were measured (Marsicano et al., 2003). The mice with active CB1 receptors showed decreased epileptic episodes and decreased cell death along with increased plasma concentrations of AEA after kainic acid was administered (Marsicano et al., 2003). This study suggests that the endocannabinoid system may be a physiological protection system for excitotoxicity (Marsicano et al., 2003).

MUSCULOSKELETAL DISORDERS

Resistance exercise, like other forms of exercise, has been shown to cause decreased pain perception in humans shortly after exercise has been completed (Galdino et al., 2014). Most other studies have shown hypoalgesia as a result of high-intensity exercise like running and cycling, but pain perception using pressure stimuli was also influenced by resistance exercise (Galdino et al., 2014). The hypoalgesic effect of resistance exercise may be of significant importance for individuals suffering from musculoskeletal disorders like osteoarthritis (Galdino et al., 2014). Musculoskeletal disorders are most often associated with both muscular atrophy and pain. Resistance exercise may prove to be important in managing these symptoms partially due to the endocannabinoid system's role in hypoalgesia (Galdino et al., 2014). The effectiveness of resistance exercise to treat certain musculoskeletal disorders has already been proven based on the theory that strengthening various muscles allows for greater function (Galdino et al., 2014). The ability of resistance exercise to cause pain reduction partially due to the endocannabinoid system has also been experimentally proven (Galdino et al., 2014). Resistance exercise seems to be an even more effective treatment for musculoskeletal disorders when considering both the effects it has on managing pain and improving motor function.

ALZHEIMER'S DISEASE

Although there are a number of different theories about the cause of Alzheimer's disease, its development has been linked to brain inflammation because of the ability of antiinflammatory drugs to decrease the rate of the disease and the increased presence of proinflammatory cytokines in individuals with Alzheimer's disease (Bonnet and Marchalant, 2015). Although the exact cause of Alzheimer's disease is unknown, chronic inflammation for many years before signs of Alzheimer's disease arise has been consistently observed (Bonnet and Marchalant, 2015). On the basis of the common theory that Alzheimer's disease is caused by an amyloid plaque that builds up in the brain, the endocannabinoid system in Alzheimer's disease patients was studied to determine what, if any, changes to the endocannabinoid system may have occurred (Bonnet and Marchalant, 2015). The antiinflammatory role of endocannabinoids may prove to be useful in preventing or slowing the development of Alzheimer's disease. In cases of Alzheimer's disease, cortical CB1 receptor presence was often decreased, but CB2 receptors were found at increased levels on microglia (Bonnet and Marchalant, 2015). In a rat study, cannabinoid receptor agonists have proven effective in improving memory function when amyloid beta was administered to cause Alzheimer's like effects, most likely due to decreased action of microglia (Bonnet and Marchalant, 2015). Although a cure to Alzheimer's disease is still not available, some drugs are efficient in blocking some of the symptoms. For example, memantine is used to control glutamatergic over activity in Alzheimer's disease patients (Marchalant et al., 2008). Endocannabinoid agonists can have similar effects on glutamate, but memantine works postsynaptically, while endocannabinoids primarily work presynaptically (Marchalant et al., 2008). A combination of both cannabinoid receptor agonists and memantine may prove to have greater benefits for Alzheimer's disease patients that memantine alone.

AMYOTROPHIC LATERAL SCLEROSIS (ALS)

ALS is a neurodegenerative disease that causes decreased motor function by damaging nerves in the brain and spinal cord. Although ALS most often occurs in the case of motor neuron dysfunction, there are certain studies that have found acetylcholine receptor dysfunction can cause ALS in some cases (Palma et al., 2016). Skeletal muscle lacking acetylcholine receptors can cause ALS even when there are no problems with motor neurons (Palma et al., 2016). A study published in January 2016 found that the endocannabinoid system may be useful in limiting the effects of acetylcholine receptor dysfunction in ALS patients (Palma et al., 2016). Muscle transplants directly from ALS patients that were placed in frogs shown to have desensitization of acetylcholine receptors. Administering the endocannabinoid palmitoylethanolamide (PEA) decreased the desensitization of acetylcholine receptors in frogs and muscle function increased (Palma et al., 2016). This study showed that acetylcholine receptors play a significant role in ALS and also that the endocannabinoid system manipulation may be useful for ALS patients (Palma et al., 2016). There is also clinical evidence of one ALS patient who experienced increased muscle force and respiratory benefits by taking medication that increased PEA concentrations (Palma et al., 2016).

STRESS-RELATED DISORDERS

Stress-related disorders that are typically associated with anxiety are often caused by flaws in the normal actions of the prefrontal cortex (Heijnen et al., 2015). The prefrontal cortex has been shown to play a large role in controlling emotional reactions, specifically due to environmental stimuli, through control of the hypothalamic-pituitary-adrenal (HPA) axis (Heijnen et al., 2015). Different components of the prefrontal cortex have shown to have both inhibitory and excitatory effects on the HPA axis (Heijnen et al., 2015). This link between the prefrontal cortex and the HPA axis has been correlated to stress-related reactions. Chronic stress can lead to dysfunction of prefrontal effects on the HPA axis and other important stress-related responses that have been shown to increase the risk of developing stress-related disorders (Heijnen et al., 2015). Autoradiography has revealed that CB1 receptors are present on prefrontal cortex neurons, dendrites, and cell bodies and the endocannabinoid system plays a role in prefrontal cortex behavior (Heijnen et al., 2015). Studies have revealed anxiolytic effects in low doses of cannabinoids due to their actions on CB1 receptors located on cortical glutamatergic neurons (Heijnen et al., 2015). It is also important to note that mice studies which removed CB1 receptors on glutamatergic neurons caused anxiogenic effects similar to chronic stress conditions (Heijnen et al., 2015). Evidence points to CB1 receptors playing a large role in stress-related neurological response, neuroendocrine response, and regulation of stress-related behavior (Heijnen et al., 2015). Although the endocannabinoid system has not been shown to be the cause of stress-related disorders originating from prefrontal cortex activity, the endocannabinoid system plays a distinct role in stress-related responses which should be further studied. The endocannabinoid system may play a key therapeutic role in protecting against the development of stress-related disorders and in coping with effects of stress-related disorders.

Posttraumatic stress disorder (PTSD) often occurs when a traumatic event is followed by the formation of a fear memory. PTSD is commonly thought of as a disease that affects veterans, but PTSD can arise from nearly any traumatic event. The exact mechanism of fear memory formation in PTSD is unknown, but patients with PTSD show alterations to biochemical amounts in the brain (McLaughlin et al., 2014). Animal tests used to determine the ability of conditioning a fear response to a certain cue has been used to test the ability of endocannabinoids to influence the development of fear memories (McLaughlin et al., 2014). Certain cannabinoid receptor agonists were able to inhibit the consolidation of fear memories in mice, while others were found to enhance fear memory consolidation (McLaughlin et al., 2014). More specifically, THC and AEA were both shown to decrease the consolidation of fear memory, while 2-AG was shown to increase the consolidation of fear memory in mice (McLaughlin et al., 2014). Decreased memory extinction of fear memories is also common in PTSD and again, endocannabinoids were shown to play a role in memory extinction (Hauer et al., 2014). Specifically, limiting reuptake of AEA was proven to cause extinction of memories (McLaughlin et al., 2014). Animal studies show that endocannabinoids play a role in memory formation and extinction. The data from these studies may be useful in treating individuals with PTSD and other similar disorders (Hauer et al., 2014). The idea that endocannabinoids play a role in memory formation and extinction in humans is supported by data collected from PTSD patients (Hauer et al., 2014). Endocannabinoid plasma concentrations, specifically AEA, were significantly changed in patients with PTSD (Hauer et al., 2014). There is no evidence to suggest that alterations in endocannabinoids cause PTSD, but there is sufficient evidence to support the theory that the endocannabinoid system can be a protective factor (Hauer et al., 2014). However, the use of exogenous cannabinoids carries risk of abuse and addiction; therefore, requiring more research before being determined efficacious in PTSD patients.

CONCLUSION

There is much to be learned through studying the endocannabinoid system and there is much potential for applying the ever increasing knowledge about the endocannabinoid system. Considerable evidence points to the possibility of implementing therapies to manage and/or treat certain chronic conditions that typically have a poor outlook through endocannabinoid regulation. Although all of the physiological actions of cannabinoid receptor agonists and antagonists are still unclear, we have discussed evidence of feasible effects that may be crucial in some circumstances. Along with appearing to have multiple effects, there are also a number of reasons why endocannabinoid system activity may increase. Even without an extensive understanding of the endocannabinoid system, there is evidence that the known effects of cannabinoid receptor activation may prove to have effective benefits for individuals with chronic conditions. Unfortunately, the incomplete knowledge of the endocannabinoid system makes it difficult to prescribe certain types of endocannabinoid stimulation to individuals with chronic conditions. Although certain drugs are effective in some chronic conditions, therapeutic treatment of the endocannabinoid system paired with current treatments may be increasingly beneficial for many patients. Exercise has an abundance of benefits that are unrelated to the endocannabinoid system, but examining the effects of exercise on the endocannabinoid system provides even more evidence for exercise as a therapy for numerous chronic diseases. This chapter presents an incomplete list of the many different possibilities of therapies for chronic diseases that focus on the endocannabinoid system. Regardless, this short summary provides ample evidence to show that further investigation would be an extremely useful investment and could be extremely beneficial for individuals suffering from a significant number of chronic diseases.

References

Boecker, H., Sprenger, T., Spilker, M.E., Henriksen, G., Koppenhoefer, M., Wagner, K.J., Valet, M., Berthele, A., Tolle, T.R., 2008. The runner's high: opioidergic mechanisms in the human brain. Cerebral Cortex 18, 2523–2531.

Bonnet, A., Marchalant, Y., 2015. Potential therapeutical contributions of the endocannabinoid system towards aging and Alzheimer's disease. Aging and Disease 6 (5), 400–405.

Bugg, J.M., Head, D., 2011. Exercise moderates age-related atrophy of medial temporal lobe. Neurobiology of Aging 32 (3), 506–514.

Bushnell, M.C., Čeko, M., Low, L.A., 2013. Cognitive and emotional control of pain and its disruption in chronic pain. Nature Reviews. Neuroscience 14 (7), 502–511.

Campos, C.A., Guimarães, F.S., 2009. Evidence for a potential role for TRPV1 receptors in the dorsolateral periaqueductal gray in the attenuation of the anxiolytic effects of cannabinoids. Progress in Neuro-Psychopharmacology and Biological Psychiatry 33 (8), 1516–1521.

Christensen, D.L., Nielsen, T.H., Schwartz, A., 2009. Herodotos and hemerodromoi: pheidippides' run from Athens to Sparta in 490 BC from historical and physiological perspectives. Hermes 137 (2), 148–169.

Dietrich, A., McDaniel, W.F., 2004. Endocannabinoids and exercise. British Journal of Sports Medicine 38, 536–541.

Fuss, J., Steinle, J., Bindila, L., Auer, M.K., Kirchherr, H., Lutz, B., Gassa, P., 2015. A runner's high depends on cannabinoid receptors in mice. Proceedings of the National Academy of Sciences of the United States of America 112 (42), 13105–13108.

Galdino, G., Romero, T., da Silva, J.F.P., Aguiar, D., de Paula, A.M., Cruz, J., Parrella, C., Piscitelli, F., Duarte, I., Marzo, V.D., Perez, A., 2014. Acute resistance exercise induces antinociception by activation of the endocannabinoid system in rats. Anesthesia and Analgesia 119 (3), 702–715.

Gaskin, D.J., Richard, P., 2011. The Economic Costs of Pain in the United States. Institute of Medicine (US) Committee on Advancing Pain Research, Care, and Education. Relieving Pain in America: A Blueprint for Transforming Prevention, Care, Education, and Research, Appendix C.

Hauer, D., Kaufmann, I., Strewe, C., Briegel, I., Campolongo, P., Schelling, G., 2014. The role of glucocorticoids, catecholamines and endocannabinoids in the development of traumatic memories and posttraumatic stress symptoms in survivors of critical illness. Neurobiology of Learning and Memory 112, 68–74.

Heijnen, S., Hommel, B., Kibele, A., Colzato, L.S., 2015. Neuromodulation of aerobic exercise. Frontiers in Psychology 6, 1890.

Heyman, E., Gamelin, F.X., Goekint, M., Piscitelli, F., Roelands, B., Leclair, E., Di Marzo, V., Meeusen, R., 2012. Intense exercise increases circulating endocannabinoid and BDNF levels in humans–possible implications for reward and depression. Psychoneuroendocrinology 37 (6), 844–851.

Jayamanne, A., Greenwood, R., Mitchell, V.A., Aslan, S., Piomelli, D., Vaughan, C.W., 2006. Actions of the FAAH inhibitor URB597 in neuropathic and inflammatory chronic pain models. British Journal of Pharmacology 147 (3), 281–288.

Katona, I., Freund, T.F., 2008. Endocannabinoid signaling as a synaptic circuit breaker in neurological disease. Nature Medicine 14, 923–930.

Kaufmann, I., Hauer, D., Huge, V., Vogeser, M., Campolongo, P., Chouker, A., Thiel, M., Schelling, G., 2009. Enhanced anandamide plasma levels in patients with complex regional pain syndrome following traumatic injury. European Surgical Research 43, 325–329.

Koltyn, K., 2000. Analgesia following exercise. Sports Medicine 29 (2), 85–98.

Di Marzo, V., Melcka, D., Bisognoa, T., De Luciano, P., 1998. Endocannabinoids: endogenous cannabinoid receptor ligands with neuromodulatory action. Trends in Neuroscience 21 (12), 521–528.

Marsicano, G., Goodenough, S., Monory, K., Hermann, H., Matthias, E., Cannich, A., Azad, S.C., Cascio, M.G., Gutiérrez, S.O., van der Stelt, M., López-Rodríguez, M., Casanova, E., Schütz, G., Zieglgänsberger, W., Di Marzo, V., Behl, C., Lutz, B., 2003. CB1 cannabinoid receptors and on-demand defense against excitotoxicity. Science 32 (5642), 84–88.

Marchalant, Y., Brothers, H.M., Wenka, G.L., 2008. Inflammation and aging: can endocannabinoids help? Biomedicine and Pharmacotherapy 62 (4), 212–217.

McLaughlin, R.J., Hill, M.N., Gorza, B.B., 2014. A critical role for prefrontocortical endocannabinoid signaling in the regulation of stress and emotional behavior. Neuroscience and Biobehavioral Reviews 42, 116–131.

Micale, V., Di Marzo, V., Sulcova, A., Wotjak, C.T., Drago, F., 2013. Endocannabinoid system and mood disorders: priming a target for new therapies. Pharmacology and Therapeutics 138 (1), 18–37.

Nagayama, T., Sinor, A.D., Simon, R.P., Chen, J., Graham, S.H., Jin, K., Greenberg, D.A., 1999. Cannabinoids and neuroprotection in global and focal cerebral ischemia and in neuronal cultures. Journal of Neuroscience 19 (8), 2987–2995.

Naugle, M.K., Fillingim, R.B., Riley, J.L., 2012. A meta-analytic review of the hypoalgesic effects of exercise. The Journal of Pain 13 (12), 1139–1150.

Palma, E., Reyes-Ruiz, J., Lopergolo, D., Roseti, C., Bertollini, C., Ruffolo, G., Cifelli, P., Onesti, E., Limatola, C., Miledi, R., Inghilleri, M., 2016. Acetylcholine receptors from human muscle as pharmacological targets for ALS therapy. Proceedings of the National Academy of Sciences of the United States of America 113 (11), 3060–3065.

Sparling, P.B., Giuffrida, A., Piomelli, D., Rosskopf, L., Dietrich, A., 2003. Exercise activates the endocannabinoid system. NeuroReport 14 (17), 2209–22111.

Taylor, A.M., Castonguay, A., Taylor, A.J., Murphy, N.P., Ghogha, A., Cook, C., Xue, L., Olmstead, M.C., De Koninck, Y., Evans, C.J., Cahill, C.M., 2015. Microglia disrupt mesolimbic reward circuitry in chronic pain. Journal of Neuroscience 35 (22), 8442.

FACTORS MODULATING EXERCISE IN AGING AND NEUROLOGICAL CONSEQUENCES

8

Changes in Cerebral Blood Flow During Steady-State Exercise

M. Hiura[1], T. Nariai[2]

[1]Hosei University, Tokyo, Japan; [2]Tokyo Medical and Dental University, Tokyo, Japan

Abstract

Physical activity and exercise have beneficial effects on brain function via multiple mechanisms. Aerobic exercise is assumed as a possible intervention for protection of age-related pathologies such as cognition impairment and stroke. For the underlying mechanisms of these preferable effects, cerebral blood flow (CBF) is a major mediator for cellular mechanisms to alter brain function. However, a limited number of studies investigated CBF during exercise. In this article, we extended and reanalyzed the data of our recent studies using the transcranial Doppler method and positron emission tomography with the oxygen-15 labeled water. The results confirmed increased CBF during steady-state exercise, demonstrating that prominent increase of global CBF at the onset of phase was contrasted to lesser increase of regional CBF at the prolonged phase. Provided that the increased CBF during exercise may facilitate neural plasticity via angiogenesis and/or vasodilation, steady-state exercise is an effective intervention for brain health.

INTRODUCTION

It is widely recognized that physical activity including exercise has beneficial effects on cardiovascular fitness and that habitual exercise mitigates the risk of cardiovascular and metabolic diseases. From the perspective of the central nervous system, exercise improves cognition and might delay age-related memory decline (Cotman et al., 2007; Hillman et al., 2008). Of note, effective roles of aerobic exercise are assumed as antidepressant (Morgan, 1985; Strohle, 2009). In addition, exercise is an important component of stroke prevention and rehabilitation (Goldstein et al., 2011). As exercise has abundance of effects on body through the cardiovascular system, brain is also influenced by exercise communicating with the other organs by the nervous, humoral, and/or immunological systems. Considering that dynamic exercise such as running and cycling with prolonged duration evokes increase in cardiac output (CO), there has been discussed how cerebral blood flow (CBF) changes during exercise (Querido and Sheel, 2007; Secher et al., 2008). As characteristics of exercise depend on the type, intensity, and amount of exercise, physiological aspects of the constant workload exercise have been observed by measurements of the pulmonary oxygen uptake (VO_2) (Jones et al., 2011; Whipp and HB, 2005). The number of the studies investigating CBF during exercise is limited, although the studies focused on cardiovascular during exercise have been well-established. To estimate changes in CBF during exercise, previous studies have applied methods of the transcranial Doppler (TCD) determined middle cerebral artery (MCA) blood velocity (V_{mean}) (Ide et al., 1999; Pott et al., 1996), single photon emission computed tomography (Williamson et al., 1999), and positron emission tomography (PET) (Christensen et al., 2000; Hiura et al., 2014).

In this article, we demonstrate two studies investigating CBF during exercise using TCD and PET, reanalyzing date from young healthy male volunteers obtained in the previous research projects (Hiura et al., 2012; Hiura et al., 2014). First, a TCD study was performed to confirm the results of a PET study in which the higher increases in CBF was identified at the onset phase compared with the prolonged phase of exercise (Hiura et al., 2014). Second, we extended our previous PET study to examine how regional CBF (rCBF) increased during exercise quantitatively using region of interest (ROI) analysis. In both studies, CBF was evaluated during moderate-intensity constant workload cycling exercise in supine position for which the kinetics of VO_2 has a steady-state without a slow component (Gaesser and Poole, 1996; Jones et al., 2011). In the following discussion, we will examine and review the possible underlying mechanisms which regulate CBF during exercise and the association between the increased CBF and beneficial effects of exercise on brain from the perspective of functional anatomy.

CBF ESTIMATED BY TCD METHOD

Since TCD apparatus was developed for evaluation of CBF by detecting beat-to-beat variation of blood flow velocity (Aaslid et al.,1982), dynamic aspects of CBF can be estimated noninvasively. TCD measures blood flow velocity in basal cerebral arteries, such as the MCA, with a time resolution of nearly 100 Hz. The velocity of blood flow in a small artery like the MCA has a characteristic in that the maximal velocity (V_{max}) is observed in the center of the vessel. Using the V_{max}, the TCD system provides the time-averaged maximum velocity (TAV_{max}) that was calculated from the peak systolic velocity (PSV) and the end-diastolic velocity (EDV) during each heart beat ($TAV_{max} = (PSV + 2EDV)/3$) (Valzueza et al., 2008). For an index of CBF, the time-averaged mean velocity of MCVA ($MCAV_{mean}$) was defined by averaging the TAV_{max} during at least 2–3 cardiac cycles.

To compare the results of TCD methods with those of our previous PET study, both of which measured changes in CBF during exercise with the similar protocol, we selected a matched sample of 11 young healthy male volunteers (age 22 ± 2 years; height 1.74 ± 0.05 m; body mass 64.6 ± 5.8 kg) for the TCD study, having given written informed consent, took part in this study. Five of 11 subjects participated in our previous PET study as well. All subjects were healthy and none reported any history of diseases. Their peak VO_2 (VO_{2peak}) was 49.4 ± 5.3 mL/min/kg, determined before the present study, as previously described (Hiura et al., 2012). All procedures used were approved by the Ethics Committee of Faculty of Sports and Health Studies of Hosei University.

Subjects performed a 15-min constant workload of exercise bout on a supine cycle ergometer (Load, Groningen, The Netherlands) with work rate of 75 or 80 W, corresponding to the level of that in our previous PET study (71 ± 11 W). The subjects breathed through a face mask (Hans Rudolph, MO, USA) connected to an online gas analyzer (CPET; Cosmed, Rome, Italy). $MCAV_{mean}$ was determined using TCD apparatus (Companion III, Nicolet Vascular, CO, USA). The proximal segment of the MCA was insonated at a depth of 48–52 mm from the temporal bone depending on the position with the best signal-to-noise ratio (Aaslid et al., 1982). $MCAV_{mean}$ was determined as 15-sec-average of TAV_{max} in the present study. Data measurements started 2 min before the onset of exercise and continued during exercise followed by 2 min after the endpoint.

Fig. 8.1 shows the time course of VO_2, end-tidal pressure of carbon dioxide ($P_{ET}CO_2$) and $MCAV_{mean}$ at the baseline (Rest) and during exercise. The constant workload exercise yielded a steady-state phase of VO_2, which corresponded to 42.2% ± 8.4% VO_{2peak} of the subjects. In addition, $P_{ET}CO_2$ also had a steady-state phase. In contrary to the steady-state kinetics of VO_2 and $P_{ET}CO_2$, it is clear that there was a decline phase during exercise for $MCAV_{mean}$. In accordance with the arrangement of CBF measurements in our previous PET study, data observed in the TCD study at Rest, 3 min (Ex1), and 13 min (Ex2) after the onset of the exercise are summarized in Table 8.1. As the duration of PET scan for each condition was 2 min, the TCD data were also averaged within 2 min at Rest (−2 to 0 min), Ex 1 (3–5 min) and Ex2 (13–15 min) using 15 s bin data. Differences in physiological data and $MCAV_{mean}$ were established using a one-way repeated-measures ANOVA with a Turkey post hoc test when appropriate. $MCAV_{mean}$ significantly increased at Ex1 by 19.2% ± 6.2% and at Ex2 as well by 9.9% ± 7.9% compared with Rest. Compared with Ex1, $MCAV_{mean}$ significantly decreased at Ex2 by 7.7% ± 5.5%. For VO_2 and $P_{ET}CO_2$, there was no significant change between Ex1 and Ex2.

Those findings suggest that respiratory and circulatory response to a 15-min constant workload cycling exercise were almost similar between the TCD and PET study. In our previous PET study, VO_2 reached 18.6 ± 4.4 and 18.8 ± 4.2 mL/min/kg at Ex1 and Ex2, respectively and $P_{ET}CO_2$ increased significantly at Ex1 and Ex2 compared with Rest, changing from 37.1 ± 2.1 to 43.9 ± 3.8 mmHg at Ex1 and to 42.2 ± 4.0 mmHg at Ex2. These data correspond to those observed in the present TCD study (Table 8.1). However, as a main finding of the present study, there is a discrepancy of data for CBF at Ex2, prolonged phase of exercise, between the TCD and PET studies. In our previous PET study, global CBF (gCBF) increased significantly at Ex1 but not at Ex2 compared with Rest. Proportional changes from Rest in gCBF were 27.9% ± 28.6% at Ex1 and 2.6% ± 13.5% at Ex2. On the other hand, $MCAV_{mean}$ increased significantly both at Ex1 and Ex2 (Table 8.1).

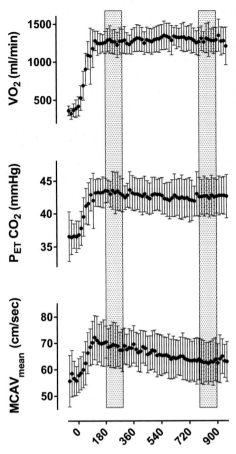

FIGURE 8.1 Time course of the indicated physiological parameters and the time-averaged mean velocity of the middle cerebral artery during a 15-min cycling ergometer exercise. *Two shaded boxes* indicate the emission scans of the oxygen-15 labeled water for positron emission tomography at the baseline, 3 and 13 min after the onset of the exercise (Hiura et al., 2014). The subjects started exercise at Time 0. Each data point represents the mean ± SD of a 15-sec epoch ($n = 11$). $MCAV_{mean}$, mean velocity of the middle cerebral artery blood flow; $P_{ET}CO_2$, end tidal pressure of carbon dioxide; VO_2, pulmonary oxygen uptake.

TABLE 8.1 Physiological Variables and Mean Velocity of the Middle Cerebral Artery Blood Flow at Rest and During Exercise

	Rest	Ex1	Ex2
VO_2 (mL/min/kg)	5.4 ± 1.5	19.9 ± 3.3***	19.6 ± 4.9***
$P_{ET}CO_2$ (mmHg)	36.6 ± 2.0	43.1 ± 2.3***	42.7 ± 2.6***
$MCAV_{mean}$ (cm/sec)	57.3 ± 6.5	68.2 ± 7.5***	62.9 ± 7.4**,††

Values are shown as mean ± SD ($n = 11$). Significance difference from Rest ***$P < .001$, **$P < .01$. Significance difference from Ex1 ††$P < .01$.
Ex1,3 min after the onset of exercise; Ex2,13 min after the onset of exercise.
$MCAV_{mean}$, mean velocity of the middle cerebral artery blood flow; $P_{ET}CO_2$, end-tidal pressure of carbon dioxide; VO_2, pulmonary oxygen uptake.

rCBF MEASUREMENT USING PET

Functional imaging with PET has been developed for investigation of normal physiology and pathology in the human brain. As a method for rapid measurement of rCBF, the $H_2^{15}O$ autoradiographic method has been established as a clinical tool (Herscovitch et al., 1983; Kanno et al., 1987; Raichle et al., 1983). Following an intravenous injection of $H_2^{15}O$, rCBF is calculated using a radioactivity–time curve of $H_2^{15}O$ in the artery and a radioactivity concentration of $H_2^{15}O$ in the brain tissue (Herscovitch et al., 1983; Kanno et al., 1987). In order to measure reactivity of rCBF by various physiological stimulations, it takes 90–120s at least for PET scan to obtain a functional image. For example, we previously investigated the alteration of rCBF during and after hyperventilation using PET to determine the circulatory response induced by daily respiratory changes in the cerebral area under chronic hemodynamic stress (Nariai et al., 1998). Since the subjects should be fixed in the scanner the scanner bed in the supine position with their heads immobilized, there is a methodological limitation for measurement of rCBF using PET during exercise. However, we recently demonstrated changes in rCBF during dynamic exercise of cycling exercise using a supine ergometer on the condition that the subjects performed low-to-moderate intensity cycling exercise so that movement of their heads occurred as little as possible (Hiura et al., 2014). To date, there has been only one PET study, except for our previous study, which described changes in rCBF during cycling exercise (Christensen et al., 2000). However, the earlier study did not show the quantitative data. Our previous study demonstrated quantitative data of rCBF during exercise for the first time and clarified that changes in rCBF elicited by exercise differed between the onset and prolonged phase.

To further examine the magnitude of changes in rCBF during exercise, we reanalyzed data from young male healthy volunteers ($n = 10$) involved in our previous study. All procedures used were approved by the Ethics Committee of Tokyo Metropolitan Institute of Gerontology and was conducted at the Tokyo Metropolitan Institute of Gerontology. As described above in the TCD study section, we engaged the exercise protocol of a 15 min constant workload of exercise bout on a supine cycle ergometer with work rate of 71 ± 11 W, which yielded a steady-state phase of VO_2 and $P_{ET}CO_2$. As did in the TCD study, the subjects breathed through a face mask connected to an online gas analyzer for measurements of physiological variables. PET scans were performed at Rest, Ex1, and Ex2, as previously described. All subjects underwent PET imaging with $H_2^{15}O$, by a bolus injection of 300 MBq averagely. Quantification of rCBF was performed with autoradiographic method (Herscovitch et al., 1983; Raichle et al., 1983). All subjects also received T1- and T2-weighted contrast magnetic resonance imaging (MRI) scan for coregistration with PET and non-linear projecting into a standard three-dimensional stereotactic space using the SPM eight and the MNI (Montreal Neurological Institute) templates, sampled at a voxel size of $2 \times 2 \times 2$ mm.

Images were analyzed using SPM 8 software. The effect of time course of exercise was evaluated on a voxel-by-voxel basis using paired (within subjects, between conditions), two-tailed t-tests (Ex1 vs. Ex2). Regions were considered significant if uncorrected significance level of $P < .005$ corresponding to Z-scores >3.24 (i.e., voxel levels of significance uncorrected for multiple analyses over the whole brain), with an extent threshold of 300 voxels. In addition, the quantitative analysis of rCBF was performed using Dr. View software (Infocom, Tokyo, Japan) based on the results from the SPM analysis. For each analysis, 10 mm² regions of interest (ROIs) at least in three consecutive slices (6 mm) were settled in each area in which significant effects were obtained in the voxel-by-voxel analyses.

The moderate-intensity constant workload cycling exercise evoked increased rCBF in great amount of areas at Ex1, as its effect was prominent in the cerebellar vermis, sensorimotor cortex for the bilateral legs ($M1_{Leg}$ and $S1_{Leg}$), bilateral supplementary motor area (SMA), bilateral inferior cerebellar hemispheres, and left insula cortex. However, these regions of increased rCBF diminished at Ex2, being confined to the vermis, $M1_{Leg}$, $S1_{Leg}$, and the SMA. To address this phenomenon precisely, the specific areas where rCBF was higher at Ex1 than Ex2 were examined by voxel-by-voxel analysis and illustrated in Fig. 8.2. These areas include the left hippocampus, pons, midbrain, vermis, cerebellum, thalamus, anterior insular cortex (AIS), anterior cingulate gyrus, SMA, $M1_{Leg}$, $S1_{Leg}$, and left middle frontal gyrus (MFG). In addition, we analyzed these changes in rCBF during exercise quantitatively. For these areas where rCBF increased prominently at Ex1, the proportional changes of rCBF at Ex1 (A) and Ex2 (B) compared with Rest are demonstrated in Fig. 8.3.

INCREASED rCBF DURING EXERCISE: UNDERLYING POSSIBLE MECHANISMS

We compared the changes of $MCAV_{mean}$ with those of gCBF measured by PET evoked by a single bout of 15-min moderate-intensity constant workload cycling exercise on a supine position. The larger increase of gCBF than $MCAV_{mean}$ may be attributable to blood flow supplied by the anterior cerebral arteries and vertebral arteries (VA). Sato et al. demonstrated the changes in blood flow velocity of the main trunk arteries for brain during 5-min constant workload cycling exercise with various intensities of 40%, 60%, and 80% VO_{2peak} (Sato et al., 2011). In that study, the increase of blood flow velocity of VA from Rest was larger than that of $MCAV_{mean}$ from rest for all of the intensities. A small amount of the increase of $MCAV_{mean}$ at Ex2 may be attributable to the increased rCBF in the AIS and thalamus. In contrary, a finding that rCBF in the AIS, ACG, and MFG did not increase at Ex2 from Rest may be attributable to the compromised gCBF at Ex2.

Although the magnitude of the increase in gCBF was different from that of $MCAV_{mean}$ at the onset phase of exercise, the steady-state exercise engaged in the present studies apparently evoked the increase in rCBF at this phase. With regards to the increased rCBF observed by neuroimaging, the possible underlying mechanism has been considered as functional hyperemia, which matches the delivery of flow to the activity level of brain (Iadecola and Nedergaard, 2007). However, it is speculated that a rapid increase in CO and some other mechanisms associated with initiating exercise, such as central command, would cause a great amount of increase in rCBF at the onset phase of exercise instead of functional hyperemia. In contrast to the onset phase, functional hyperemia would occur in competition within the brain at the prolonged phase of exercise where rCBF recovers to nearly resting state. As it is clear that exercise elicits increased rCBF, we will review the beneficial effects of exercise on brain in the next section.

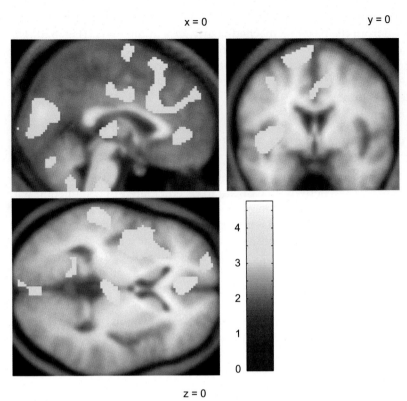

FIGURE 8.2 Brain regions showing higher rCBF at 3 min than 13 min after the onset of exercise. Areas of significant common activation above $P < .005$ (uncorrected for multiple analyses over the whole brain) with an extent threshold of 300 voxels are color-scaled according to the T-score (scale given in the Figure). Group data are presented on an averaged T1-weighted structural image derived from the 10 subjects and normalized to the MNI standard space. MNI coordinates in the x dimension and y dimension are given for parasagittal and coronal slices, respectively. *MNI*, Montreal Neurological Institute.

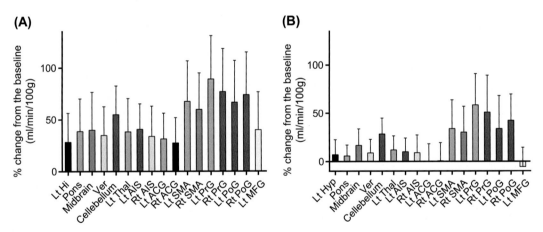

FIGURE 8.3 Quantitative data of the proportional (%) changes at 3 min (A) and 13 min (B) from the baseline for region of interests (ROI) analysis. ROIs were selected based on results of the voxel-by-voxel analysis in which brain regions showing higher rCBF at 3 min than 13 min after the onset of exercise. *ACG*, anterior cingulate gyrus; *AIS*, anterior insular cortex; *Hi*, hippocampus; *Lt*, left; *MFG*, middle frontal gyrus; *PoG*, postcentral gyrus; *PrG*, precentral gyrus; *Rt*, right; *SMA*, supplementary motor area; *Thal*, thalamus; *Ver*, vermis.

At the onset of dynamic cycling exercise, a rapid increase in CO evoked the concomitant change in blood pressure (BP). Changes in mean arterial pressure (MAP) scans were 10–15 mmHg, which were measured during PET scans in our laboratory. As described so far, CBF apparently increased in this phase. It seems that this phenomenon might be inconsistent with cerebral autoregulation, which has been defined as the ability of the brain vessels to maintain a constant blood flow within a perfusion pressure range, i.e., the difference MAP and intracranial pressure of ~60 to ~150 mmHg (Lassen, 1959; Paulson et al., 1990,). However, cerebral autoregulation has been assessed by the static methodologies such as the Kety-Schmidt technique or ^{133}Xe measurements, manipulating BP using vasoactive medications. Consequently, cerebral autoregulation is not a single regulating mechanism for the relationship between BP and CBF during exercise. Another major regulatory mechanism is cerebrovascular response (CVR) to CO_2, which was defined as the vasodilatory response of cerebral resistance vessels to increases in $P_{ET}CO_2$ during inhalation of CO_2 (Ainslie and Duffin, 2009; Lassen, 1959). At the onset phase of exercise in the present studies, the proportional change in rCBF from the baseline reached nearly 75% in the $M1_{Leg}$ (Fig. 8.3). This large increase seems to be out of range for the CVR to CO_2 even if the heterogeneous nature of the brain regions involved in the CVR to CO_2 is considered (Ito et al., 2000). Thus multiple underlying mechanisms are to be considered for regulating CBF during exercise. As it is clear that exercise elicits increased rCBF, we will review the beneficial effects of exercise on brain in the next section.

INCREASED rCBF DURING EXERCISE AND BENEFICIAL EFFECTS OF BRAIN

Functional brain imaging is based on mapping the changes in the rCBF that are rCBF induced by neuronal activity. Although the underlying mechanisms coupling neural activity to CBF are to be elucidated in conjunction with oxidative and nonoxidative metabolisms in astrocytes (Gjedde et al., 2002; Iadecola and Nedergaard, 2007), increased CBF to various regions of the brain during exercise may be associated with the beneficial effects of exercise on brain health. Increased CBF induced by administration of citicoline, the cholinergic agonist (Alvarez et al., 1999), milameline, the alpha-2A adrenergic agonist, (Schwarz et al., 1999) and estrogen (Maki and Resnick, 2001) have shown to enhance cognitive performance. Consequently, aerobic exercise engaged in the present study might be associated with enhancing cognition. Furthermore, increased CBF to the brain via angiogenesis and/or vasodilation facilitates synaptic plasticity via multiple mechanisms (Christie et al., 2008). Recent studies which investigated underlying mechanisms of the beneficial effects of exercise on brain, such as learning and memory, protection from neurodegeneration and alleviation of depression, has focused on changes in neurotransmission, neurotrophins and vasculature, which contribute to neural plasticity (Cotman et al., 2007).

As present PET study demonstrated various areas where rCBF increased at the onset of exercise (Fig. 8.3), the hippocampus has been recognized as a key structure for cognitive function and stress-related pathologies such as depression (Kim and Diamond, 2002). One aspect of hippocampal plasticity that has received considerable attention is adult neurogenesis, which has been associated with cognition and emotion and is hypothesized to mediate, at least in part, the beneficial effects of exercise (Abrous et al., 2005). Indeed, running enhances hippocampal neurogenesis in animal studies via vascular endothelial growth factor (Fabel et al., 2003) and β-endorphin (Koehl et al., 2008). More precisely, a previous MRI study using measurements of cerebral blood volume (CBV) demonstrated that exercise was found to have a primary effect on CBV of dentate gyrus in the hippocampus, suggesting that exercise may induce neurogenesis in the dentate gyrus (Pereira et al., 2007).

Neuroanatomical evidence showed that cardiovascular fitness was related with age-related declines in cortical tissues density and these effects were greatest in the frontal, prefrontal, and parietal cortices (Colcombe et al., 2003). In the present study, rCBF in the MFG increased only in Ex1 and rather tended to decrease at Ex2. A previous neuroimaging study demonstrated that the MFG was consistently implicated in attentional selection and the resolution of response conflict elicited by incongruent response cues (Casey et al., 2000). In addition, Colcombe et al. (2004) demonstrated that older adults with higher cardiovascular fitness demonstrated significantly greater activation in the MFG, which established a direct link between the extant animal and human literature on aging, brain, and cardiovascular fitness. They concluded that even moderate cardiovascular activity of the sort that is within reach of most healthy older adult population results in improved neural functioning, and may help to extend or enhance independent living in older adult populations. A moderate-intensity 15-min cycling exercise engaged in our studies is in accordance with this perspective. Although we focused on young healthy subjects in the present studies, our results may be regarded as a fundamental data for elderly or poststroke population in future study unraveling the underlying mechanism for exercise-induced changes in rCBF.

Furthermore, we suggest possible role of the increased rCBF during exercise for poststroke rehabilitation and prevention of stroke. A prospective population study of stroke incidence, that lack of exercise was an independent risk factor for poor outcome postischemic insult (Wadley et al., 2007). Ivey et al. (2011) showed that treadmill aerobic exercise training for stroke survivors induced improved CVR to CO_2 in that study, CVR to CO_2 was measured using the changes in the $MCAV_{mean}$ obtained by TCD method. The results demonstrated that change in aerobic capacity induced by 6-month exercise intervention was implicated as a partial mediator of adaptation in cerebral vasomotor function after stroke. On the basis of our previous PET study in normal volunteers and on previous reports on the feasibility of aerobic exercise for stroke survivors, we are conducting clinical PET studies to investigate the time course of rCBF during and after the exercise around the ischemic lesions among poststroke patients with mild disability. Such approach may contribute to establish feasible exercise protocol for poststroke patients.

CONCLUSION

The present article confirmed increased CBF during steady-state exercise which is a possible candidate for the underlying mechanism for beneficial effects of physical activity and exercise on brain function. As we briefly introduced the methodological aspects of TCD and PET methods and the results of our recent studies using the both methods, the $MCAV_{mean}$ does not represent gCBF but rCBF perfused by these arteries. Particularly, despite the steady-state of circulatory and respiratory response between the onset and prolonged phase of exercise, prominent increase of gCBF at the onset of phase was contrasted to lesser increase of rCBF at the prolonged phase. Although the underlying mechanisms are to be elucidated, literature from animal and human studies reviewed here demonstrated increased CBF evoked by exercise has roles for protective effects on aging brain function and rehabilitation for stroke survivors. Provided that the increased CBF during exercise may facilitate neural plasticity via angiogenesis and/or vasodilation, steady-state exercise is an effective intervention for brain health. For a clinical application, we are conducting a PET study examining changes in rCBF during steady-state exercise among ischemic stroke survivors to establish feasible exercise protocol for their hemodynamic conditions. Future research that investigates possible mechanisms mediating increased CBF and neural plasticity may prove valuable.

Acknowledgments

This work was supported in part by Grant–in Aid for Scientific Research (C) No. 24500478 from the Japan Society for the Promotion of Science 2012–14 (to M. Hiura) and Grant for Scientific Research from the Nakatomi Foundation for Health Promotion Focusing on Physical Exercise 2012–13 (to M. Hiura).

Disclosure/Conflict of Interest

The authors declare no conflict of interest.

References

Aaslid, R., Markwalder, T.M., Nornes, H., 1982. Noninvasive transcranial Doppler ultrasound recording of flow velocity in basal cerebral arteries. Journal of Neurosurgery 57 (6), 769–774. http://dx.doi.org/10.3171/jns.1982.57.6.0769.

Abrous, D.N., Koehl, M., Le Moal, M., 2005. Adult neurogenesis: from precursors to network and physiology. Physiological Reviews 85 (2), 523–569. http://dx.doi.org/10.1152/physrev.00055.2003.

Ainslie, P.N., Duffin, J., 2009. Integration of cerebrovascular CO_2 reactivity and chemoreflex control of breathing: mechanisms of regulation, measurement, and interpretation. American Journal of Physiology Regulatory Integrative and Comparative Physiology 296 (5), R1473–R1495. http://dx.doi.org/10.1152/ajpregu.91008.2008.

Alvarez, X.A., Mouzo, R., Pichel, V., Perez, P., Laredo, M., Fernandez-Novoa, L., et al., 1999. Double-blind placebo-controlled study with citicoline in APOE genotyped Alzheimer's disease patients. Effects on cognitive performance, brain bioelectrical activity and cerebral perfusion. Methods and Findings in Experimental and Clinical Pharmacology 21 (9), 633–644.

Casey, B.J., Thomas, K.M., Welsh, T.F., Badgaiyan, R.D., Eccard, C.H., Jennings, J.R., Crone, E.A., 2000. Dissociation of response conflict, attentional selection, and expectancy with functional magnetic resonance imaging. Proceedings of the National Academy of Sciences of the United States of America 97 (15), 8728–8733.

Christensen, L.O., Johannsen, P., Sinkjaer, T., Petersen, N., Pyndt, H.S., Nielsen, J.B., 2000. Cerebral activation during bicycle movements in man. Experimental Brain Research 135 (1), 66–72.

Christie, B.R., Eadie, B.D., Kannangara, T.S., Robillard, J.M., Shin, J., Titterness, A.K., 2008. Exercising our brains: how physical activity impacts synaptic plasticity in the dentate gyrus. Neuromolecular Medicine 10 (2), 47–58. http://dx.doi.org/10.1007/s12017-008-8033-2.

Colcombe, S.J., Erickson, K.I., Raz, N., Webb, A.G., Cohen, N.J., McAuley, E., Kramer, A.F., 2003. Aerobic fitness reduces brain tissue loss in aging humans. The Journals of Gerontology Series A Biological Sciences and Medical Sciences 58 (2), 176–180.

Colcombe, S.J., Kramer, A.F., Erickson, K.I., Scalf, P., McAuley, E., Cohen, N.J., et al., 2004. Cardiovascular fitness, cortical plasticity, and aging. Proceedings of the National Academy of Sciences of the United States of America 101 (9), 3316–3321. http://dx.doi.org/10.1073/pnas.0400266101.

Cotman, C.W., Berchtold, N.C., Christie, L.A., 2007. Exercise builds brain health: key roles of growth factor cascades and inflammation. Trends in Neurosciences 30 (9), 464–472. http://dx.doi.org/10.1016/j.tins.2007.06.011.

Fabel, K., Fabel, K., Tam, B., Kaufer, D., Baiker, A., Simmons, N., et al., 2003. VEGF is necessary for exercise-induced adult hippocampal neurogenesis. The European Journal of Neuroscience 18 (10), 2803–2812.

Gaesser, G.A., Poole, D.C., 1996. The slow component of oxygen uptake kinetics in humans. Exercise and Sport Sciences Reviews 24, 35–71.

Gjedde, A., Marrett, S., Vafaee, M., 2002. Oxidative and nonoxidative metabolism of excited neurons and astrocytes. Journal of Cerebral Blood Flow and Metabolism 22 (1), 1–14. http://dx.doi.org/10.1097/00004647-200201000-00001.

Goldstein, L.B., Bushnell, C.D., Adams, R.J., Appel, L.J., Braun, L.T., Chaturvedi, S., et al., 2011. Guidelines for the primary prevention of stroke: a guideline for healthcare professionals from the American Heart Association/American Stroke Association. Stroke 42 (2), 517–584. http://dx.doi.org/10.1161/STR.0b013e3181fcb238.

Herscovitch, P., Markham, J., Raichle, M.E., 1983. Brain blood flow measured with intravenous $H_2(15)O$. I. Theory and error analysis. Journal of Nuclear Medicine 24 (9), 782–789.

Hillman, C.H., Erickson, K.I., Kramer, A.F., 2008. Be smart, exercise your heart: exercise effects on brain and cognition. Nature Reviews Neuroscience 9 (1), 58–65. http://dx.doi.org/10.1038/nrn2298.

Hiura, M., Kinoshita, N., Izumi, S., Nariai, T., 2012. Comparison of the kinetics of pulmonary oxygen uptake and middle cerebral artery blood flow velocity during cycling exercise. Advances in Experimental Medicine and Biology 737, 25–31. http://dx.doi.org/10.1007/978-1-4614-1566-4_4.

Hiura, M., Nariai, T., Ishii, K., Sakata, M., Oda, K., Toyohara, J., Ishiwata, K., 2014. Changes in cerebral blood flow during steady-state cycling exercise: a study using oxygen-15-labeled water with PET. Journal of Cerebral Blood Flow and Metabolism 34 (3), 389–396. http://dx.doi.org/10.1038/jcbfm.2013.220.

Iadecola, C., Nedergaard, M., 2007. Glial regulation of the cerebral microvasculature. Nature Neuroscience 10 (11), 1369–1376. http://dx.doi.org/10.1038/nn2003.

Ide, K., Horn, A., Secher, N.H., 1999. Cerebral metabolic response to submaximal exercise. Journal of Applied Physiology (1985) 87 (5), 1604–1608.

Ito, H., Yokoyama, I., Iida, H., Kinoshita, T., Hatazawa, J., Shimosegawa, E., et al., 2000. Regional differences in cerebral vascular response to $PaCO_2$ changes in humans measured by positron emission tomography. Journal of Cerebral Blood Flow and Metabolism 20 (8), 1264–1270. http://dx.doi.org/10.1097/00004647-200008000-00011.

Ivey, F.M., Ryan, A.S., Hafer-Macko, C.E., Macko, R.F., 2011. Improved cerebral vasomotor reactivity after exercise training in hemiparetic stroke survivors. Stroke 42 (7), 1994–2000. http://dx.doi.org/10.1161/STROKEAHA.110.607879.

Jones, A.M., Grassi, B., Christensen, P.M., Krustrup, P., Bangsbo, J., Poole, D.C., 2011. Slow component of VO_2 kinetics: mechanistic bases and practical applications. Medicine and Science in Sports and Exercise 43 (11), 2046–2062. http://dx.doi.org/10.1249/MSS.0b013e31821fcfc1.

Kanno, I., Iida, H., Miura, S., Murakami, M., Takahashi, K., Sasaki, H., et al., 1987. A system for cerebral blood flow measurement using an $H_2^{15}O$ autoradiographic method and positron emission tomography. Journal of Cerebral Blood Flow and Metabolism 7 (2), 143–153. http://dx.doi.org/10.1038/jcbfm.1987.37.

Kim, J.J., Diamond, D.M., 2002. The stressed hippocampus, synaptic plasticity and lost memories. Nature Reviews Neuroscience 3 (6), 453–462. http://dx.doi.org/10.1038/nrn849.

Koehl, M., Meerlo, P., Gonzales, D., Rontal, A., Turek, F.W., Abrous, D.N., 2008. Exercise-induced promotion of hippocampal cell proliferation requires beta-endorphin. FASEB Journal 22 (7), 2253–2262. http://dx.doi.org/10.1096/fj.07-099101.

Lassen, N.A., 1959. Cerebral blood flow and oxygen consumption in man. Physiological Reviews 39 (2), 183–238.

Maki, P.M., Resnick, S.M., 2001. Effects of estrogen on patterns of brain activity at rest and during cognitive activity: a review of neuroimaging studies. NeuroImage 14 (4), 789–801. http://dx.doi.org/10.1006/nimg.2001.0887.

Morgan, W.P., 1985. Affective beneficence of vigorous physical activity. Medicine and Science in Sports and Exercise 17 (1), 94–100.

Nariai, T., Senda, M., Ishii, K., Wakabayashi, S., Yokota, T., Toyama, H., et al., 1998. Posthyperventilatory steal response in chronic cerebral hemodynamic stress: a positron emission tomography study. Stroke 29 (7), 1281–1292.

Paulson, O.B., Strandgaard, S., Edvinsson, L., 1990. Cerebral autoregulation. Cerebrovascular and Brain Metabolism Reviews 2 (2), 161–192.

Pereira, A.C., Huddleston, D.E., Brickman, A.M., Sosunov, A.A., Hen, R., McKhann, G.M., et al., 2007. An in vivo correlate of exercise-induced neurogenesis in the adult dentate gyrus. Proceedings of the National Academy of Sciences of the United States of America 104 (13), 5638–5643. http://dx.doi.org/10.1073/pnas.0611721104.

Pott, F., Jensen, K., Hansen, H., Christensen, N.J., Lassen, N.A., Secher, N.H., 1996. Middle cerebral artery blood velocity and plasma catecholamines during exercise. Acta Physiologica Scandinavica 158 (4), 349–356. http://dx.doi.org/10.1046/j.1365-201X.1996.564325000.x.

Querido, J.S., Sheel, A.W., 2007. Regulation of cerebral blood flow during exercise. Sports Medicine 37 (9), 765–782.

Raichle, M.E., Martin, W.R., Herscovitch, P., Mintun, M.A., Markham, J., 1983. Brain blood flow measured with intravenous $H_2(15)O$. II. Implementation and validation. Journal of Nuclear Medicine 24 (9), 790–798.

Sato, K., Ogoh, S., Hirasawa, A., Oue, A., Sadamoto, T., 2011. The distribution of blood flow in the carotid and vertebral arteries during dynamic exercise in humans. The Journal of Physiology 589 (Pt 11), 2847–2856. http://dx.doi.org/10.1113/jphysiol.2010.204461.

Schwarz, R.D., Callahan, M.J., Coughenour, L.L., Dickerson, M.R., Kinsora, J.J., Lipinski, W.J., et al., 1999. Milameline (CI-979/RU35926): a muscarinic receptor agonist with cognition-activating properties: biochemical and in vivo characterization. The Journal of Pharmacology and Experimental Therapeutics 291 (2), 812–822.

Secher, N.H., Seifert, T., Van Lieshout, J.J., 2008. Cerebral blood flow and metabolism during exercise: implications for fatigue. Journal of Applied Physiology (1985) 104 (1), 306–314. http://dx.doi.org/10.1152/japplphysiol.00853.2007.

Strohle, A., 2009. Physical activity, exercise, depression and anxiety disorders. Journal of Neural Transmission 116 (6), 777–784. http://dx.doi.org/10.1007/s00702-008-0092-x.

Valzueza, J.M., Schreiber, S.J., Roehl, J.E., Klingebiel, R., 2008. Neurosonology and Neuroimaging of Stroke. Thieme, New York.

Wadley, V.G., McClure, L.A., Howard, V.J., Unverzagt, F.W., Go, R.C., Moy, C.S., et al., 2007. Cognitive status, stroke symptom reports, and modifiable risk factors among individuals with no diagnosis of stroke or transient ischemic attack in the REasons for Geographic and Racial Differences in Stroke (REGARDS) Study. Stroke 38 (4), 1143–1147. http://dx.doi.org/10.1161/01.STR.0000259676.75552.38.

Whipp, B.J., Rossiter, H.B., 2005. The Kinetics of Oxygen Uptake: Physiological Inferences from the Parameters. Routledge, London.

Williamson, J.W., McColl, R., Mathews, D., Ginsburg, M., Mitchell, J.H., 1999. Activation of the insular cortex is affected by the intensity of exercise. Journal of Applied Physiology (1985) 87 (3), 1213–1219.

9

Biochemical Mechanisms Associated With Exercise-Induced Neuroprotection in Aging Brains and Related Neurological Diseases

M.S. Shanmugam, W.M. Tierney, R.A. Hernandez, A. Cruz, T.L. Uhlendorf, R.W. Cohen

California State University Northridge, Northridge, CA, United States

Abstract

Population studies in the United States indicate that there are over 40 million people over 65 years of age. Age-related cognitive decline and their associated neuronal disorders have been shown to disturb neurological processes such as memory, learning, and the ability to perform spatial tasks. While there have been countless drugs created to reduce or mask symptoms associated with aging, there are also various physical therapies that improve memory by augmenting the brain's own neuroprotective mechanisms. Numerous studies attest to the observation that physical exercise significantly improves cognition, memory, learning, and motor function diminished both by aging and disease. Exercise appears to induce neuroprotection by targeting multiple biochemical and genetic pathways, and by triggering morphological and physiological changes in various cells throughout the brain. Exercise, by promoting such alterations, plays a strategic role both in reversing cognitive deficits and in preventing such damage from occurring due to age or disease.

INTRODUCTION

Current demographic studies in the United States indicate that there are over 40 million people over 65 years of age. Due to the graying of America's population and an increase in their life spans, the medical community is searching for more innovative practices to meet the challenges of aging. The aging human brain is highly susceptible to severe cognitive decline and neurodegenerative disease, significantly affecting neurological processes such as learning, memory, and the ability to perform spatial tasks (Jagust, 2013; Ojo et al., 2015). Although there have been countless drugs and homeopathic remedies created to reduce these symptoms related to aging, there are also various physical therapies that utilize the brain's own neuroprotective mechanisms to reduce or mask these clinical manifestations.

Neuroplasticity, the ability of brain cells to alter both structure and function throughout the life span of the individual, is an endogenous process that targets the cognitive decline associated with aging (Voss et al., 2013). One method to augment and expand neuronal connections throughout the brain is through physical exercise. Numerous studies conducted both on human and animal models of aging subjected to various exercise regimens show a causal relationship between exercise and significant improvements in cognition (Churchhill et al., 2002; van Praag, 2009; Baker et al., 2010; Voss et al., 2013; Vivar et al., 2013).

Exercise benefits the brain through various mechanisms, including the enhancement of memory, cognitive function, improved neurotransmission, and neuronal plasticity (Gyorkos et al., 2014; Noble et al., 2014; Revilla et al., 2014). The exact mechanisms of how these exercise-induced effects transpire have been studied extensively. These studies reveal changes at the cellular level that induce modifications that reverse age-related neurodegeneration (Vivar et al., 2013), and has been shown to be coupled with increased release of neurotrophic factors that regulate neuroprotective pathways (Vianney et al., 2013). In addition, the neuroprotective effects of exercise on increased antioxidant activity as well as discrete changes to phenotypic expression at the epigenetic level (Kaliman et al., 2011) have also been shown to contribute significantly to the improvements in cognitive function.

EXERCISE EFFECTS: NEUROTROPHIC FACTORS

Neurological growth factors such as brain-derived-neurotrophic factor (BDNF) and glial-cell-derived-neuro-trophic factor (GDNF) are crucial to maintain proper functioning of neurons. Studies have shown that downregu-lation of BDNF and GDNF are linked to the cognitive decline associated with age and related neurodegenerative diseases (Kleim et al., 2003). In contrast, upregulation of these same neurotrophic factors supplemented by increased exercise supports the idea that exercise improves cognitive function.

BDNF is known to promote neuronal plasticity, and GDNF is critical in maintaining neuromuscular synapses (Vianney et al., 2013), identifying both chemicals as essential to normal brain function by preserving synaptic integ-rity. In aging and many related neurological disorders, reduced levels of BDNF and GDNF have been recognized as key contributors to neurodegeneration and the resultant symptoms (Coelho et al., 2012). Specifically, the decline in BDNF levels has been associated with hippocampal shrinkage, decreased cell signaling, and concomitant memory loss (Luellen et al., 2007; Erickson et al., 2010; Calabrese et al., 2013). Alternatively, increased BDNF expression has been linked to the improvements in motor function (Kim et al., 2005), while decreased BDNF levels have been associ-ated with a decline in cognitive function (Ploughman et al., 2005, 2007).

Many studies have shown that exercise-induced upregulation of BDNF and GDNF (McCollough et al., 2013) alleviate age-associated cognitive decline. Studies suggest that exercise may be a natural way to increase BDNF pro-duction as an alternative to drug administration. Animal studies have shown that moderate exercise is sufficient to increase the levels of BDNF in the brain by preserving neuroprotective pathways (Van Kummer and Cohen, 2015), building synaptic connections (Côté et al., 2011), and preventing brain injury (Di Loreto et al., 2014). BDNF effects have been shown to enhance neural plasticity and induce recovery function in animal models of aging (Kleim et al., 2003), corresponding with improvements in cognitive function and faster neural processing speed after exercise (Chin et al., 2015). Aged mice placed on a 4-month exercise regimen showed improvements in cognitive function through the activation of neuroprotective pathways initiated by BDNF, facilitating synaptic survival and preserva-tion (Di Loreto et al., 2014).

In addition, GDNF has been shown to act as a mediator, activating other brain proteins that help maintain neuronal plasticity. Plasticity of neuromuscular synapses is sustained in rats by activity-dependent GDNF expression result-ing from minimal slow and fast twitch muscle fiber activity (Gyorkos et al., 2014). Recent animal studies showed that exercise increased GDNF expression in the spinal cord (McCollough et al., 2013) as well as in skeletal muscle (Vianney et al., 2013; Gyorkos and Spitsbergen, 2014), enhancing neural plasticity.

Numerous studies looking into the effects of forced exercise regimes were used to determine whether this proce-dure is more effective in producing neuroprotective effects through GDNF compared to voluntary exercise regimes. Forced exercise has been shown to have both positive and negative effects. Forced, low-intensity exercise has proven to enhance the integrity of neuro-muscular connectivity in aged rats by increasing spinal cord GDNF (McCullough et al., 2013) and improve general cardiovascular health. However, this forced exercise methodology has also been shown to diminish the trophic effects of GDNF through increased release of the stress hormone, corticosterone (Ploughman et al., 2005). In contrast, daily voluntary exercise displayed the greatest benefit to brain health through decreased stress and downregulation of the inflammatory response associated with increased GDNF levels (Revilla et al., 2014).

EXERCISE EFFECTS: EPIGENETICS

Epigenetics is a regulatory mechanism that elicits precise modifications of the genome via activation or suppres-sion of transcription. Epigenetic alterations in genotypic expression can be influenced by environmental, biochemical or physiological changes. Obviously, aging has been shown to contribute considerably to these modifications in gene expression, including increased DNA demethylation, decreased histone regulation, and miRNA changes.

Many studies have highlighted the direct effects of exercise on the epigenome, including increase in histone acety-lation (Elsner et al., 2011) and decrease in DNA methylation (Gomez-Pinilla et al., 2011; Abel and Rissman, 2013; Elsner et al., 2013). The results of these studies support the idea that exercise can be used to alter epigenetic factors thus creating novel therapies for age and disease-related cognitive decline. In addition, the increased expression of specific miRNAs (Bao et al., 2014), the epigenetic suppression of pro-apoptotic genes (Bao et al., 2014) and the activation of antiapoptotic genes (Zhao et al., 2015) as a consequence of exercise suggest that these mechanisms can help prevent neuronal cell damage.

Particular to this chapter, research has shown that exercise can induce these epigenetic changes directly within neurons. Studies with mice show that exercise correlates directly with epigenetic changes in hippocampal neurons, starting 3h after onset of an exercise regime (Kaliman et al., 2011). In addition, these exercise-induced epigenetic modifications in the hippocampus have been shown to increase neuroplasticity and improve cognitive responses. Finally, research suggests that epigenetic effects in exercised mice may last up to 2weeks posttreatment (Kaliman et al., 2011).

As discussed previously, decreased levels of BDNF have been identified in aging brains (Silhol et al., 2005; Erickson et al., 2010) while other studies have correlated increased BDNF expression with exercise (Shen et al., 2013), making BDNF regulation an important link between both exercise and epigenetic alterations (Denham et al., 2014). In related research, the mRNAs of both BDNF and its receptor have been determined to be epigenetically regulated via exercise (Ntanasis-Stathopoulos et al., 2013). DNA methylation was found to be decreased on the BDNF promoter in exercised rats (Gomez-Pinilla et al., 2011); specifically, epigenetic changes in methyl-CpG-binding protein led to the observed DNA demethylation of the BDNF promoter (Gomez-Pinilla and Hillman, 2013). In addition, this epigenetic effect of increased BDNF mRNA expression was also observed within hippocampi of neonate rats whose dams exercised during pregnancy (Parnpiansil et al., 2003).

Histone modifications have been shown to be responsible for a large proportion of observed epigenetic alterations, and subsequent research has indicated an increase in histone acetylation correlated with exercise. Elsner and colleagues found a decrease in neuronal histone deacetylase (HDAC) activity and a corresponding increase in histone acetyltransferase activity within the rat hippocampus with just a single bout of exercise, but no change with chronic exercise (Elsner et al., 2011). Decreased DNA methylation and histone modification were also noted in hippocampi and cerebellums of mice after 1week of exercise (Abel and Rissman, 2013). Increased acetylation of histone H3 (Gomez-Pinilla et al., 2011; Denham et al., 2014) and decreased levels of HDAC were found in moderately exercised rats (Ntanasis-Stathopoulos et al., 2013). Collins et al. (2009) determined that exercise evoked an increase in acetylation of the histone H3 which was correlated with increased c-Fos expression (Collins et al., 2009).

Researchers examined the effects of single-session exercise (SSE) and chronic-exercise (CE) rats on epigenetic changes of DNA methyltransferase (DNMT) 1 and DNMT3b, and H3–K9 histone methylation levels in the hippocampus of young (3months) and old (20months) rats (Elsner et al., 2013). SSE young rats were found to have decreased methylation levels of DNMT1 and DNMT3 after 1-h exercise sessions. After 18h, the CE young rats displayed increased methylation levels of DNMT1 and DNMT3 comparable to unexercised rats. Aged rats saw no DMNT3 methylation changes due to either exercise parameter, but were found to have decreased DMNT1 levels comparable to controls. Young SSE rats were found to have decreased methylation of H3–K9 after 1h of exercise while the methylation of H3–K9 dropped even more after 18h. Interestingly, aged SSE rats had an increase in methylation of H3–K9 levels at 1h and also at 18h. Yet, aged CE rats saw no change in methylation of H3–K9 levels, suggesting that moderate not chronic exercise can significantly reduce aging effects via epigenetic changes.

The epigenetic activity of RNA silencing via miRNA is another avenue of research as miRNA alterations are common epigenetic modifications, resulting in reduced transcription. Bao et al. (2014) found that there were significant differences in miRNAs in the hippocampus between sedentary and exercised rats that were subjected to traumatic brain injury (TBI). Specifically, miR-21 and miR-34a were found to be upregulated in sedentary TBI but downregulated in the exercised TBI groups (Bao et al., 2014). Another study showed upregulation of miRNAs known to be involved in neural protection and antiapoptotic activity as well as the downregulation of pro-apoptotic miRNAs in TBI mice subjected to an exercise regimen (Miao et al., 2015). Thus, inducing epigenetic change as a positive consequence of exercise appears to help reduce neuronal cell damage without the further need for expensive drug therapy.

EXERCISE EFFECTS: APOPTOSIS

Apoptosis, or programmed cell death, is a major contributor to the cognitive decline in the aging brain and age-related disorders. Zhao et al. (2015) illustrated that TBI mice displayed many indicators of apoptosis, including increased expression of pro-apoptotic molecules, Bid, PUMA, and AIF-1, in both the cytosol and nucleus of damaged neurons, increased release of cytochrome C from mitochondria and cleaved alpha-spectrin. Yet, TBI mice that were exercised on a running wheel exhibited significantly decreased levels of these apoptosis markers. Experiments with an ischemia animal model showed that exercised rats had significant decreases in neuron loss and lesion volume in the hippocampus, cortex, and thalamus compared to their sedentary counterparts and were correlated with decreases in AIF expression (Liebelt et al., 2010). In addition, these exercised rats displayed significantly increased expression of two types of heat shock proteins, HSP70a1a and HSP70a1b, that directly alleviate apoptosis by associating with Bcl-xL, an antiapoptosis molecule, compared to nonexercised TBI rats which had a significantly lower expression of these heat shock proteins (Liebelt et al., 2010). These researchers subsequently blocked the expression of both HSP70 proteins in exercised rats and confirmed that without HSP70, Bcl-xL-induced apoptosis proceeded normally (Liebelt et al., 2010). Itoh et al. (2011) discovered that single stranded DNA (ssDNA), associated with concurrent apoptosis, was found in abundance near TBI infarcts in treated rats. Yet, Itoh et al. (2011) found that ssDNA amounts were significantly lower surrounding these same infarcts in TBI rats after 1, 3, and 7 days of exercise.

EXERCISE EFFECTS: OXIDATIVE STRESS

Another positive effect of exercise on aging is alterations to oxidative stress metabolism. Oxidative stress is an imbalance of harmful reactive oxygen species (ROS) that have the capacity to overwhelm detoxifying mechanisms commonly associated with aging and neurodegenerative disorders. Because neurons utilize large amounts of oxygen for energy production, these cells have the potential to produce large amounts of ROS such as hydroxyl radicals, the superoxide anion, and nitric acid via aerobic respiration. These free radicals make neurons more susceptible to damage from oxidative stress, causing disturbances in signaling pathways that affect the entire cellular microenvironment (Kim et al., 2014; Chalimoniuk et al., 2015).

Increased oxygen consumption though moderate exercise increases the production of ROS in susceptible neurons; however, exercise has been shown to have the paradoxical effect of over-expressing antioxidant enzymes such as superoxide dismutase, catalase, and glutathione peroxidase that convert the abundant, newly-produced ROS into less toxic molecules. Under the effects of exercise, these enzymes reduce oxidative stress, theoretically decreasing the cognitive decline associated with aging (Falone et al., 2012; Chalimoniuk et al., 2015). In addition to neurodegeneration, neuronal synapses have also been shown to be affected negatively by oxidative stress, leading to the loss of synaptic connections concomitant with age-related, cognitive deficits (Sambe, 2009).

Studies indicate that exercise exerts its effects on oxidative metabolism through regulation of mitochondrial biochemical pathways. Functional mitochondria are essential to the survival of neurons and necessary for efficient energy production via aerobic respiration. Exercise has been shown to upregulate molecules such as optic dominant atrophy 1 (OPA1) involved in processes crucial to maintaining dynamic mitochondria. In contrast, decreased levels of OPA1 can help initiate apoptosis by inducing mitochondrial destruction (Zhang et al., 2014). Molecules involved in mitochondrial biogenesis such as peroxisome proliferator-activated receptor gamma coactivator 1 (Steiner et al., 2011; Zhang et al., 2012; Lezi et al., 2014), nuclear respiratory factor 1 (Zhang et al., 2012), and sirtuin 1 (Falone et al., 2012) have been found in elevated levels in exercised animal models. Exercised rats were also observed to have increased levels of mitochondrial respiratory chain complexes II, III, and IV molecules, suggesting that exercise plays a direct role in enhancing cellular metabolism. Other exercise studies observed decreased levels of lipid and DNA perioxidation (oxidative stress markers) compared to their sedentary counterparts (Cui et al., 2009). Mitochondrial dysfunction via oxidative stress has also been found in mice models for Alzheimer's Disease (AD) (Bo et al., 2014). Here, Bo et al. (2014) found that 20 weeks of treadmill exercise served to improve long-term memory, short-term memory, and spatial perception. These results were associated with markers of enhanced mitochondrial function, including increased activation of respiratory chain enzymes and upregulation of antioxidant enzymes (Bo et al., 2014). Four months of treadmill exercise in aged mice drastically reduced oxidative stress markers while upregulating neuroprotective pathways (Falone et al., 2012). Studies indicate that epileptic seizures trigger neuronal tissue damage via free radial formation (Kim et al., 2014, 2015); yet, low-intensity exercise, in combination with nutritional supplements, can prevent this form of neuronal damage by accelerating the expression of antioxidant enzymes (Kim et al., 2015). Because increased oxidative stress and reduced functionality of antioxidant defenses are associated with decreased cognitive function in aging, the positive effects of exercise on combating oxidative stress continue to implicate exercise as a viable means to improve neurological function.

EXERCISE EFFECTS: NEUROGENESIS

Neuronal circuitry modifications in the adult brain are important areas for studying age-related cognitive deficits. Some neural circuits that can be affected by aging or age-related disease have been shown to compensate for these deteriorating connections, improving overall cognitive function and mask further cognitive decline

(Foster et al., 2011). Exercise has been shown to increase cardiac output which augments cerebral blood flow, triggering neurogenesis and subsequent synaptogenesis in the hippocampus (Paillard, 2015). The connection between exercise and synthesis of new neurons in the adult hippocampus has been studied extensively, thus, it is intuitive that increased bouts of regular exercise can decrease the risk of cognitive decline associated with aging (Paillard, 2015).

The subgranular zone (SGZ) of the dentate gyrus region of the hippocampus is one of the few regions of the adult mammalian brain where neurogenesis continues throughout adulthood (Pereira et al., 2007). Hippocampal neurogenesis in the adult brain has been shown to be crucial to amplify memory function and to prevent cognitive decline (Periera et al., 2007). Studies have shown that hippocampal plasticity linked to SGZ neurogenesis is sensitive to environmental enrichment such as physical exercise (Foster et al., 2011). MRI scans of aging subjects has revealed that exercise increases hippocampal volume (Periera et al., 2007; Erickson et al., 2010) as well as the plasticity of the neural networks (Foster et al., 2011), suggesting improvements in spatial memory in aged individuals who exercise frequently (Erickson et al., 2009).

The rate and duration of exercise can have a direct influence on neurogenesis. Choi et al. (2016) showed that after 30 min exercise bouts per day for 4 weeks, adult rats displayed a significantly greater rate of neurogenesis. In addition, this increased rate of neurogenesis continued for 1 week after exercise treatment had concluded. Experiments conducted by Redila and Christie (2006) showed that voluntary exercise increased cell proliferation in multiple regions of adult rat brains, including the dentate gyrus, inner granule zone, and outer granule cell zone. These areas of neurogenesis were characterized by large quantities of newly-formed immature neurons as well as glial cells.

Glial cells are common nonneuronal cells that support brain activity. Astrocytes, the most abundant glial cells, play a significant role in neurotransmission, and are important for synaptic plasticity and overall neuronal health (Bernardi et al., 2013). One treadmill study showed that moderate exercise had significant effects on the morphology of rat astrocytes: increased cell size and plasticity (Bernardi et al., 2013). These astrocyte modifications culminated in improved cognitive function in the medial prefrontal cortex, helping to decipher object discrimination and increase long-term memory storage. The effects of exercise on microglia, the immune cells of the brain, are also of significance as increased activation of immune response have been linked with aging (Littlefield et al., 2015). An elevated microglia response is correlated with increased expression of major histocompatibility complex II (MHC II). Decreased MHC II expression on microglia isolated from the hippocampi of aged-male mice was observed after only 1 month of wheel running (Kohman et al., 2013). Results also show that exercise may contribute to reducing the negative effects of excessive neuroinflammatory microglia on age-related cognition decline (Littlefield et al., 2015).

EXERCISE EFFECTS: SYNAPTOGENESIS

Studies performed on animal models of aging have shown that in addition to promoting neurogenesis, exercise has also been shown to increase the number of synaptic connections among neurons (Foster et al., 2011). This post-exercise increase in synaptogenesis is correlated with increased dendritic spine density and dendritic outgrowth in various regions of the brain. Increased spine density and length of the dendrites of pyramidal neurons in the hippocampus (Nam et al., 2014), medial frontal and orbitofrontal cortex (Brockett et al., 2015), entorhinal cortex, and CA1 hippocampal region (Stranahan et al., 2007) were observed after moderate exercise. Exercise-related synaptogenesis has been shown to reverse some symptoms of various neurological diseases by increasing dendritic spine density in the Purkinje cells of the cerebellum, the pyramidal cells of the hippocampus, and layer III cortical neurons (Petzinger et al., 2015). In addition, exercise after peripheral nerve injury has been shown to aid in axonal survival, regeneration (English et al., 2014), and sprouting (Sabatier et al., 2008).

In addition to inducing morphological changes in neurons, prolonged exercise also has definitive effects on strengthening synapses. Voluntary exercise has been noted to increase levels of cAMP response element binding protein (Vaynman et al., 2003) and synapsin I (Vaynman et al., 2003; Chae et al., 2014), chemicals known to play crucial roles in synaptic transmission. Synapsin I plays a major role in regulating presynaptic neurotransmitter release by initiating synaptic vesicle formation, leading to increases in neurotransmitter release in exercised mice (Chae et al., 2014); a possible mode through which exercise may improve cognitive function (Vaynman et al., 2003). Moderate treadmill running appeared to induce increased expressions of other synaptic proteins such as the presynaptic marker, synaptophysin, and the postsynaptic marker, PSD-95 (Brockett et al., 2015). Studies indicate that decreased synaptic function may play a role in many of the motor deficits noted in progressive neuro-diseases like Parkinson's disease which may be restored by intensive exercise therapy (Petzinger et al., 2013).

The exact mechanism through which exercise promotes synaptogenesis is unclear, but various pathways, including the Wnt/beta-catenin pathway, have been linked to synaptic plasticity (Stranahan et al., 2010; Chen and Do, 2012; Bayod et al., 2014). Dickkopf-related protein 1 (DKK-1) is a naturally occurring Wnt/beta-catenin pathway antagonist often found in increased levels in dementia and AD patients and has been linked directly to the neuronal degeneration seen in these disorders (Stranahan et al., 2010). In addition, DKK-1 has been associated with suppression of synaptogenesis in aging individuals, potentially contributing to the observed cognitive decline associated with age. Studies have shown that experimentally reducing DKK-1 levels can significantly improve the cognitive decline associated with age (Seib et al., 2013). Of interest to this review, significantly lower levels of DKK-1 were observed in animal models of aging subjected to increased levels of exercise (Bayod et al., 2014).

EXERCISE EFFECTS: AGE-RELATED NEURODEGENERATIVE DISEASES

As the human brain ages, various neurological diseases such as AD, Parkinson's disease, Huntington's disease, stroke, and amyotrophic lateral sclerosis can accelerate the cognitive-deteriorating symptoms of natural aging (Davis et al., 2014). When combined, these neurological diseases affect nearly one billion people around the globe. While numerous companies are currently working to develop drugs to cure these diseases, unfortunately none have shown effectiveness to cure or stabilize these neuro-disorders.

Similar to aging studies described previously, exercise has been established to ameliorate the cognitive effects of many age-related, progressive neurodegenerative disorders (Radak et al., 2010; Ojo et al., 2015). It has been established that exercise renders patients suffering from these ailments with improved cognitive function, sustained motor capabilities, and improved quality of life. As mentioned previously, the decline in cognitive function has been correlated with the physiological deterioration in the hippocampus in aged individuals and those suffering from a range of progressive neuro-disorders. A clinical MRI study with older adults showed that exercise sustained hippocampus volumes over a 1-year period (Erickson et al., 2011). On average, the aged adult exercise group increased hippocampal volume by 2% compared to sedentary control groups. This increase of hippocampus size was correlated with overall improvements in memory function (Erickson et al., 2011). In another study, older adults aged 55–85 who were suffering from mild cognitive impairments were given a 6-month, high-intensity aerobic exercise regimen (Baker et al., 2010). Besides a significant improvement in cognition, this study also illustrated slight gender differences associated with exercise. Aged females showed improvements in executive memory functioning correlated with decreased levels of the hormone cortisol. Aged males also showed a significant manifestation of improved memory without change in cortisol levels (Baker et al., 2010).

The most common disorder related to the cognitive decline seen in aging is AD. AD patients show memory impairment, particularly affecting short-term memory (Baker et al., 2010; Budni et al., 2015). Various brain markers signal the presence of AD, such as the tissue shrinkage in the cortex involved in planning, and in the hippocampus involved in new memory formation (Baker et al., 2010). One research study used four sets of transgenic AD mice to study the effects of exercise on the expression of known AD markers, beta-amyloid peptides $A\beta_{40}$ and $A\beta_{42}$ (Hampel et al., 2010; Radak et al., 2010). The exercise protocol used treadmill training for 9 weeks and resulted in improvements in the structure and function of hippocampal neurons by enhancing the BDNF pathway, and by reducing the $A\beta$ markers. In another randomized control study using AD patients (Pitkälä et al., 2013), a set of three treatments were initiated: one group received normal care but did not exercise, another underwent group-based exercise regime (4 h, weekly twice), and an individualized home exercise group (1 h weekly twice). The outcome of the study concluded that both groups that exercised showed a significant delay in the onset of Alzheimer's symptoms compared to normal care group that showed faster deterioration in cognition (Pitkälä et al., 2013). A 4-month intervention with Alzheimer's patients, who attended a 1-h, exercise session 3 times a week, showed definitive improvements in postural balance and frontal cortex cognitive function (de Andrade et al., 2013).

Prescribing daily physical exercise is highly suggested in elderly adults to prevent and even reverse the symptoms associated with many neurological diseases like AD. Physical exercise improves cognitive processes such as planning, scheduling, coordination, inhibition, and working memory (Churchill et al., 2002). There has also been additional evidence that cardiorespiratory fitness is associated with brain and gray matter volume increases as measured by MRI (Hayes et al., 2013). The US. Department of Health and Human Services recommends 150 min of aerobic exercise and 75 min of strength exercise weekly. These recommendations can help battle both age and neurological diseases associated with mental and physical deficits while successful drug therapies are still being developed.

CONCLUSIONS

Exercise triggers neuronal changes such as neuroplasticity by targeting multiple different pathways throughout brain tissue. Multiple pathways, including the upregulation of crucial neurotrophic factors, synaptic and cellular plasticity, antioxidant defenses, and epigenetics have been extensively studied, indicating that the effects of exercise on the mammalian brain and body are quite complex. The ability of a neuron to change its structure and function even in adulthood allows the brain to combat successfully age-related physiological and environmental changes. Numerous studies can attest to the observation that exercise significantly improves cognition, memory, learning, and motor function diminished by aging and disease. One thing, however, is almost certain: Exercise is efficient at inducing positive changes to cognitive function and should be used as a method to stall or even reverse the neurological decline associated with aging.

References

Abel, J., Rissman, E., 2013. Running-induced epigenetic and gene expression changes in the adolescent brain. International Journal of Developmental Neuroscience 31, 382–390.

Baker, L., Frank, L., Foster-Schubert, K., Green, P., Wilkinson, C., McTiernan, A., Plymate, S., Fishel, M., Watson, G., Cholerton, B., Duncan, G., Mehta, P., Craft, S., 2010. Effects of aerobic exercise on mild cognitive impairment: a controlled trial. Archives of Neurology 67, 71–79.

Bao, T., Miao, W., Han, J., Yin, M., Yan, Y., Wang, W., Zhu, Y., 2014. Spontaneous running wheel improves cognitive functions of mouse associated with miRNA expressional alteration in hippocampus following traumatic brain injury. Journal of Molecular Neuroscience 54, 622–629.

Bayod, S., Menella, I., Sanchez-Roige, S., Lalanza, J., Escorihuela, R., Camins, A., Pallas, M., Canudas, A., 2014. Wnt Pathway regulation by long-term moderate exercise in rat hippocampus. Brain Research 1543, 38–48.

Bernardi, C., Tramontina, A., Nardin, P., Biasibetti, R., Costa, A., Vizueti, A., Batassini, C., Tortorelli, L., Wartchow, K., Dutra, M., Bobermin, L., Sesterheim, P., Quincozes-Santos, A., de Souza, J., Goncalves, C., 2013. Treadmill exercise induces hippocampal astroglial alterations in rats. Neural Plasticity. http://dx.doi.org/10.1155/2013/709732.

Bo, H., Kang, W., Jiang, N., Wang, X., Zhang, Y., Ji, L., 2014. Exercise-induced neuroprotection of hippocampus in APP/PS1 transgenic mice via upregulation of mitochondrial 8-oxoguanine DNA glycosylase. Oxidative Medicine and Cellular Longevity. http://dx.doi.org/10.1155/2014/834502.

Brockett, A., LaMarca, E., Gould, E., 2015. Physical exercise enhances cognitive flexibility as well as astrocytic and synaptic markers in the medial prefrontal cortex. PLoS One. http://dx.doi.org/10.137/journal.pone.0124859.

Budni, J., Bellettini-Santos, T., Mina, F., Garcez, M., Zugno, A., 2015. The involvement of BDNF, NGF and GDNF in aging and Alzheimer's disease. Aging and Disease 6, 331–341.

Calabrese, F., Guidotti, G., Racagni, G., Riva, M., 2013. Reduced neuroplasticity in aged rats: a role for the neurotrophin brain-derived neurotrophic factor. Neurobiology of Aging 34, 2768–2776.

Chae, C., Jung, S., An, S., Park, B., Kim, T., Wang, S., Kim, J., Lee, H., Kim, H., 2014. Swimming exercise stimulates neurogenesis in the subventricular zone via increase in synapsin I and nerve growth factor levels. Biology of Sport 31, 309–314.

Chalimoniuk, M., Jagsz, S., Sadowska-Krepa, E., Chrapusta, S., Klapcinska, B., Langfort, J., 2015. Diversity of endurance training effects on antioxidant defenses and oxidative damage in different brain regions of adolescent male rats. Journal of Physiological Pharmacology 66, 539–547.

Chen, M., Do, H., 2012. Wnt signaling in neurogenesis during aging and physical activity. Brain Sciences 2, 745–768.

Chin, L., Keyser, R., Dsurney, J., Chan, L., 2015. Improved cognitive performance following aerobic exercise training in people with traumatic brain injury. Archives of Physical Medicine and Rehabilitation 96, 754–759.

Choi, D., Lee, K., Lee, J., 2016. Effect of exercise-induced neurogenesis on cognitive function deficit in a rat model of vascular dementia. Molecular Medicine Reports. http://dx.doi.org/10.3892/mmr.2016.4891.

Churchill, J., Galvez, R., Colcombe, S., Swain, R., Kramer, F., Greenough, W., 2002. Exercise, experience and the aging brain. Neurobiology of Aging 23, 941–955.

Coelho, F., Pereira, D., Lustosa, L., Silva, J., Dias, J., Dias, R., Queiroz, B., Texeira, A., Pereira, L., 2012. Physical therapy intervention (PTI) increases plasma brain-derived neurotrophic factor (BDNF) levels in non-frail and pre-frail elderly women. Archives of Gerontology and Geriatrics 54, 415–420.

Collins, A., Hill, L., Chandramohan, Y., Whitcomb, D., Droste, S., Reul, J., 2009. Exercise improves cognitive responses to psychological stress through enhancement of epigenetic mechanisms and gene expression in the dentate gyrus. PLoS One. http://dx.doi.org/10.1371/journal.pone.0004330.

Côté, M., Azzam, G., Lemay, M., Zhukareva, V., Houlé, J., 2011. Activity-dependent increase in neurotrophic factors is associated with an enhanced modulation of spinal reflexes after spinal cord injury. Journal of Neurotrauma 28, 299–309.

Cui, L., Hofer, T., Rani, A., Leeuwenburgh, C., Foster, T., 2009. Comparison of lifelong and late life exercise on oxidative stress in the cerebellum. Neurobiology of Aging 30, 903–909.

Davis, M., Keene, C., Jayadev, S., Bird, T., 2014. The co-occurrence of Alzheimer's disease and Huntington's disease: a neuropathological study of 15 elderly Huntington's disease subjects. Journal of Huntington's Disease 3, 209–217.

de Andrade, L., Gobbi, L., Coelho, F., Christofoletti, G., Costa, J., Florindo, S., Stella, F., 2013. Benefits of multimodal exercise intervention for postural control and frontal cognitive functions in individuals with Alzheimer's disease: a controlled trial. Journal of the American Geriatrics Society 61, 1919–1926.

Denham, J., Marques, F., O'Brien, B., Charchar, F., 2014. Exercise: putting action into our epigenome. Sports Medicine 44, 189–209.

Di Loreto, S., Falone, S., D'Alessandro, A., Santini, S., Sebastiani, P., Cacchio, M., Amicarelli, F., 2014. Regular and moderate exercise initiated in middle age prevents age-related amyloidogenesis and preserves synaptic and neuroprotective signaling in mouse brain cortex. Experimental Gerontology 57, 57–65.

Elsner, V., Lovatel, G., Bertoldi, K., Vanzella, C., Moysés, F., Spindler, C., Almeida, E., Nardin, P., Siqueira, I., 2011. Effect of different exercise protocols on histone acetyltransferases and histone deacetylases activities in rat hippocampus. Neuroscience 192, 580–587.

Elsner, V., Lovatel, G., Moyses, F., Bertoldi, K., Spindler, C., Cechinel, L., Muotri, A., Siqueira, I., 2013. Exercise induces age-dependent changes on epigenetic parameters in rat hippocampus: a preliminary study. Experimental Gerontology 48, 136–139.

English, A., Wilhelm, J., Ward, P., 2014. Exercise, neurotrophins, and axon regeneration in the PNS. Physiology 29, 437–445.

Erickson, K., Prakash, R., Voss, M., Chaddock, L., Hu, L., Morris, K., White, S., Wojcicki, R., McAuley, E., Kramer, A., 2009. Aerobic fitness is associated with hippocampal volume in elderly humans. Hippocampus 19, 1030–1039.

Erickson, K., Prakash, R., Voss, M., Chaddock, L., Heo, S., 2010. Brain-derived neurotrophic factor is associated with age-related decline in hippocampal volume. Journal of Neuroscience 30, 5368–5375.

Erickson, K., Voss, M., Prakash, R., Basak, C., Szabo, A., Chaddock, L., Kim, J., Heo, S., Alves, H., White, S., Wojcicki, T., Mailey, E., Vieira, V., Martin, S., Pence, B., Woods, J., McAuley, E., Kramer, A., 2011. Exercise training increases size of hippocampus and improves memory. Proceedings of the National Academy of Sciences of the United States of America 108, 3017–3022.

Falone, S., D'Alessandro, A., Mirabilio, A., Cacchio, M., Di Ilio, C., Di Loreto, S., Amicarelli, F., 2012. Late-onset running biphasically improves redox balance, energy- and methylglyoxal-related status, as well as SIRT1 expression in mouse hippocampus. PLoS One. http://dx.doi.org/10.1371/journal.pone.0048334.

Foster, P., Rosenblatt, K., Kuljis, R., 2011. Exercise-induced cognitive plasticity, implications for mild cognitive impairment and Alzheimer's disease. Frontiers in Neurology. http://dx.doi.org/10.3389/fneur.2011.00028.

Gomez-Pinilla, F., Hillman, C., 2013. The influence of exercise on cognitive abilities. Comprehensive Physiology 3, 403–428.

Gomez-Pinilla, F., Zhuang, Y., Feng, J., Ying, Z., Fan, G., 2011. Exercise impacts brain-derived neurotrophic factor plasticity by engaging mechanisms of epigenetic regulation. European Journal of Neuroscience 33, 383–390.

Gyorkos, A., Spitsbergen, J., 2014. GDNF content and NMJ morphology are altered in recruited muscles following high-speed and resistance wheel training. Physiological Reports. http://dx.doi.org/10.1002/phy2.235.

Gyorkos, A., McCullough, M., Spitsbergen, J., 2014. Glial cell line-derived neurotrophic factor (GDNF) expression and NMJ plasticity in skeletal muscle following endurance exercise. Neuroscience 257, 111–118.

Hampel, H., Shen, Y., Walsh, D., Aisen, P., Shaw, L., Zetterberg, H., Trojanowski, J., Blennow, K., 2010. Biological markers of amyloid β-related mechanisms in Alzheimer's disease. Experimental Neurology 223, 334–346.

Hayes, S., Hayes, J., Cadden, M., Verfaellie, M., 2013. A review of cardiorespiratory fitness-related neuroplasticity in the aging brain. Frontiers in Aging Neuroscience. http://dx.doi.org/10.3389/fnagi.2013.0031.

Itoh, T., Imano, M., Nishida, S., Tsubaki, M., Hashimoto, S., Ito, A., Satou, T., 2011. Exercise inhibits neuronal apoptosis and improves cerebral function following rat traumatic brain injury. Journal of Neural Transmission 118, 1263–1272.

Jagust, W., 2013. Vulnerable neural systems and the borderland of brain aging and neurodegeneration. Neuron 77, 219–234.

Kaliman, P., Párrizas, M., Lalanza, J., Camins, A., Escorihuela, R., Pallàs, M., 2011. Neurophysiological and epigenetic effects of physical exercise on the aging process. Ageing Research Reviews 10, 475–486.

Kim, M., Bang, M., Han, T., Ko, Y., Yoon, B., Kim, J., Kang, L., Lee, K., Kim, M., 2005. Exercise increased BDNF and trkB in the contralateral hemisphere and of the ischemic rat brain. Brain Research 1052, 16–21.

Kim, H., Song, W., Kim, J., Jin, E., Kwon, M., Park, S., 2014. Synergistic effect of exercise and lipoic acid on protection against kainic acid induced seizure activity and oxidative stress in mice. Neurochemical Research 39, 1579–1584.

Kim, H., Song, W., Jin, E., Kim, J., Chun, Y., An, E., Park, S., 2015. Combined low-intensity exercise and ascorbic acid attenuates kainic acid-induced seizure and oxidative stress in mice. Neurochemical Research. http://dx.doi.org/10.1007/s11064-015-1789-5.

Kleim, J., Jones, T., Schallert, T., 2003. Motor enrichment and the induction of plasticity before or after brain injury. Neurochemical Research 28, 1757–1769.

Kohman, R., Bhattacharya, T., Wojcik, E., Rodes, J., 2013. Exercise reduces activation of microglia isolated from hippocampus and brain of aged mice. Journal of Neuroinflammation. http://dx.doi.org/10.1186/1742-2094-10-114.

Lezi, E., Burns, J., Swerdlow, R., 2014. Effect of high-intensity exercise on aged mouse brain mitochondria, neurogenesis, and inflammation. Neurobiology of Aging 35, 2574–2583.

Liebelt, B., Papapetrou, P., Ali, A., Guo, M., Ji, X., Peng, C., Rogers, R., Curry, A., Jimenez, D., Ding, Y., 2010. Exercise preconditioning reduces neuronal apoptosis in stroke by up-regulating heat shock protein-70 (heat shock protein-72) and extracellular-signal-regulated-kinase 1/2. Neuroscience 166, 1091–1100.

Littlefield, A., Setti, S., Priester, C., Kohman, R., 2015. Voluntary exercise attenuates LPS-induced reductions in neurogenesis and increases microglia expression of a proneurogenic phenotype in aged mice. Journal of Neuroinflammation. http://dx.doi.org/10.1186/s12974-015-0362-0.

Luellen, B., Bianco, L., Schneider, L., Andrews, A., 2007. Reduced brain-derived neurotrophic factor is associated with a loss of serotonergic innervation in the hippocampus of aging mice. Genes, Brain, and Behavior 6, 482–490.

McCullough, M., Gyorkos, A., Spitsbergen, J., 2013. Short-term exercise increases GDNF protein levels in the spinal cord of young and old rats. Neuroscience 240, 258–268.

Miao, W., Bao, T., Han, J., Yin, M., Yan, Y., Wang, W., Zhu, Y., 2015. Voluntary exercise prior to traumatic brain injury alters miRNA expression in the injured mouse cerebral cortex. Brazilian Journal of Medical and Biological Research 48, 433–439.

Nam, S., Kim, J., Yoo, D., Yim, H., Kim, D., Choi, J., Kim, W., Jung, H., Won, M., Hwang, I., Seong, J., Yoon, Y., 2014. Physical exercise ameliorates the reduction of neural stem cell, cell proliferation, and neuroblast differentiation in senescent mice induced by D-galactose. BMC Neuroscience. http://dx.doi.org/10.1186/s12868-014-0116-4.

Noble, E., Mavanji, V., Little, M., Billington, C., Kotz, C., Wang, C., 2014. Exercise reduces diet-induced cognitive decline and increases hippocampal brain-derived neurotrophic factor in CA3 neurons. Neurobiology of Learning and Memory 114, 40–50.

Ntanasis-Stathopoulos, J., Tzanninis, J., Philippou, A., Koutsilieris, M., 2013. Epigenetic regulation on gene expression induced by physical exercise. Journal of Musculoskeletal and Neuronal Interaction 13, 133–146.

Ojo, J., Rezaie, P., Gabbott, P., Stewart, M., 2015. Impact of age-related neuroglial cell responses on hippocampal deterioration. Frontiers in Aging Neuroscience. http://dx.doi.org/10.3389/fnagi.2015.00057.

Paillard, T., 2015. Preventive effects of regular exercise against cognitive decline and the risk of dementia with age advancement. Sports Medicine. http://dx.doi.org/10.1186/s40798-015-0016-x.

Parnpiansil, P., Jutapakdeegul, N., Chentanez, T., Kotchabhakdi, N., 2003. Exercise during pregnancy increases hippocampal brain-derived neurotrophic factor mRNA expression and spatial learning in neonatal rat pup. Neuroscience Letters 352, 45–48.

Pereira, A., Huddleston, D., Brickman, A., Sosunov, A., Hen, R., McKhann, G., Sloan, R., Gage, F., Brown, T., Small, S., 2007. An *in vivo* correlate of exercise-induced neurogenesis in the adult dentate gyrus. Proceedings of the National Academy of Sciences of the United States of America. 104, 5638–5643.

Petzinger, G., Fisher, B., McEwen, S., Beeler, J., Walsh, J., Jakowec, M., 2013. Exercise-enhanced neuroplasticity targeting motor and cognitive circuitry in Parkinson's disease. The Lancet Neurology 12, 716–726.

Petzinger, G., Holschneider, D., Fisher, B., McEwen, S., Kintz, N., Halliday, W., Toy, W., Walsh, J., Beeler, J., Jakowec, M., 2015. The effects of exercise on dopamine neurotransmission in Parkinson's disease: targeting neuroplasticity to modulate basal ganglia circuitry. Brain Plasticity 1, 29–39.

Pitkälä, K., Pöysti, M., Laakkonen, M., Tilvis, R., Savikko, N., Kautiainen, H., Strandberg, T., 2013. Effects of the Finnish Alzheimer disease exercise trial (FINALEX): a randomized controlled trial. JAMA Internal Medicine 173, 894–901.

Ploughman, M., Granter-Button, S., Chernenko, G., Tucker, B., Mearow, K., Corbett, D., 2005. Endurance exercise regimens induce differential effects on brain-derived neurotrophic factor, synapsin-I and insulin-like growth factor I after focal ischemia. Neuroscience 136, 991–1001.

Ploughman, M., Granter-Button, S., Chernenko, G., Attwood, Z., Tucker, B., Mearow, K.M., Corbett, D., 2007. Exercise intensity influences the temporal profile of growth factors involved in neuronal plasticity following focal ischemia. Brain Research 1150, 207–216.

Radak, Z., Hart, N., Sarga, L., Koltai, E., Atalay, M., Ohno, H., Boldogh, I., 2010. Exercise plays a preventive role against Alzheimer's disease. Journal of Alzheimer's Disease 20, 777–783.

Redila, V., Christie, B., 2006. Exercise induced changes in dendritic structure and complexity in the adult hippocampus and dentate gyrus. Neuroscience 137, 1299–1307.

Revilla, S., Sunol, C., Garcia-Mesa, Y., Gimenez-Llort, L., Sanfeliu, C., Cristofol, R., 2014. Physical exercise improves synaptic dysfunction and recovers the loss of survival factors in 3xTg-AD mouse brain. Neuropharmacology 81, 55–63.

Sabatier, M., Redmon, N., Schwartz, G., English, A., 2008. Treadmill training promotes axon regeneration in injured peripheral nerves. Experimental Neurology 211, 489–493.

Sambe, A.D., 2009. Aging brain: prevention of oxidative stress by vitamin E and exercise. The Scientific World Journal 9, 366–372.

Seib, D., Corsini, N., Ellwanger, K., Plaas, C., Mateos, A., Pitzer, C., Niehrs, C., Celikel, T., Martin-Villalba, A., 2013. Loss of Dickkopf-1 restores neurogenesis in old age and counteracts cognitive decline. Cell Stem Cell 12, 204–214.

Shen, X., Li, A., Zhang, Y., Dong, X., Shan, T., 2013. The effect of different intensities of treadmill exercise on cognitive function deficit following a severe controlled cortical impact in rats. International Journal of Molecular Sciences 14, 21598–21612.

Silhol, M., Bonnichon, V., Rage, F., Tapia-Arancibia, L., 2005. Age-related changes in brain-derived neurotrophic factor and tyrosine kinase receptor isoforms in the hippocampus and hypothalamus in male rats. Neuroscience 132, 613–624.

Steiner, J., Murphy, E., McClellan, J., Carmichael, M., Davis, J., 2011. Exercise training increases mitochondrial biogenesis in the brain. Journal of Applied Physiology 111, 1066–1071.

Stranahan, A., Khalil, D., Gould, E., 2007. Running induces widespread structural alterations in the hippocampus and entorhinal cortex. Hippocampus 17, 1017–1022.

Stranahan, A., Lee, K., Becker, K., Zhang, Y., Maudsley, S., Martin, B., Cutler, R., Mattson, M., 2010. Hippocampal gene expression patterns underlying the enhancement of memory by running in aged mice. Neurobiology of Aging 31, 1937–1949.

Van Kummer, B., Cohen, R., 2015. Exercise-induced neuroprotection in the spastic Han Wistar rat: the possible role of brain-derived neurotrophic factor. BioMed Research International. http://dx.doi.org/10.1155/2015/834543.

van Praag, H., 2009. Exercise and the brain: something to chew on. Trends in Neurosciences 32, 283–290.

Vaynman, S., Ying, Z., Gomez-Pinilla, F., 2003. Interplay between brain-derived neurotrophic factor and signal transduction modulators in the regulation of the effects of exercise on synaptic-plasticity. Neuroscience 122, 647–657.

Vianney, J., McCullough, M., Gyorkos, A., Spitsbergen, J., 2013. Exercise-dependent regulation of glial cell line-derived neurotrophic factor (GDNF) expression in skeletal muscle and its importance for the neuromuscular system. Frontiers in Biology 8, 101–108.

Vivar, C., Potter, M., van Praag, H., 2013. All about running: synaptic plasticity, growth factors and adult hippocampal neurogenesis. Current Topics in Behavioral Neurosciences 15, 189–210.

Voss, M., Vivar, C., Kramer, A., van Praag, H., 2013. Bridging animal and human models of exercise-induced brain plasticity. Trends in Cognitive Sciences 17, 525–544.

Zhang, Q., Wu, Y., Sha, H., Zhang, P., Jia, J., Hu, Y., Zhu, J., 2012. Early exercise affects mitochondrial transcription factors expression after cerebral ischemia in rats. International Journal of Molecular Sciences 13, 1670–1679.

Zhang, L., Zhijie, H., Zhang, Q., Wu, Y., Yang, X., Niu, W., Hu, Y., Jia, J., 2014. Exercise pretreatment promotes mitochondrial dynamic protein *OPA1* expression after cerebral ischemia. International Journal of Molecular Science 15, 4453–4463.

Zhao, Z., Sabirzhanov, B., Wu, J., Faden, A., Stoica, B., 2015. Voluntary exercise preconditioning activates multiple antiapoptotic mechanisms and improves neurological recovery after experimental traumatic brain injury. Journal of Neurotrauma 32, 1347–1360.

10

Role of Melatonin Supplementation During Strenuous Exercise

J. Díaz-Castro, M. Pulido-Morán, J. Moreno-Fernández, N. Kajarabille, S. Hijano, J.J. Ochoa

University of Granada, Granada, Spain

Abstract

The beneficial effects of regular, nonexhaustive physical exercise are well-known, however, these beneficial effects are lost with strenuous exercise. High-intensity exercise induces inflammatory reactions together with high production of free radicals, muscle damage, and subsequent inflammation indicated by muscle soreness and swelling, prolonged loss of muscle function, and the leakage of muscle proteins, such as creatine kinase and myoglobin, into the circulation. The pineal hormone, melatonin (N-acetyl-5-methoxytryptamine), is a potent, endogenously produced and diet-derived free radical scavenger and broad-spectrum antioxidant, consequently, it might have positive effects on the recovery following the exercise session. Among other effects, several studies have shown that oral supplementation of melatonin during high-intensity exercise is efficient in reducing the degree of oxidative stress (decreasing lipid peroxidation, with a significant increase of antioxidant enzymes activity), which lead to the maintenance of the cell integrity and the reduction of secondary tissue damage. Data also indicate that melatonin has potent protective effects, preventing over-expression of pro-inflammatory mediators and inhibiting the effects of several pro-inflammatory cytokines. The aim of this chapter is to review the most relevant studies focused on the effect of melatonin on diverse negative aspects associated with strenuous exercise, such as oxidative stress or the inflammatory signaling, in human, animals, and in vitro assays. Melatonin supplementation can decrease muscle damage through modulation of oxidative stress, inflammatory signaling, improving recovery, and performance efficiency associated to the physical challenge.

MELATONIN: SOURCES, BIOSYNTHESIS, AND PHYSIOLOGICAL EFFECTS

Melatonin is the main hormone secreted by the pineal gland and was first discovered and isolated from the bovine pineal gland by Aaron Lerner (Lerner et al., 1958). This methoxyindole compound (N-acetyl-5-methoxytryptamine) is synthesized from serotonin. Its name is indicative of melatonin's first identified function, namely its skin-lightening properties in some fish and amphibians. However, alteration in skin coloring was not applicable to mammals, whose melanocytes do not contain physiologically controlled, mobile melanosomes. Molecular biology techniques and highly sensitive antibodies against melatonin allowed to identify melatonin in extra-pineal tissues such as retina and cerebellum (Cardinali and Rosner, 1971; Bubenik et al., 1974), gastrointestinal tract, Harderian gland, testes, and lymphocytes (Reiter et al., 2013) including, gut mucosa, airway epithelium, liver, kidney, adrenals, thymus, thyroid, pancreas, ovary, carotid body, placenta, endometrium, mast cells, natural killer cells, eosinophilic leukocytes, platelets, and endothelial cells (Kvetnoy, 1999; Sanchez-Hidalgo et al., 2009; Acuña-Castroviejo et al., 2014). Indeed, melatonin has been detected in all organs which have been examined, where often high concentrations of this indoleamine have been measured.

Melatonin is synthesized in a four step process. First, the precursor L-tryptophan is taken up from the circulation (blood) and is converted to 5-hydroxy-tryptophan in the mitochondria by trp-5-mono-oxygenase/hydroxylase and then it is decarboxylated in the cytosol by L-aromatic amino acid decarboxylase to form serotonin (5-hydroxytryptamine), which after that is acetylated (N-acetylation) into N-acetyl serotonin by arylalkylamine-N-acetyltransferase (AANAT) (Voisin et al., 1984; Mukherjee and Maitra, 2015). This step is considered as the rate-limiting enzyme in melatonin biosynthetic pathway. Finally, N-acetyl serotonin is O-methylated by hydroxyindole-O-methyltransferase

Physical Activity and the Aging Brain
http://dx.doi.org/10.1016/B978-0-12-805094-1.00010-1

to form melatonin (Axelrod and Weissbach, 1960; Mukherjee and Maitra, 2015). Its synthesis starts by the binding of norepinephrine to adrenergic β1receptors, subsequent activation of pineal adenylate cyclase, increase in cyclic AMP and de novo synthesis of AANAT (Claustrat and Leston, 2015). Availability of tryptophan is a limiting factor in the synthesis of melatonin (Zimmermann et al., 1993). Nutritional factors could also influence melatonin synthesis, such as folate status (Fournier et al., 2002) and B6 vitamin, a coenzyme in tryptophan decarboxylation, which is able to stimulate melatonin production in prepubertal children but not in adults (Munoz-Hoyos et al., 1996; Luboshitzky et al., 2002; Claustrat and Leston, 2015).

The main original effect of this hormone was the regulation, influence, and reset of circadian and circannual rhythms (Marczynski et al., 1964; Reiter, 1991a,b, 1993) and, its secretion is related with the duration of darkness. In species responding to photoperiodic changes, to be involved in the measurement of day length, an environmental variable used for seasonal timing of reproduction, metabolism, and behavior (Tamarkin et al., 1985; Arendt, 1986; Reiter, 1991a,b, 1993).

The direct effects in regions containing high densities of melatonin receptors, such as the circadian pacemaker, the suprachiasmatic nucleus, or the pars tuberalis, a site of particular relevance to photoperiodically controlled reproduction (Fraschini and Stankov, 1994; Gauer et al., 1994; Masson-Pévet et al., 2000; Pévet et al., 2002; Stehle et al., 2003) strongly supported the premier significance of this physiological role. In the perception of many investigators, the control of circadian and seasonal rhythmicities represents melatonin's main physiological function (Hardeland et al., 2011). Although this view is not generally disputed, the actions of the methoxyindole are by no means restricted to areas of high receptor density.

During the recent decades, melatonin has been shown to possess numerous additional functions and to act in tissues or cells that express melatonin receptors at much lower levels (Dubocovich and Markowska, 2005; Pandi-Perumal et al., 2006; Hardeland and Poeggeler, 2008; Hardeland, 2009b). The classic membrane-associated melatonin receptors, in mammals MT1 and MT2 (Reppert et al., 1994, 1995; Jin et al., 2003; Korf and von Gall, 2006; Dubocovich et al., 2010), transduces numerous chronobiological actions of the hormone and are, in particular, responsible for circadian phase shifting, the "chronobiotic" effects of melatonin (Dawson and Armstrong, 1996). In addition, various other melatonin binding sites have been identified, but whose roles are either poorly understood or almost unknown (Hardeland, 2009b). Melatonin has gained many additional functions in the course of evolution (Hardeland et al., 1995; Tan et al., 2010).

Besides the regulation of sleep cycle, melatonin takes part in a variety of other molecular pathways, such as apoptotic, antiproliferative, antimetastasis, antiangiogenesis, antiinflammatory, and even (nuclear erythroid-related factor 2) Nrf2-mediated antioxidant response element (Rushworth and Macewan, 2011; Di Bella et al., 2013; Perepechaeva et al., 2014; Zamfir Chiru et al., 2014; Tuli et al., 2015). Furthermore, due to its potent antioxidative activity, it has been recognized as an organ protective and as an antiaging agent.

From these other sites of formation, melatonin is either poorly or only released in response to specific stimuli, e.g., as a postprandial surge from the gastrointestinal tract (Huether et al., 1992; Huether, 1993, 1994; Bubenik, 2002). Relative to the amounts present in the pineal gland and the circulation, the quantities of melatonin in extrapineal tissues are by no means negligible, but, owing to the total size these organs, are orders of magnitude greater (Huether, 1993; Bubenik, 2002). Melatonin displays an exceptional multiplicity of actions. These can only be understood on the basis of an integrative, orchestrating role by which melatonin is distinguished from many other important signal molecules. Deficiencies in melatonin production or melatonin receptor expression, and decrease in melatonin levels (such as those occurring during aging) are likely to cause numerous dysfunctions. In these cases, insufficient amounts of melatonin or poor melatonergic signaling can be associated with a multitude of pathophysiological changes, which, again, reflect the pleiotropy of this molecule.

EXERCISE: OXIDATIVE STRESS AND INDUCED INFLAMMATORY SIGNALING

Increased production of reactive oxygen species (ROS) leading to cellular oxidative stress is linked to several pathologies such as cancer, diabetes, and neurological diseases (Xie and Huang, 2003; Valko et al., 2006; Wei et al., 2009; Thanan et al., 2015; Marseglia et al., 2015). Therefore, it seems paradoxical that although exercise promotes oxidative stress, a routine of regular nonexhaustive exercise is associated with numerous health benefits including a lower risk of all-cause mortality stemming a reduced threat of cardiovascular disease, cancer, diabetes, and dementia (Blair and Wei, 2000; Blair et al., 2001; Hayes and Kriska, 2008; Kraus and Slentz, 2009; Shay et al., 2015; Burton et al., 2015). Furthermore, according to the evidences, exercise changes the gene expression of thousands of subcutaneous white adipose tissue (WAT) genes and an altered adipokine profile in both subcutaneous WAT and visceral cavity

WAT. Human and rodent studies based on training, have shown that exercise can modify circulating adipokine concentration as well as adipokine expression in adipose tissue. Therefore, those deep changes to WAT in response to exercise training might be a part of the mechanism by which exercise improves whole body metabolic health (Stanford et al., 2015). Growing evidence indicates that although high levels of ROS production can damage cellular components, low-to-moderate levels of cellular oxidants play important regulatory roles in the modulation of skeletal muscle force production and contraction-induced adaptive responses of muscle fibers to exercise training, control of cell signaling pathways, and regulation of gene expression. This oxidant-mediated change in gene expression involves changes at transcriptional, mRNA stability, and signal transduction levels. Moreover, several products associated with oxidant-modulated genes have been identified and include antioxidant enzymes, stress proteins, DNA repair proteins, and mitochondrial electron transport proteins. In this sense, low and physiological levels of ROS are required for normal force production in skeletal muscle, however, high levels of ROS promote contractile dysfunction resulting in muscle weakness and fatigue (Droge, 2002; McClung et al., 2009, 2010; Powers and Jackson, 2008; Powers et al., 2010). A persistent pro-oxidant environment can modify redox-sensitive targets in the cell. The most common approach used to assess exercise-induced oxidative stress involves the measurement of the increase in one or more molecular biomarkers of oxidative damage. Specifically, many studies have documented exercise-induced oxidant stress by measurement of oxidative damage to cellular components (lipids, proteins, DNA). Many studies using both animal and human subjects have demonstrated that a variety of exercise intensities and exercise modes (e.g., cycling, running, and resistance exercise) result in increased biomarkers of oxidative damage in both blood and skeletal muscle (Davies et al., 1982; Lawler et al., 1994; Nikolaidis et al., 2008; Powers et al., 2010). Based on the literature, the oxidative stress response of skeletal muscle to exercise is generally independent of muscle fiber type. Most of the changes in oxidative stress/damage appeared are sustained for days after muscle-damaging exercise (Nikolaidis et al., 2008). Those primary sources of ROS production during exercise remain a hot topic of debate and are discussed in the next segment.

Many tissues can produce ROS during exercise (Powers and Jackson, 2008; Aoi et al., 2013). However, to date, few studies have investigated that organs are primarily responsible for ROS production in exercising humans because of restricted access to most tissues. The lack of studies on this topic is due to the fact that it is a challenging one to investigate in humans and other animals because of the multifaceted nature of exercise involving many organ systems that are connected through the increased energy requirement of contracting skeletal muscles (Powers and Jackson, 2008; Aoi et al., 2013). Although the discovery that contracting skeletal muscles produce ROS (Davies et al., 1982), many investigators have assumed that skeletal muscle provides the major source of free radical and ROS generation during exercise (Powers and Jackson, 2008; Powers et al., 2010). Nonetheless, other tissues such as the heart, lungs, or blood may also contribute to the total body generation of ROS during exercise (Powers and Jackson, 2008; Nikolaidis and Jamurtas, 2009; Powers et al., 2010). For example, phagocytic white cells can play a major role in modifying muscle redox state after exercise-induced muscle damage. Indeed, substantial injury to muscle fibers is accompanied by invasion of the injured areas with macrophages and other phagocytic cells (McArdle et al., 2004) and although this process could be essential for effective muscle repair, it also involves the release of substantial amounts of ROS from the phagocytic cells (Malech and Gallin, 1987; Brar et al., 1999, 2002).

MELATONIN AND INFLAMMATORY SIGNALING

Several studies with animal models show that melatonin plays an important role in improving several diseases through multiple mechanisms of action, based on recognized antioxidant and antiinflammatory capacity. Among other effects, melatonin inhibits oxidant damage and inflammatory ácytokines (Sánchez et al., 2015). The role of melatonin as an immune modulator has been reported several times (Carrillo-Vico et al., 2005, Hardeland et al., 2011; Hardeland, 2013). Its functions are diverse. Melatonin is produced by and acts on various types of leukocytes. Melatonin formation has been demonstrated in monocytes, where it enhances ROS formation and cytotoxicity, representing one of the strongest direct pro-oxidant effects of melatonin reported (Morrey et al., 1994).

During inflammation in mammals, melatonin affects the vascular permeability, the recruitment of leukocytes (Lotufo et al., 2006), and the expression of pro- and antiinflammatory mediators (García-Mauriño et al., 1999). Melatonin moreover upregulates the synthesis of many cytokines, e.g., interleukins: IL-1, IL-2, IL-6, IL-12, interferon gamma (IFN-γ), and tumor necrosis factor alfa (TNF-α) (Garcia-Mauriño et al., 1997, 1999; Barjavel et al., 1998). The positive effect on IFN-γ and IL-6 synthesis indicates that melatonin acts on T-helper cells in favor of the cellular Th1 response (Carrillo-Vico et al., 2005). This effect is even further boosted by melatonin-induced increase of IL-12 production (García-Mauriño et al., 1999). In contrast, IL-4, the cytokine specific for the Th2 response is not stimulated

FIGURE 10.1 Effects of melatonin on antioxidant status and inflammatory signaling.

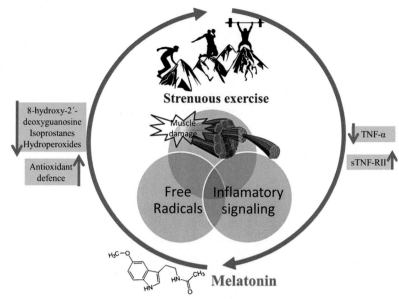

by melatonin (García-Mauriño et al., 1999), while IL-10 is even downregulated (Kühlwein and Irwin, 2001). Also antibody production may be modulated by melatonin (Cernysiov et al., 2010).

However, these results seem to largely depend on cells, systems studied, and especially conditions relevant to the grade of inflammation. In particular, downregulations of IL-1β, IL-6, IL-8, IL-12, and TNF-α have been repeatedly documented under conditions of high oxidative stress, ischemia/reperfusion, brain trauma, hemorrhagic shock, and various forms of high-grade inflammation including sepsis (Hardeland, 2013). Two additional antiinflammatory effects have to be taken into consideration. First, cyclooxygenase-2 expression has been shown to be downregulated by melatonin in macrophages via nuclear factor-kB (NF-kB) (Mayo et al., 2005; Korkmaz et al., 2012). The same signaling pathway seems to be involved in the suppression of inducible nitric oxide synthase (iNOS) in macrophages (Korkmaz et al., 2012).

The effects of melatonin on oxidative stress and inflammatory signaling are summarized in Fig. 10.1.

EFFECTS OF MELATONIN IN STRENUOUS EXERCISE

Melatonin interacts with many endocrine and nonendocrine tissues to effect their metabolic activity. High doses of melatonin (1 g orally and 0.4 mg/kg intravenously) have been observed to have a stimulatory effect on basal GH concentrations (Valcavi et al., 1993). A short period of exercise is a stimulus for endogenous GH secretion. It is very well-known that the GH response increases with both duration (Raynaud et al., 1983) and intensity of exercise (Näveri, 1985). Meeking et al. (1999) studied the effects of a single dose of oral melatonin (5 mg) on the exercise-induced GH secretion in men. They concluded that the effect of melatonin is to increase exercise-induced GH secretion. This would suggest that it has an effect on the central hypothalamic regulation through either the GH releasing hormone or the somatostatin release. The exercise studied by Meeking et al. (1999) was short and low in intensity, however, other authors (Ochoa et al., 2011) were interested in the effects of oral ingestion of melatonin with a high intensity resistance exercise session. This high intensity resistance exercise strongly increases GH response but with the oral ingestion of melatonin the exercise-induced increase is greater and the effect might be mediated predominantly through a hypothalamic pathway, having positive effects on the recovery following the exercise session.

Ochoa et al. (2011) observed a decrease in the bilirubin concentrations in the runners taking oral supplements of melatonin, before and after the run, indicating a protective effect of melatonin (Dubbels et al., 1995). Bilirubin is a natural antioxidant; therefore, there would be a lower need in the melatonin supplemented runners, given the radical scavenger and antioxidant effects of melatonin (Tan et al., 1993; Reiter et al., 2009; Jou et al., 2010; Paradies et al., 2010). In addition, this study reported that melatonin is able to protect against hepatotoxicity, as demonstrated by the lower total bilirubin concentration found in rats with induced liver injury, not only through its direct antioxidant action but also by inhibiting the infiltration of polymorphonuclear neutrophils into the liver tissue (Sewerynek et al., 1996; Calvo et al., 2001).

Physical activity, especially strenuous and high-intensity exercise, promotes free radical generation and oxidative stress as mentioned previously. CAT and GPx erythrocyte activities, together with the TAS increased significantly in the after melatonin supplementation in male runners after the physical performance (Ochoa et al., 2011). Therefore, the melatonin supplement can be beneficial because of its antioxidant action. Melatonin is an endogenous radical scavenger and also acts as an indirect antioxidant through the activation of the major antioxidant enzymes including SOD, CAT, and GPx (Rodriguez et al., 2004). In addition, the significant increase in the TAS in melatonin-supplemented groups after strenuous exercise (Ochoa et al., 2011) documents that plasma antioxidant capacity with the melatonin supplement is higher as compared to the control group even before starting the physical test, which from the point of view of the oxidative damage, would suppose a benefit for the sportsman.

Melatonin provided protection against oxidative stress as the isoprostanes and 8-OHdG were reduced in sportsman taking oral supplements of melatonin, again documenting the antioxidant action of melatonin (Ochoa et al., 2011). Mitochondrial DNA is a major target for oxygen radicals because of its location near the inner mitochondrial membrane where oxidants are formed and DNA repair activity is lacking. Mitochondria have been identified as a target for melatonin actions, and melatonin lowers mitochondrial protein damage, improving electron transport chain activity and reducing mitochondrial DNA damage (Acuña Castroviejo et al., 2011). Melatonin also functions as an indirect antioxidant by stimulating the activities of GPx and CAT (Rodriguez et al., 2004). Elevated activities of these enzymes have an important protective role in reducing lipid peroxidation and molecular damage. Besides these direct and indirect beneficial actions, it was reported that melatonin has the ability to bind Fe^{3+} (Limson et al., 1998), thus preventing it from being reduced to Fe^{2+} which promotes the formation of the hydroxyl radical via the Fenton reaction. Thus, removal of Fe^{3+} by melatonin would reduce hydroxyl generation from its precursor H_2O_2; important recent discoveries also show that metabolites of melatonin are formed when it scavenges toxic reactants are themselves potent detoxifiers of ROS (Hardeland et al., 2009a,b,c). Thus, not only the parent molecule, melatonin, but also its metabolites sequentially neutralize toxic reactants. This greatly increases the efficacy of melatonin as a protector against oxygen and nitrogen-based reactants. There is also evidence that melatonin promotes intracellular glutathione levels; glutathione is an important antioxidant and the fact that melatonin stimulates its synthesis (Urata et al., 1999) contributes to melatonin's protective actions against oxidative damage.

Acute exercise increases oxidative stress, especially when the exercise intensity is high, a fact that can be correlated with the over-expression of inflammatory cytokines and C-reactive protein (Kasapis and Thompson, 2005). Ochoa et al. (2011) found a significant rise in the pro-inflammatory cytokine TNF-α, after competition in runners with and without melatonin supplementation, which is in agreement with previous results (Veneroso et al., 2009) and they are induced by the ROS generation during the exercise. In the study performed by Ochoa et al. (2011), melatonin reduced oxidative stress parameters, and significantly decreased the levels of pro-inflammatory cytokine TNF-α. Alonso et al. (2006) investigated the effects of melatonin on the expressions of iNOS and NF-jB in rat skeletal muscle after high-intensity exercise, leading to an induction of the pro-inflammatory cytokines TNF-α and IL-6. These results indicate that melatonin had potent protective effects against damage caused by acute exercise by preventing oxidative stress, NF-jB activation, and iNOS over-expression.

TNF-α seems to have a biphasic effect on muscle: high levels of the cytokine promote muscle catabolism, probably by an NF-kB-mediated effect, whereas low levels of TNF-α, which do not induce NF-kB, stimulate myogenesis (Reid and Li, 2001). Protective roles of melatonin have been reported in various experimental models of tissue damage including exercise-induced skeletal muscle degeneration, by reducing oxidative stress and lipid peroxidation (Ghosh et al., 2007), and several studies have demonstrated that melatonin exerts important antiinflammatory actions (Kireev et al., 2008; Caballero et al., 2008). Ochoa et al. (2011) also found a significant increase in the IL-6, after strenuous exercise, while melatonin supplementation significantly decreased the levels of IL-6.

Ochoa et al. (2011) reported an increase in sTNF-RII after melatonin supplementation, and the over-expression of this molecule limits the detrimental, pro-inflammatory effects of TNF as it has been postulated that, by sequestering TNF, the soluble form of TNF-RII limits TNF availability and binding to TNF-RI, the receptor subtype which mediates the classic pro-inflammatory activities of the cytokine.

A balanced and effective antioxidant defense system is vital for the prevention of exhaustive exercise damage and melatonin molecule is a safe and nontoxic, even at high doses. In addition, the amphiphilic characteristics of melatonin allows it to act as both intra- and extracellularly. Because exercise produces free radicals, melatonin's intracellular half-life is shortened as it is rapidly used as a free radical scavenger (Reiter and Richardson, 1992). In addition, attention has also been focused on the antioxidant properties of melatonin catabolites, which are generated by oxidative cleavage of the melatonin indole ring, are even more effective than melatonin as antiinflammatory and antioxidant agents (Mayo et al., 2005; Galano et al., 2013). Borges Lda et al. (2015) suggest that melatonin treatment may reverse the skeletal muscle inflammation and oxidative stress induced by strenuous exercise, improving the recovery of athletes after exhaustive exercise. In addition, the inflammation (systemic and muscular) and oxidative stress resulting from exhaustive exercise is reduced in the muscles of melatonin-treated animal models.

In the study conducted by Favero et al. (2015), they demonstrated that heme oxygenase 1 (HO-1) activity is stimulated by both free radicals and especially by melatonin in skeletal myotubes and that this activation is associated with a concomitant important reduction in oxidative stress. These results supported the finding of Essig et al. (1997) in which it was postulated that HO-1 is stimulated in rat skeletal muscle and mediates cell adaptation to oxidative stress during muscle contraction. HO-1 is a strong candidate as a key player in protecting against skeletal muscle damage and has been reported to perform this action in other cell types as well (Hirai et al., 2003; Lee et al., 2003).

Finally, the results reported by Leonardo-Mendonça et al. (2015) support the beneficial effects of the supplementation with melatonin not only to adjust the circadian clock, but also to modulate the circadian components of the sleep–wake cycle, improving sleep efficiency in athletes, fact that could improve exercise performance.

References

Acuña Castroviejo, D., López, L.C., Escames, G., López, A., García, J.A., Reiter, R.J., 2011. Melatonin- mitochondria interplay in health and disease. Current Topics in Medicinal Chemistry 11, 221–240.

Acuña-Castroviejo, D., Escames, G., Venegas, C., Díaz-Casado, M.E., Lima-Cabello, E., López, L.C., Rosales-Corral, S., Tan, D.-X., Reiter, R.J., 2014. Extrapineal melatonin: sources, regulation, and potential functions. Cellular and Molecular Life Sciences 71 (16), 2997–3025.

Alonso, M., Collado, P.S., Gonza´lez-Gallego, J., 2006. Melatonin inhibits the expression of the inducible isoform of nitric oxide synthase and nuclear factor kappa B activation in rat skeletal muscle. Journal of Pineal Research 41, 8–14.

Aoi, W., Naito, Y., Yoshikawa, T., 2013. Role of oxidative stress in impaired insulin signaling associated with exercise-induced muscle damage. Free Radical Biology and Medicine 65, 1265–1272.

Arendt, J., 1986. Role of the pineal gland and melatonin in seasonal reproductive function in mammals. Oxford Reviews of Reproductive Biology 8, 266–320.

Axelrod, J., Weissbach, H., 1960. Enzymatic O-methylation of N-acetylserotonin to melatonin. Science 131, 1312.

Barjavel, M.J., Mamdouh, Z., Raghbate, N., Bakouche, O., 1998. Differential expression of the melatonin receptor in human monocytes. Journal of Immunology 160, 1191–1197.

Blair, S.N., Wei, M., 2000. Sedentary habits, health, and function in older women and men. American Journal of Health Promotion 15 (1), 1–8.

Blair, S.N., Cheng, Y., Holder, J.S., 2001. Is physical activity or physical fitness more important in defining health benefits? Medicine and Science in Sports and Exercise 33, S379–S399.

Borges Lda, S., Dermargos, A., da Silva Junior, E.P., Weimann, E., Lambertucci, R.H., Hatanaka, E., 2015. Melatonin decreases muscular oxidative stress and inflammation induced by strenuous exercise and stimulates growth factor synthesis. Journal of Pineal Research 58 (2), 166–172.

Brar, S.S., Kennedy, T.P., Whorton, A.R., Murphy, T.M., Chitano, P., Hoidal, J.R., July 9, 1999. Requirement for reactive oxygen species in serum-induced and platelet-derived growth factor-induced growth of airway smooth muscle. The Journal of Biological Chemistry 274 (28), 20017–20026.

Brar, S.S., Kennedy, T.P., Sturrock, A.B., Huecksteadt, T.P., Quinn, M.T., Murphy, T.M., Chitano, P., Hoidal, J.R., 2002. NADPH oxidase promotes NF-B activation and proliferation in human airway smooth muscle. American Journal of Physiology Lung Cellular and Molecular Physiology 282, L782–L795.

Bubenik, G.A., Brown, G.M., Uhlir, I., Grota, L.J., 1974. Immunohistological localization of N-acetylindolealkylamines in pineal gland, retina and cerebellum. Brain Research 81, 233–242.

Bubenik, G.A., 2002. Gastrointestinal melatonin: localization, function, and clinical relevance. Digestive Diseases and Sciences 47, 2336–2348.

Burton, E., Cavalheri, V., Adams, R., Browne, C.O., Bovery-Spencer, P., Fenton, A., Campbell, B.W., Hill1, K.D., 2015. Effectiveness of exercise programs to reduce falls in older people with dementia living in the community: a systematic review and meta-analysis. Clinical Interventions in Aging 421–434.

Caballero, B., Vega-Naredo, I., Sierra, V., Huidobro-Fernández, C., Soria-Valles, C., De Gonzalo-Calvo, D., Tolivia, D., Gutierrez-Cuesta, J., Pallas, M., Camins, A., Rodríguez-Colunga, M.J., Coto-Montes, A., 2008. Favorable effects of a prolonged treatment with melatonin on the level of oxidative damage and neurodegeneration in senescence-accelerated mice. Journal of Pineal Research 45, 302–311.

Calvo, J.R., Reiter, R.J., García, J.J., Ortiz, G.G., Tan, D.X., Karbownik, M., 2001. Characterization of the protective effects of melatonin and related indoles against alpha-naphthylisothiocyanate-induced liver injury in rats. Journal of Cellular Biochemistry 80, 461–470.

Cardinali, D.P., Rosner, J.M., 1971. Retinal localization of the hydroxyindole-O-methyl transferase (HIOMT) in the rat. Endocrinology 89, 301–303.

Carrillo-Vico, A., Guerrero, J.M., Lardone, P.J., Reiter, R.J., 2005. A review of the multiple actions of melatonin on the immune system. Endocrine 27 (2), 189–200.

Cernysiov, V., Gerasimcik, N., Mauricas, M., Girkontaite, I., 2010. Regulation of T-cell-independent and T-cell-dependent antibody production by circadian rhythm and melatonin. International Immunology 22, 25–34.

Claustrat, B., Leston, J., 2015. Melatonin: physiological effects in humans. Neurochirurgie 61, 77–84.

Davies, K.J., Quintanilha, A.T., Brooks, G.A., Packer, L., 1982. Free radicals and tissue damage produced by exercise. Biochemical and Biophysical Research Communications 107, 1198–1205.

Dawson, D., Armstrong, S.M., 1996. Chronobiotics—drugs that shift rhythms. Pharmacology & Therapeutics 69, 15–36.

Di Bella, G., Mascia, F., Gualano, L., Di Bella, L., 2013. Melatonin anticancer effects: review. International Journal of Molecular Sciences 14, 2410–2430.

Droge, W., 2002. Free radicals in the physiological control of cell function. Physiological Reviews 82, 47–95.

Dubbels, R., Reiter, R.J., Klemke, E., Goebel, A., Schnakenberg, E., Ehlers, C., Schiwara, H.W., Schloot, W., 1995. Melatonin in edible plants identified by radioimmunoassay and by high performance liquid chromatography-mass spectrometry. Journal of Pineal Research 18, 28–31.

Dubocovich, M.L., Markowska, M., 2005. Functional MT_1 and MT_2 melatonin receptors in mammals. Endocrine 27, 101–110.

Dubocovich, M.L., Delagrange, P., Krause, D.N., Sugden, D., Cardinali, D.P., Olcese, J., 2010. International Union of Basic and Clinical Pharmacology. LXXV. Nomenclature, classification, and pharmacology of G protein-coupled melatonin receptors. Pharmacological Reviews 62, 343–380.

Essig, D.A., Borger, D.R., Jackson, D.A., 1997. Induction of heme oxygenase-1 (HSP32) mRNA in skeletal muscle following contractions. Amercian Journal of Physiology 272, C59–C67.

Favero, G., Rodella, L.F., Nardo, L., Giugno, L., Cocchi, M.A., Borsani, E., Reiter, R.J., Rezzani, R., 2015. A comparison of melatonin and α-lipoic acid in the induction of antioxidant defences in L6 rat skeletal muscle cells. Age (Dordrecht) 37 (4), 9824.

Fournier, I., Ploye, F., Cottet-Emard, J.M., Brun, J., Claustrat, B., 2002. Folate deficiency alters melatonin secretion in rats. The Journal of Nutrition 132, 2781–2784.

Fraschini, F., Stankov, B., 1994. High affinity melatonin receptors in the vertebrate brain: implications for the control of the endogenous oscillatory systems. Chronobiologia 21, 89–92.

Galano, A., Tan, D.X., Reiter, R.J., 2013. On the free radical scavenging activities of melatonin's metabolites, AFMK and AMK. Journal of Pineal Research 54, 245–257.

Garcia-Mauriño, S., Gonzalez-Haba, M.G., Calvo, J.R., Rafii-El-Idrissi, M., Sanchez- Margalet, V., Goberna, R., Guerrero, J.M., 1997. Melatonin enhances IL-2, IL-6, and IFN-gamma production by human circulating CD4+ cells: a possible nuclear receptor-mediated mechanism involving T helper type 1 lymphocytes and monocytes. Journal of Immunology 159, 574–581.

García-Mauriño, S., Pozo, D., Carrillo-Vico, A., Calvo, J.R., Guerrero, J.M., 1999. Melatonin activates Th1 lymphocytes by increasing IL-12 production. Life Sciences 65, 2143–2150.

Gauer, F., Masson-Pévet, M., Stehle, J., Pévet, P., 1994. Daily variations in melatonin receptor density of rat pars tuberalis and suprachiasmatic nuclei are distinctly regulated. Brain Research 641, 92–98.

Ghosh, G., De, K., Maity, S., Bandyopadhyay, D., Bhattacharya, S., Reiter, R.J., Bandyopadhyay, A., 2007. Melatonin protects against oxidative damage and restores expression of GLUT4 gene in the hyperthyroid rat heart. Journal of Pineal Research 42, 71–82.

Hardeland, R., Poeggeler, B., 2008. Melatonin beyond its classical functions. The Open Physiology Journal 1, 1–23.

Hardeland, R., Balzer, I., Poeggeler, B., Fuhrberg, B., Uri´a, H., Behrmann, G., Wolf, R., Meyer, T.J., Reiter, R.J., 1995. On the primary functions of melatonin in evolution: mediation of photoperiodic signals in a unicell, photooxidation, and scavenging of free radicals. Journal of Pineal Research 18, 104–111.

Hardeland, R., Tan, D.X., Reiter, R.J., 2009a. Kynuramines, metabolites of melatonin and other indoles: the resurrection of an almost forgotten class of biogenic amines. Journal of Pineal Research 47, 109–126.

Hardeland, R., Poeggeler, B., Pappolla, M.A., 2009b. Mitochondrial actions of melatonin – an endeavor to identify their adaptive and cytoprotective mechanisms, Abhandlungen der Akademie der Wissenschaften in Göttingen. Mathematisch-Naturwissenschaftliche Klasse 65 (Pt. 3), 14–31.

Hardeland, R., Cardinali, D.P., Srinivasan, V., Spence, D.W., Brown, G.M., Pandi-Perumal, S.R., March 2011. Melatonin—a pleiotropic, orchestrating regulator molecule. Progress in Neurobiology 93 (3), 350–384.

Hardeland, R., 2009c. Melatonin: signaling mechanisms of a pleiotropic agent. BioFactors 35, 183–192.

Hardeland, R., 2013. Melatonin and the theories of aging: a critical appraisal of melatonin's role in antiaging mechanisms. Journal of Pineal Research 55, 325–356.

Hayes, C., Kriska, A., 2008. Role of physical activity in diabetes management and prevention. Journal of the American Dietetic Association 108, S19–S23.

Hirai, H., Kubo, H., Yamaya, M., Nakayama, K., Numasaki, M., Kobayashi, S., Suzuki, S., Shibahara, S., Sasaki, H., 2003. Microsatellite polymorphism in heme oxygenase-1 gene promoter is associated with susceptibility to oxidant-induced apoptosis in lymphoblastoid cell lines. Blood 102, 1619–1621.

Huether, G., Poeggeler, B., Reimer, A., George, A., 1992. Effect of tryptophan administration on circulating melatonin levels in chicks and rats: evidence for stimulation of melatonin synthesis and release in the gastrointestinal tract. Life Sciences 51, 945–953.

Huether, G., 1993. The contribution of extrapineal sites of melatonin synthesis to circulating melatonin levels in higher vertebrates. Experientia 49, 665–670.

Huether, G., 1994. Melatonin synthesis in the gastrointestinal tract and the impact of nutritional factors on circulating melatonin. Annals of the New York Academy of Sciences 31 (719), 146–158.

Jin, X., von Gall, C., Pieschl, R.L., Gribkoff, V.K., Stehle, J.H., Reppert, S.M., Weaver, D.R., 2003. Targeted disruption of the mouse Mel_{1b} melatonin receptor. Molecular and Cellular Biology 23, 1054–1060.

Jou, M.J., Peng, T.I., Hsu, L.F., Jou, S.B., Reiter, R.J., Yang, C.M., Chiao, C.C., Lin, Y.F., Chen, C.C., 2010. Visualization of melatonin's multiple mitochondrial levels of protection against mitochondrial Ca^{2+} -mediated permeability transition and beyond in rat brain astrocytes. Journal of Pineal Research 48, 20–38.

Kasapis, C., Thompson, P.D., 2005. The effects of physical activity on serum C-reactive protein and inflammatory markers: a systematic review. Journal of the American College of Cardiology 45, 1563–1569.

Kireev, R.A., Tresguerres, A.C.F., Garcia, C., Ariznavarreta, C., Vara, E., Tresguerres, J.A., 2008. Melatonin is able to prevent the liver of old castrated female rats from oxidative and pro-inflammatory damage. Journal of Pineal Research 45, 394–402.

Korf, H.W., von Gall, C., 2006. Mice, melatonin and the circadian system. Molecular and Cellular Endocrinology 252, 57–68.

Korkmaz, A., Rosales-Corral, S., Reiter, R.J., 2012. Gene regulation by melatonin linked to epigenetic phenomena. Gene 503 (1), 1–11.

Kraus, W.E., Slentz, C.A., 2009. Exercise training, lipid regulation, and insulin action: a tangled web of cause and effect. Obesity (Silver Spring) 17 (Suppl. 3), S21–S26.

Kühlwein, E., Irwin, M., 2001. Melatonin modulation of lymphocyte proliferation and Th1/Th2 cytokine expression. Journal of Neuroimmunology 117, 51–57.

Kvetnoy, I.M., 1999. Extrapineal melatonin: location and role within diffuse neuroendocrine system. The Histochemical Journal 31, 1–12.

III. FACTORS MODULATING EXERCISE IN AGING AND NEUROLOGICAL CONSEQUENCES

Lawler, J.M., Powers, S.K., Van Dijk, H., Visser, T., Kordus, M.J., Ji, L.L., 1994. Metabolic and antioxidant enzyme activities in the diaphragm: effects of acute exercise. Respiration Physiology 96, 139–149.

Lee, H.T., Xu, H., Ota-Setlik, A., Emala, C.W., 2003. Oxidant preconditioning protects human proximal tubular cells against lethal oxidant injury via p38 MAPK and heme oxygenase-1. American Journal of Nephrology 23, 324–333.

Leonardo-Mendonça, R.C., Martinez-Nicolas, A., de Teresa Galván, C., Ocaña-Wilhelmi, J., Rusanova, I., Guerra-Hernández, E., Escames, G., Acuña-Castroviejo, D., September 11, 2015. The benefits of four weeks of melatonin treatment on circadian patterns in resistance-trained athletes. Chronobiology International 1–10.

Lerner, A.B., Case, J.D., Takahashi, Y., Lee, T.H., Mori, N., 1958. Isolation of melatonin, a pineal factor that lightens melanocytes. Journal of the American Chemical Society 80, 2587.

Limson, J., Nyokong, T., Daya, S., 1998. The interaction of melatonin and its precursors with aluminium, cadmium, copper, iron, lead, and zinc: an adsorptive voltammetric study. Journal of Pineal Research 24, 15–21.

Lotufo, C.M., Yamashita, C.E., Farsky, S.H., Markus, R.P., 2006. Melatonin effect on endothelial cells reduces vascular permeability increase induced by leukotriene B$_4$. European Journal of Pharmacology 534, 258–263.

Luboshitzky, R., Ophir, U., Nave, R., Epstein, R., Shen-Orr, Z., Herer, P., 2002. The effect of pyridoxine administration on melatonin secretion in normal men. Neuroendocrinology Letters 23, 213–217.

Malech, H.L., Gallin, J.I., 1987. Current concepts: immunology. Neutrophils in human diseases. The New England Journal of Medicine 317, 687–694.

Marczynski, T.J., Yamaguchi, N., Ling, G.M., Grodzinska, L., 1964. Sleep induced by the administration of melatonin (5-methoxy-N-acetyltryptamine) to the hypothalamus in unrestrained cats. Experientia 20, 435–437.

Marseglia, L., Manti, L., D'Angelo, G., Nicotera, A., Parisi, E., Di Rosa, G., Gitto, E., Arrigo, T., 2015. Oxidative stress in obesity: a critical component in human diseases. International Journal of Molecular Sciences 16, 378–400.

Masson-Pévet, M., Gauer, F., Schuster, C., Guerrero, H.Y., 2000. Photic regulation of mt$_1$ melatonin receptors and 2-iodomelatonin binding in the rat and Siberian hamster. Biological Signals and Receptors 9, 188–196.

Mayo, J.C., Sainz, R.M., Tan, D.X., Hardeland, R., Leon, J., Rodriguez, C., Reiter, R.J., 2005. Anti-inflammatory actions of melatonin and its metabolites, N1-acetyl-N2-formyl-5-methoxykynuramine (AFMK) and N1-acetyl-5-methoxykynuramine (AMK), in macrophages. Journal of Neuroimmunology 165, 139–149.

McArdle, A., Dillmann, W.H., Mestril, R., Faulkner, J.A., Jackson, M.J., 2004. Overexpression of HSP70 in mouse skeletal muscle protects against muscle damage and age-related muscle dysfunction. FASEB Journal 18, 355–357.

McClung, J.M., Judge, A.R., Talbert, E.E., Powers, S.K., 2009. Calpain-1 is required for hydrogen peroxide-induced myotube atrophy. American Journal of Physiology Cell Physiology 296, C363–C371.

McClung, J.M., Judge, A.R., Powers, S.K., Yan, Z., 2010. p38 MAPK links oxidative stress to autophagy-related gene expression in cachectic muscle wasting. American Journal of Physiology Cell Physiology 298, C542–C549.

Meeking, D.R., Wallace, J.D., Cuneo, R.C., Forsling, M., Russell-Jones, D.I., 1999. Exercise-induced GH secretion is enhanced by the oral ingestion of melatonin in healthy adult male subjects. European Journal of Endocrinology 141, 22–26.

Morrey, K.M., McLachlan, J.A., Serkin, C.D., Bakouche, O., 1994. Activation of human monocytes by the pineal hormone melatonin. Journal of Immunology 153, 2671–2680.

Mukherjee, S., Maitra, S.K., 2015. Gut melatonin in vertebrates: chronobiology and physiology. Frontiers in Endocrinology 6, 112. http://dx.doi.org/10.3389/fendo.2015.00112.

Munoz-Hoyos, A., Amoros-Rodriguez, I., Molina-Carballo, A., Uberos-Fernández, J., Acuña-Castroviejo, D., 1996. Pineal response after pyridoxine test in children. Journal of Neural Transmission 103, 833–842.

Näveri, H., 1985. Blood hormone and metabolite levels during graded cycle ergometer exercise. Scandinavian Journal of Clinical and Laboratory Investigation 45, 599–603.

Nikolaidis, M.G., Jamurtas, A.Z., 2009. Blood as a reactive species generator and redox status regulator during exercise. Archives of Biochemistry and Biophysics 490, 77–84.

Nikolaidis, M.G., Jamurtas, A.Z., Paschalis, V., Fatouros, I.G., Koutedakis, Y., Kouretas, D., 2008. The effect of muscle-damaging exercise on blood and skeletal muscle oxidative stress: magnitude and time-course considerations. Sports Medicine. 38 (7), 579–606.

Ochoa, J.J., Díaz-Castro, J., Kajarabille, N., García, C., Guisado, I.M., De Teresa, C., Guisado, R., 2011. Melatonin supplementation ameliorates oxidative stress and inflammatory signaling induced by strenuous exercise in adult human males. Journal of Pineal Research 51, 373–380.

Pandi-Perumal, S.R., Srinivasan, V., Maestroni, G.J.M., Cardinali, D.P., Poeggeler, B., Hardeland, R., 2006. Melatonin: nature's most versatile biological signal? FEBS Journal 273, 2813–2838.

Paradies, G., Petrosillo, G., Paradies, V., Reiter, R.J., Ruggiero, F.M., 2010. Melatonin, cardiolipin and mitochondrial bioenergetics in health and disease. Journal of Pineal Research 48, 297–310.

Perepechaeva, M., Stefanova, N., Grishanova, A., 2014. Expression of genes for AhR and Nrf2 signal pathways in the retina of OXYS rats during the development of retinopathy and melatonin-induced changes in this process. Bulletin of Experimental Biology and Medicine 157, 424–429.

Pévet, P., Bothorel, B., Slotten, H., Saboureau, M., 2002. The chronobiotic properties of melatonin. Cell and Tissue Research 309, 183–191.

Powers, S.K., Jackson, M.J., 2008. Exercise-induced oxidative stress: cellular mechanisms and impact on muscle force production. Physiological Reviews 88, 1243–1276.

Powers, S.K., Duarte, J., Kavazis, A.N., Talbert, E.E., 2010. Reactive oxygen species are signalling molecules for skeletal muscle adaptation. Experimental Physiology 95, 1–9.

Raynaud, J., Capderou, A., Martineaud, J.P., Bordachar, J., Durand, J., 1983. Intersubject variability in growth hormone time course during different types of work. Journal of Applied Physiology 55, 1682–1687.

Reid, M.B., Li, Y.P., 2001. Cytokines and oxidative signalling in skeletal muscle. Acta Physiologica Scandinavica 171, 225–232.

Reiter, R.J., Richardson, B.A., 1992. Some perturbations that disturb the circadian melatonin rhythm. Chronobiology International 9, 314–321.

Reiter, R.J., Paredes, S.D., Manchester, L.C., Tan, D.X., 2009. Reducing oxidative/nitrosative stress: a newly-discovered genre for melatonin. Critical Reviews in Biochemistry and Molecular Biology 44, 175–200.

Reiter, R.J., Tan, D.X., Rosales-Corral, S., Manchester, L.C., 2013. The universal nature, unequal distribution and antioxidant functions of melatonin and its derivatives. Mini Reviews in Medicinal Chemistry 13, 373–384.

Reiter, R.J., 1991a. Melatonin: the chemical expression of darkness. Molecular and Cellular Endocrinology 9, C153–C158.

Reiter, R.J., 1991b. Pineal melatonin: cell biology of its synthesis and of its physiological interactions. Endocrine Reviews 12, 151–180.

Reiter, R.J., 1993. The melatonin rhythm: both a clock and a calendar. Experientia 49, 654–664.

Reppert, S.M., Weaver, D.R., Ebisawa, T., 1994. Cloning and characterization of a mammalian melatonin receptor that mediates reproductive and circadian responses. Neuron 13, 1177–1185.

Reppert, S.M., Godson, C., Mahle, C.D., Weaver, D.R., Slaugenhaupt, S.A., Gusella, J.F., 1995. Molecular characterization of a second melatonin receptor expressed in human retina and brain: the Mel_{1b} melatonin receptor. Proceedings of the National Academy of Sciences of the United States of America 92, 8734–8738.

Rodriguez, C., Mayo, J.C., Sainz, R.M., Antolín, I., Herrera, F., Martin, V., Reiter, R.J., 2004. Regulation of antioxidant enzymes: a significant role for melatonin. Journal of Pineal Research 36, 1–9.

Rushworth, S.A., Macewan, D.J., 2011. The role of Nrf2 and cytoprotection in regulating chemotherapy resistance of human leukemia cells. Cancers (Basel) 3, 1605–1621.

Sánchez, A., Calpena, A.C., Clares, B., 2015. Evaluating the oxidative stress in inflammation: role of melatonin. International Journal of Molecular Sciences 16 (8), 16981–17004.

Sanchez-Hidalgo, M., de la Lastra, C.A., Carrascosa-Salmoral, M.P., Naranjo, M.C., Gomez-Corvera, A., Caballero, B., Guerrero, J.M., 2009. Age-related changes in melatonin synthesis in rat extrapineal tissues. Experimental Gerontology 44, 328–334.

Sewerynek, E., Reiter, R.J., Melchiorri, D.A., Ortiz, G.G., Lewinski, A., 1996. Oxidative damage in the liver induced by ischemia- reperfusion: protection by melatonin. Hepatogastroenterology 43, 898–905.

Shay, C.M., Gooding, H.S., Murillo, R., Forakerd, R., 2015. Understanding and improving cardiovascular health: an update on the American Heart Association's Concept of Cardiovascular Health. Progress in Cardiovascular Disease 58, 41–49.

Stanford, K.I., Middelbeek, R.J., Goodyear, L.J., 2015. Exercise effects on white adipose tissue: Beiging and metabolic adaptations. Diabetes 64 (7), 2361–2368.

Stehle, J.H., vonGall, C., Korf, H.W., 2003. Melatonin: a clock-output, a clock-input. Journal of Neuroendocrinology 15 (4), 383–389.

Tamarkin, L., Baird, C.J., Almeida, O.F., 1985. Melatonin: a coordinating signal for mammalian reproduction? Science 227, 714–720.

Tan, D.X., Pöeggeler, B., Reiter, R.J., Chen, L.D., Chen, S., Manchester, L.C., Barlow-Walden, L.R., 1993. The pineal hormone melatonin inhibits DNA-adduct formation induced by the chemical carcinogen safrole in vivo. Cancer Letters 70, 65–71.

Tan, D.X., Manchester, L.C., Hardeland, R., Lopez-Burillo, S., Mayo, J.C., Sainz, R.M., Reiter, R.J., 2003. Melatonin: a hormone, a tissue factor, an autocoid, a paracoid, and an antioxidant vitamin. Journal of Pineal Research 34, 75–78.

Tan, D.X., Hardeland, R., Manchester, L.C., Paredes, S.D., Korkmaz, A., Sainz, R.M., Mayo, J.C., Fuentes-Broto, L., Reiter, R.J., 2010. The changing biological roles of melatonin during evolution: from an antioxidant to signals of darkness, sexual selection and fitness. Biological Reviews of the Cambridge Philosophical Society 85, 607–623.

Thanan, R., Oikawa, S., Hiraku, Y., Ohnishi, S., Ma, N., Pinlaor, S., Yongvanit, P., Kawanishi, P., Murata, M., 2015. Oxidative stress and its significant roles in neurodegenerative diseases and cancer. International Journal of Molecular Sciences 16, 193–217.

Tuli, H.S., Kashyap, D., Sharma, A.K., Sandhu, S.S., 2015. Molecular aspects of melatonin (MLT)-mediated therapeutic effects. Life Sciences. http://dx.doi.org/10.1016/j.lfs.2015.06.004.

Urata, Y., Honma, S., Goto, S., Todoroki, S., Iida, T., Cho, S., Honma, K., Kondo, T., 1999. Melatonin induces gamma-glutamylcysteine synthetase mediated by activator protein-1 in human vascular endothelial cells. Free Radical Biology & Medicine 27, 838–847.

Valcavi, R., Zini, M., Maestroni, G.J., Conti, A., Portioli, I., 1993. Melatonin stimulates growth hormone secretion through pathways other than the growth hormone-releasing hormone. Clinical Endocrinology 39, 193–199.

Valko, M., Rhodes, C.J., Moncol, J., Izakovic, M., Mazur, M., March 10, 2006. Free radicals, metals and antioxidants in oxidative stress-induced cancer. Chemico Biological Interactions 160 (1), 1–40.

Veneroso, C., Tuñón, M.J., Gonza´lez-Gallego, J., Collado, P.S., 2009. Melatonin reduces cardiac inflammatory injury induced by acute exercise. Journal of Pineal Research 47, 184–191.

Voisin, P., Namboodiri, M.A.A., Klein, D.C., 1984. Arylamine N-acetyltransferase and arylalkylamine N-acetyltransferase in the mammalian pineal gland. The Journal of Biological Chemistry 259, 10913–10918.

Wei, W., Liu, Q., Tan, Y., Liu, L., Li, X., Cai, L., 2009. Oxidative stress, diabetes, and diabetic complications. Hemoglobin 33, 370–377.

Xie, K., Huang, S., 2003. Regulation of cancer metastasis by stress pathways. Clinical & Experimental Metastasis 20, 31–43.

Zamfir Chiru, A.A., Popescu, C.R., Gheorghe, D.C., 2014. Melatonin and cancer. Journal of Medicinal and Life 7, 373–374.

Zimmermann, R.C., McDougle, C.J., Schumacher, M., Olcese, J., Mason, J.W., Heninger, G.R., Price, L.H., 1993. Effects of acute tryptophan depletion on nocturnal melatonin secretion in humans. Journal of Clinical Endocrinology and Metabolism 76, 1160–1164.

EXERCISE AS THERAPY FOR NEUROLOGICAL DISEASES

Mechanisms of Functional Recovery With Exercise and Rehabilitation in Spinal Cord Injuries

M. Cowan[1,2], R.M. Ichiyama[1]

[1]University of Leeds, Leeds, United Kingdom; [2]Imperial College London, London, United Kingdom

Abstract

A spinal cord injury can result in significant motor, sensory, and autonomic impairments. Despite extensive research, physical rehabilitation is currently the most widely used treatment employed in an attempt to regain some of the lost motor function. However, the underlying mechanisms behind rehabilitation still remain to be solidified. Furthermore, the key parameters of rehabilitation programs such as their intensity, frequency, duration, and onset are still to be optimized. Here we compare and contrast what is currently known about the underlying mechanisms of two different types of movement-based therapy; continuous exercise and skill training. We then discuss how the key parameters of rehabilitation programs may affect outcomes differently, depending on whether they comprise continuous exercise, or motor skills training. A more complete understanding of such underlying mechanisms is necessary to advance treatment efficacy, especially in light of developing pharmaceutical and cell replacement strategies in spinal cord injury.

INTRODUCTION

Spinal cord injury (SCI) can be a devastating event, leaving an individual with significant motor, sensory, and autonomic impairments. Currently "rehabilitation" training is the most widely prescribed treatment following an SCI, which often results in some recovery of motor function especially in the less severely injured (AIS C and D) (Behrman and Harkema, 2000; Curt et al., 1998; Dobkin et al., 2003; Wessels et al., 2010). However, the efficacy of such interventions can be limited and variable, likely due to the fact that the underlying mechanisms associated with its effects are poorly understood. In animal models of SCI, a wide range of activity-based treatments designed to improve motor function have been tested. Terms such as rehabilitation, physical therapy, exercise, and training are often used interchangeably; referring to movement-based interventions that aim to improve motor function after SCI. This lack of specificity may be an important factor contributing to the general misleading, and at times contradictory results.

A variety of types of continuous exercise training have been shown to enhance functional recovery following an SCI. This includes swimming, cycling, and running, the effects of which have all been examined in animal SCI models (Engesser-Cesar et al., 2007; Ganzer et al., 2016; Smith et al., 2006). The fundamental question, here, is whether a nonspecific enhancement in physiological function and capacity may have beneficial systemic effects which could positively affect central nerve system (CNS) function and repair. Clearly, it is important for exercise to be more specifically defined in experimental designs, particularly since there is a large volume of evidence demonstrating that factors such as modality, intensity, and duration, produce different effects in different physiological systems, both in healthy individuals and those with pathological conditions (Boussana et al., 2001; Cheetham et al., 2002; Davidson et al., 2009; Shephard, 1968; Tiidus and Lanuzzo, 1982; Wenger and Bell, 1986). Unfortunately, these parameters have not always been addressed within the field of SCI research.

Another movement-based therapy that has been investigated is motor skill training; defined as training that involves a precise movement carried out with the intention of achieving a specific goal. Examples of skill training that have been shown to enhance recovery in animal SCI models include reaching and grasping tasks, as well as body weight supported treadmill-stepping. Skill training can be further divided into fine motor skills and gross motor skills; the former comprising movements that require precise accurate control by the small muscles of the body (e.g., grasping) and the latter functional movements that involve large muscle groups (e.g., treadmill-stepping locomotion). In this regard it is important to appreciate that, depending on duration and intensity, activities such as treadmill training can be considered to be a combination of both motor skill training and continuous exercise. Another approach to gross motor skill training occurs by enriching the environment of animals with apparatuses such as ladders, ropes, and beams. Obviously, it is essential to evaluate what types of apparatus have actually been used in these studies. For example, Lankhorst et al. (2001) included a running wheel along with ladders and beams; this particular environmental enrichment would facilitate training of gross motor tasks along with continuous voluntary exercise. One difficulty with interpretation of results from enriched environment studies is the fact that usually there is no control over which and how much activity is actually being performed on the different apparatuses.

As far as we are aware no study has directly compared the effects of exercise and skill training in an SCI animal model. However, the different effects of exercise and skill training in stroke animal models have been investigated. Maldonado et al. (2008) showed that in an ischemic stroke rat model, training in a single-pellet retrieval task improved reaching, whereas exercise alone (access to a running wheel for 5 weeks 6 h/day) did not. Furthermore, compared to skill training in isolation, when the two types of intervention were combined no functional improvements were seen. However, Ploughman et al. (2009) reported that in a rat stroke model the combination of exercise training via a motorized running wheel prior to skill training in a single-pellet retrieval task had a synergistic effect, resulting in improved reaching performance. Although the findings discussed previously were generated from stroke models, understanding how motor skill-based training and exercise interact is just as relevant to SCI, and as such is an area that warrants investigation.

In this chapter, we aim to compare and contrast the underlying mechanisms behind the recovery of function in SCI after continuous exercise and motor skill training. We hypothesize that exercise will result in general systemic unspecific adaptation within the CNS, whereas skill training will cause specific reorganization of neuronal networks leading to recovery of specific functions. Furthermore, we will review how key parameters of rehabilitation programs may influence motor outcomes differently, depending on whether the training is continuous exercise, or training of fine or gross motor skills.

MECHANISMS UNDERLYING OF REHABILITATION

Currently, the underlying mechanisms responsible for the improvement in motor control after rehabilitation training are still to be solidified. Moreover, better understanding could lead to identification of potentially novel interventions. Importantly, due to the multitude of adaptive changes occurring following SCI and rehabilitation, estimating the contribution of specific adaptation changes to motor recovery remains challenging.

This section will review the known neural mechanisms associated with functional recovery after skill training and exercise within both the spinal cord and the motor cortex.

Exercise

Trophic Factors Within the Spinal Cord

A variety of exercise modalities have been shown to increase a number of different neurotrophic factors within the spinal cord of both intact and SCI animals; these include, for example, brain-derived neurotrophic factor (BDNF), neurotrophic-3 (NT3), and glial cell line-derived neurotrophic factor (GDNF) (Detloff et al., 2014; Gómez-Pinilla et al., 2001, 2002; Hutchinson et al., 2004; Ying et al., 2005). BDNF is currently the most studied neurotrophic factor in relation to SCI. Ying et al. (2008) reported that blocking TrkB (the high-affinity receptor for BDNF) through injecting inhibitor TrkB IgG into the cervical spinal cord below the lesion, reduced the recovery of stepping in rats with a thoracic hemi-section lesion that underwent running wheel training. Furthermore, it has been reported that treating spinal cats with BDNF releasing fibroblasts results in similar gate kinematics to treadmill training (Boyce et al., 2007). In addition, cats that received both interventions demonstrated a step length that was similar to intact animals, suggesting that the two treatments may be additive. In rats with complete thoracic transections, injecting adeno-associated-virus encoding BDNF into the spinal cord, caudal to the lesion site, enhanced hindlimb stepping (Boyce et al., 2012). Notably, BDNF treated rats also developed hindlimb spasticity, making this intervention unviable as a potential treatment in humans. By contrast, running wheel trained SCI rats have reduced muscle spasms compared to their untrained counterparts (Gonzenbach et al., 2010). There are several potential explanations for these differences in outcome; including, for example, that the levels of BDNF produced varied to such an extent that they caused differences in spasticity, or that other adaptations occurring as a result of exercise caused a net reduction in spasticity. As spasticity itself is a complex phenomenon not well characterized it is probably premature to come to specific conclusions.

Elevated levels of BDNF within lumbar motor pools have also been found in the absence of motor recovery after treadmill walking training in SCI rats (Macias et al., 2009). Importantly, the treadmill belt speed was kept relatively slow in this study (0.05–0.1 m/s), with short 4 min sessions separated by ~30 min of rest. Whereas, Wang et al. (2015) reported that when SCI rats were stepped at a faster belt speed (5–12 m/min) for a longer continuous period (15 min), a parallel increase in BDNF within lumbar motor pools with improvement in open-field locomotion and grid walking occurred. Taken together, these results indicate that although low-intensity short-duration exercise may evoke increased BDNF within the spinal cord, it is not sufficient in itself to induce increased motor performance; and for functional improvement to occur, exercise needs to be carried out at higher levels of intensity and/or duration.

Another neurotrophic factor that has been shown to be upregulated as a result of exercise within the spinal cord is NT-3 (Hutchinson et al., 2004). Increasing levels of NT-3 within the spinal cord has been shown to enhance motor recovery after an SCI; in rats with incomplete SCI grafting fibroblast that produce NT-3 to the lesion site improved performance on a grid walking task, correlating with increased corticospinal tract (CST) axon growth distal to the lesion site (Grill et al., 1997). Furthermore, Giehl and Tetzlaff (1996) showed that intraparenchymal application of NT-3 (or BDNF) into the cortex resulted in reduced cell death after axotomy of corticospinal neurons. Overall, these results indicate that the upregulation of NT-3 is likely to be a contributing factor to the recovery seen after exercise, and that a potential mechanism for this is via increased CST axonal growth and cell survival. Hutchinson et al. (2004) reported that in SCI rats, treadmill training and swimming increased levels of NT-3 equally within the spinal cord. Considering caudal levels of NT-3 were not increased by standing training, it appears NT-3 expression may be sensitive to continuous rhythmic exercise activity. As NT-3 has been associated with maintaining proprioception sensation, potentially the lack of limb movement in standing training was insufficient to induce an upregulation of NT-3 (Ernfors et al., 1994; Liebl et al., 1997; Tessarollo et al., 1994).

In addition to reducing painful muscle spasms, exercise within animal models of SCI has been shown to reduce both allodynia and hyperalgesia; Detloff et al. (2014) reported that in rats with incomplete cervical lesions, development of neuropathic pain correlated with a significant decrease in levels of artemin and GDNF in the lower cervical spinal cord and dorsal root ganglia. However, forced wheel training resulted in a reduction in the frequency of allodynia, which was accompanied by maintenance of normal levels of both artemim and GDNF. In addition to the increased levels of trophic factors, there was also a reduction in afferent sprouting in the dorsal horn. Interestingly, Côté et al. (2011) found that in rats with complete SCI, GDNF was upregulated after bipedal stepping training, but not after bicycle training; indicating that GDNF may be sensitive to specific movements rather than the effect of exercise per se.

Hoffman Reflex Normalization and Intraspinal Circuitry

The Hoffman Reflex (H-reflex) is a monosynaptic reflex brought about by electrical stimulation of Ia afferent fibers that project signals directly onto the homologous alpha motor neurons. The H-reflex is the most extensively studied reflex in both intact and CNS lesioned animal. After an SCI, the H-reflex has been shown to significantly increase in excitability; and it has been reported that in rats with a complete transection (T10), excitability of the H-reflex is normalized after a period of continuous exercise training via a motorized bicycle (Skinner et al., 1996). Due to the lack of descending input, it is likely that the continuous exercise preserved or caused the reorganization of spinal neural circuitry that maintained the overall level of presynaptic inhibition of the motor neurons, resulting in an H-reflex that had normal excitability. Furthermore, Ollivier-Lanvin et al. (2010) reported that in rats with complete spinal transection, removal of proprioceptive input (group I and group II afferents) via pyridoxine neurotoxicity prevented bicycle exercise training normalizing the H-reflex; indicating that normal afferent input is a critical mechanism behind exercise reversing the hyperreflexia of the H-reflex seen after SCI. The effect of continuous exercise has also been shown to affect H-reflex excitability in humans; single bout bicycle training has been reported to normalize the soleus H-reflex in human participants with incomplete SCIs (Phadke et al., 2009).

As previously stated, SCI can significantly affect an individual's autonomic function resulting in a number of severe complications. Perhaps the most dangerous of which is autonomic dysreflexia, an acute reflex-evoked uncontrolled hypertension (Krassioukov and Claydon, 2006). It is thought that changes in spinal networks and sprouting of central branches of calcitonin-gene-related peptide (CGRP) in lamina III/IV in the lumber regions of the spinal cord play a key role in the development of autonomic dysreflexia after an SCI (Cameron et al., 2006; Krenz et al., 1999; Krenz and Weaver, 1998). In this context, it has recently been shown that rats with a complete transection that underwent hind-limb cycling training experienced a significant reduction in the severity of autonomic dysreflexia, which correlates with the reduction in CGRP density within the L4/5 region of the spinal cord (West et al., 2015).

Cell Signalling Pathways

Recent studies have investigated intracellular changes that occur as a result of exercise in SCI models. Alterations in the regulation of the PTEN/mTOR pathways are thought to be a key to the prevention of axonal regeneration after an SCI (Sandrow-Feinberg and Houlé, 2015). Once an injury has occurred in the CNS the mTOR pathway becomes deregulated and suppressed, and a critical negative regulator of the PTEN pathway has been shown to play a role in the prevention of axonal regeneration. Park et al. (2008) used a virus-assisted in vivo conditional knockout approach to delete PTEN in mice to promote axonal regrowth after optic nerve injury; and it has subsequently been shown that knocking down PTEN using the same method results in CST sprouting and regeneration after a neonatal SCI in mice (Liu et al., 2010). Furthermore, the regenerated CST axons have the ability to form synapses caudal to the lesion.

When rats with a complete transection at T10 underwent passive cycling, Liu et al. (2012) demonstrated changes in expression of microRNAs (miRs) associated with PTEN/mTOR signalling within the lumbar region of the SCI. This signalling pathway has been shown to be a key regulator of regeneration and synaptic plasticity within neurons after damage to the CNS; mTOR has been strongly associated with facilitating cell growth, regeneration, and synaptic plasticity, whereas PTEN is an upstream inhibitor of mTOR, and thus suppresses mTOR's effects. Liu et al. (2012) reported an increase in the expression of miR21 and a decrease in miR199a-3p in the lumbar region; correlating respectively with a decrease in PTEN mRNA/protein and an increase in mTOR mRNA/protein. These results suggest that the increased plasticity associated with exercise after an SCI may be modulated, at least in part, through miRs that regulate the PTEN/mTOR signalling pathway.

Cell Membrane Proteins

It has been documented that after an SCI there is a change in the makeup of specific receptors on the surface of motor neurons, which ultimately leads to an alteration in functional motor output. For example, the potassium-chloride cotransporter (KCC2) has been shown to be downregulated in a mouse model of SCI. This downregulation of KCC2 leads to a reduction in the strength of postsynaptic inhibition; the downregulation of KCC2 is therefore likely to be a key contributor to the spasticity commonly seen in SCI patients (Boulenguez et al., 2010). Furthermore, Murray et al. (2010) reported that in rats that received a staggered-hemisection lesion, changes in posttranscriptional editing of 5-HT2C receptor mRNA resulted in upregulation of spontaneously activating 5-HT2C receptors on motor neurons. Again this upregulation of 5-HT2C receptors is thought to contribute to the muscle spasticity of SCI patients. The oral administration of the 5-HT antagonist cyproheptadine, reduced muscle spasticity in a human SCI patient (Wainberg et al., 1990).

But does exercise prevent/reverse these changes in surface receptor expression? In the case of KCC2, Boulenguez et al. (2010) reported that administration of BDNF prevented its early downregulation; suggesting a potential link between exercise and reversal of KCC2 downregulation. Subsequently, this link has been independently tested by two different research groups. First, in completely transected rats that underwent bicycle training, levels of KCC2 and the sodium-potassium-chloride cotransporter (NKCC1) returned toward normal levels in the lumbar spinal cord (Côté et al., 2014). Furthermore, the effect of exercise on the tibial nerve H-reflex was masked when KCC2 was blocked, whereas blocking NKCC1 resulted in excitability of the H-reflex that was moving toward intact levels. Tashiro et al. (2015) showed that the positive effect (reduced spasticity and allodynia) of treadmill training in rats with a moderate lower thoracic contusion injury was prevented by inhibiting the function of BDNF using TrkB-Fc chimera; and that blocking BDNF also prevented the upregulation of KCC2. Overall, these results indicate that the restoration of KCC2 levels and subsequent reduction in muscle spasticity seen after exercise in SCI animals is BDNF mediated. Similarly, Engesser-Cesar et al. (2007) showed significantly increased 5-HT and CST fiber sprouting in the lumbar region in response to wheel running in mice with an incomplete SCI. This increased 5-HT fiber sprouting may result in the reestablishment of hierarchical control over the 5-HT2C, and could be a possible mechanism behind the reduction in muscle spasms reported after exercise training.

Motor and Somatosensory Cortex Adaptations

Cortical adaptations as a result of exercise in both lesioned and intact animals are less well studied than changes that occur due to skill training. However, Graziano et al. (2013) reported that in completely transected rats, passive bicycle training caused the primary somatosensory representation area associated with the forelimb to expand into the area previously dedicated to the hindlimb. In a more recent study, rats with a complete mid-thoracic transection underwent the combined treatment of bicycle training and intraperitoneal injections of quipazine (5-HT agonist), this caused the area within the motor cortex associated with the axial trunk to expand into the deafferented hindlimb motor cortex area (Ganzer et al., 2016). Furthermore, the magnitude of the axial trunk area expansion correlated with enhanced open-field locomotion. Interestingly, there was also a reorganization of the forelimb motor cortex areas.

By contrast, access to a free running wheel in intact rats for 30 days failed to induce changes in the motor cortical representation associated with forelimb movements (Kleim et al., 2004). Nonetheless, it has been reported that intact rats that have free access to running wheels for 30 days have increased blood flow and angiogenesis in the forelimb regions of the motor cortex (Kleim et al., 2004; Swain et al., 2003). Moreover, similar changes were not identified in other regions of the cortex; indicating that these adaptations may be specific to the motor cortex region involved in the control of the continuous movement (Swain et al., 2003). Interestingly, changes in the motor cortex were not detected at the preceding 20-day measurement time point, suggesting that for these changes to occur exercise needs to be of a sufficient intensity, duration, and/or frequency. Furthermore, we have shown that exercise via free access to running wheels causes a downregulation of perineuronal nets in the somatosensory cortex in intact rat models; perineuronal nets are extracellular matrix structures made up of chondroitin sulfate proteoglycans that inhibit plasticity (Smith et al., 2015). Interestingly, this is in contrast to an observed upregulation of perineuronal nets within the lumbar region of the spinal cord. Overall, the effects of exercise training on motor and somatosensory cortex is largely unknown, and further research is required in order to establish if the effect seen in intact animal models also occurs after SCI.

Skill Training

Spinal Networks

One potential mechanism of skill training that results in motor recovery after SCI is the instigation of use dependent adaptations of spinal networks caudal to the lesion involved in controlling locomotion. This was originally hypothesized as a result of the observation that completely spinalized cats can recover weight supported stepping on a treadmill after a period of training (Lovely et al., 1986). Furthermore, in completely transected rats (T7-9) we have shown that treadmill training in combination with 5-HT agonists and epidural stimulation results in recovery of stepping ability accompanied by a reduction in the number of active neurons within the lumbar region of the spinal cord in response to locomotion (Courtine et al., 2009; Ichiyama et al., 2008). Because of the lack of descending input, the modulation of interneuronal activity due to locomotor training was most likely a result of changes in afferent input to central pattern generator circuitry. However, a direct test of this hypothesis remains elusive.

We have also demonstrated that locomotor training following a complete mid-thoracic neonatal transection (postnatal day 5) decreases the ratio of inhibitory to excitatory synapses apposing both alpha and gamma motor neurons back to intact control levels (Ichiyama et al., 2011). Similarly, we have shown that locomotor training after PN5 transection, modulates the amplitude of excitatory postsynaptic potentials and action potentials after the hyperpolarizing of motor neurons in response to peripheral and ventral lateral funiculus stimulation (Petruska et al., 2007). These results suggest that locomotor training induces intraspinal segmental reorganization, both anatomically and functionally, which is highly correlated with improvements in stepping. In addition, Barrière et al. (2008) found that when cats were trained to recover after a hemisection lesion and then received a complete transection caudal to the first injury, they recovered significantly faster than cats that only received a complete transection; suggesting that recovery of locomotion after partial lesions is in part due to an intrinsic reorganization of the spinal locomotor network below the lesion.

Motor Cortex Plasticity

The representation area within the motor cortex that is dedicated to controlling movement has been shown to vary in size in a use-dependent manner (Sanes and Donoghue, 2000). Hence, unsurprisingly after an SCI there is a corresponding reduction in the area of the motor cortex controlling movement in denervated areas of the body (Fouad and Tetzlaff, 2012). By contrast, both monkeys trained in a precision grasping task and rats who underwent reaching training, an increase in the area of the motor cortex associated with control of these trained movements has been demonstrated (Kleim et al., 1998; Nudo et al., 1996). This increase in representation area of the motor cortex involved in the control of a trained movement also occurs after training in SCI animal models. For example, in rats with incomplete cervical lesions, functional improvement after reaching task training has been shown to correlate with an increase in the cortical area where wrist movement could be evoked by micro-stimulation (Girgis et al., 2007).

In addition to changing overall motor cortex representation, reaching skill training has been shown to result in other adaptations within the motor cortex of intact rats and stroke models, notably increased complexity and density of dendritic processes of forelimb associated neurons and increased total synapses per neuron (Allred and Jones, 2004; Bury and Jones, 2002; Greenough et al., 1985; Withers and Greenough, 1989). These plastic changes within the motor cortex are thought to represent a reorganization in the cortical circuitry that encodes for the corresponding trained movement (Adkins et al., 2006). As far as we are aware no attempt has been made to observe if these plastic changes occur in the motor cortex of SCI animals as a result of skill training, and hence this area warrants further research.

In regards to trophic factors, Girgis et al. (2007) found increased level of growth associated protein 43, but not elevated levels of BDNF in the motor cortex of SCI rats that were trained in a single pellet retrieval task. Furthermore, as previously noted, walking ability appears to be enhanced by increasing BDNF expression using adeno-associated-virus (AAV) injected into the spinal cord (Boyce et al., 2012). Interestingly, however, Weishaupt et al. (2012) using AAV to increase BDNF expression, reported that this only had an effect on reaching ability in combination with single pellet retrieval training in an SCI rat model. By contrast, elevated levels of BDNF have been shown to correlate with improved performance after reaching training in both intact and stroke models; and blocking the function of BDNF in stroke models has been demonstrated to prevent recovery (Griesbach et al., 2009; Ploughman et al., 2009; Swain et al., 2003). Hence, it would be premature to conclude that BDNF upregulation in the motor cortex does not play a role in functional recovery after skill training in SCI.

Descending Tract Plasticity

Training inducing CST plasticity has been put forward as another potential mechanism for recovery of function after an SCI. Goldshmit et al. (2008) reported that quadrupedal treadmill training mice that had a hemisection lesion to T12 resulted in increased axonal regrowth, maintenance of synaptic markers on motor neurons, and increased collateral sprouting proximal to the lesion site. Notably, there was no axonal regeneration into or across the lesion site. As previously stated, wheel running mice that have an incomplete SCI has been reported to induce increased 5-HT and CST fiber sprouting in the lumbar region (Engesser-Cesar et al., 2007). Notably, Maier et al. (2009) reported no increase in either CST or 5-HT fiber sprouting after treadmill training in rats with T-shaped lesions to T8. Similarly, quadrupedal treadmill training rats with a moderate contusion injury did not show increases in 5-HT terminals within the lumbar motoneuron pools (Wang et al., 2015). In addition, Krajacic et al. (2010) reported that reaching training did not significantly increase cortical sprouting in rats C2/C3 dorsal lateral lesions. However, the data showed a correlation between collateral sprouting and cortical map changes; suggesting that cortical map changes may be influenced by alternative connections of injured axons. Overall, due to the inconsistency and small number of studies, it is not possible to characterize the role that descending tract plasticity plays in the motor recovery seen after physical rehabilitation. Furthermore, whether descending tract plasticity has a greater association with motor skill training or exercise is currently unclear.

Summary

We originally hypothesized that exercise would cause general systemic unspecific adaptations throughout the CNS, and that skill training would cause specific reorganization of neuronal networks leading to recovery of specific functions. With regard to some aspects, this statement can be accepted. For example, exercise does appear to cause an upregulation of neurotrophic factors within the CNS, and the evidence suggests that skill training causes the reorganization of neuronal networks within the spinal cord and cortex. However, exercise has also been shown to cause specific adaptations such has H-reflex normalization. Furthermore, some adaptations of exercise have been shown to be activity specific rather than general; GDNF, for example, is upregulated after bipedal stepping training but not after bicycle training. Undoubtedly, studies would benefit if the parameters of rehabilitation modalities were consistently defined, but currently there is often a lack of information on factors such as intensity of exercise, making the results difficult to interpret. Future studies should consider directly comparing the adaptations that occur after exercise, motor skill training, and modality that is a combination of both (e.g., treadmill training, obstacle course running).

REFINING REHABILITATION PROGRAMS

Although rehabilitation has been shown to enhance motor function clinically, a number of key parameters are still to be optimized, including the type of activity, as well as the frequency, duration, and time of onset of training. While some of these issues have been previously reviewed, typically all movement-based rehabilitations have been grouped together. Here we discuss the different factors in the context of distinguishing between exercise, as well as fine and gross motor skill training.

Motor Skill Transfer

The ultimate goal of any rehabilitation training is the transfer of motor skills (the change in capability of performing a motor task as a result of practising a different task). A rehabilitation program is deemed successful if exercises and drills practiced during training are transferred to activities of daily living. Animal studies of SCI have provided evidence of both negative and positive transfer; these studies are summarized in Table 11.1.

Inclined ladder stepping has been demonstrated to improve in SCI rats that had been previously trained in bipedal treadmill locomotion (Maier et al., 2009). It is important to note that both these tasks involve coordination of limbs, but that successful performance on the inclined ladder stepping apparatus requires rats to integrate visual and proprioceptive information, using information from forelimb placement to guide hindlimb placement. Furthermore, quadrupedal treadmill and running-wheel training results in improved performance in over-ground locomotion in rats and mice with incomplete SCIs (Engesser-Cesar et al., 2007; Multon et al., 2003). Lankhorst et al. (2001), also reported improved open-field locomotion and performance in a grid walking test, in rats with a mild thoracic contusion injury that were given access to running wheels and objects such as climbing frames and tubes. Interestingly, in completely transected rats, it has also been reported that training backwards or sideways stepping under epidural stimulation yields a greater improvement in forward stepping than training forward step-training alone (Shah et al., 2012).

In addition, gross motor training through enriching the environment of rats with contusion injuries facilitated improvement in the gross motor task of ladder climbing (García-Alías et al., 2009). In the same study, rats trained in the fine motor task of picking up food from a small container, exhibited enhanced performance in a similar grasping task (Whishaw test). However, gross motor training (enriched environment) did not positively transfer to fine motor skill tasks, and fine motor training (reaching task) did not transfer positively to gross motor tasks. Moreover, compared to rats that had no rehabilitation, rats that were exposed to the enriched environment had inferior performance on a staircase reaching task. This negative transfer was further exacerbated when the enriched environment was combined with the pharmacological agent chondroitinase ABC. Girgis et al. (2007) also reported negative transfer between tasks; when untrained rats that received an incomplete cervical lesion, had significantly better horizontal ladder scores than rats who had undergone 6 weeks of grasping training. In addition, cats with complete SCIs that were trained to step could not stand, and likewise cats that were trained to stand could not step (De Leon et al., 1998). Moreover, spinalized cats that were first trained to step and then trained to stand lost the ability to step (De Leon et al., 1999) Interestingly, when standing training was intermittently combined with step training (i.e., 1 min stand followed by step training until failure and repeating stand/step cycles for 20 min) no negative transfer was observed in a several contusion model (Ichiyama et al., 2009) Trained rats had superior stand and step ability especially when combined with irradiation therapy. With respect to clinical application, the negative transfer findings from animal studies underscore the need for careful consideration in designing rehabilitation programs in SCI patients.

In addition to evidence showing transfer (positive or negative), other studies have reported no associations between training in one task and performance in others. For example, Smith et al. (2006) found no relationship between swimming training (with and without increased afferent feedback) and over-ground locomotion in a rat model with a contusion SCI at T9. Also, when rats with an incomplete lesion to C4–C5 were trained in reaching and grid walking, as well as being exposed to an enriched environment that contained a variety of apparatus including a running wheel, motor improvement was only seen in the trained tasks and not in a novel cylinder test or in over-ground locomotion (Dai et al., 2009). Furthermore, in human SCI patients (ASIA A–D) who underwent 3–5 months of body weight supported treadmill training, no improvement in backwards stepping was observed (Grasso et al., 2004).

In summary, it appears that motor training in one task is more likely to have a positive effect on motor performance of a different task if the two tasks are similar. Hence, positive transfer will typically occur between gross motor skill training in one task and another gross motor skill, rather than to a fine motor skill. Similarly, positive transfer is more likely to occur between fine motor tasks. By contrast negative transfer, or no transfer at all, occurs when tasks require very different motor outputs. To date, continuous exercise has only been shown to positively transfer to tasks that share similar motor actions, for example, wheel running and open-field locomotion.

Frequency and Duration

Studies have shown that training frequency and duration also affects recovery in animal models. For example, in completely transected rats that were bipedally treadmill stepped with the aid of a robotic device, those that were stepped 1000 times during a single session had superior kinematic step profiles to those that were only stepped 100 times (Cha et al., 2007). Furthermore, it has also been reported that in mice with incomplete thoracic SCIs recovery

TABLE 11.1   Studies That Have Found Positive or Negative Transfer Between Motor Tasks in Animal Models of SCI

Study	Model	Injury	Training	Positive Transfer to
Maier et al. (2009)	Rat	T10–T-lesion	Bipedal treadmill stepping (exercise/gross motor)	Inclined ladder (gross motor)
Engesser-Cesar et al. (2005)	Mouse	T9–Contusion injury	Wheel running (exercise)	Open-field locomotion (gross motor) and ladder beam crossing (gross motor)
Engesser-Cesar et al. (2007)	Mouse	T9–Contusion injury	Wheel running (exercise)	Open-field locomotion (gross motor) and treadmill stepping (gross motor)
García-Alías et al. (2009)	Rat	C4–Dorsal funiculus transection	Reaching training (fine motor)	Whishaw reaching test (grasping fine motor)
García-Alías et al. (2009)	Rat	C4–Dorsal funiculus transection	Enriched environment (gross motor)	Ladder (gross motor)
Multon et al. (2003)	Rat	T9–Dorsal column compression-injury	Quadruped treadmill (exercise/gross motor)	Open-field locomotion (gross motor)
Lankhorst et al. (2001)	Rat	T8–Contusive injury	Enriched environment (gross motor)/Running wheel (exercise)	Open-field locomotion (gross motor) and gridwalk (gross motor)
Goldshmit et al. (2008)	Mouse	T12–Hemiscection	Quadrupedal treadmill training (exercise/gross motor)	Open-field locomotion (gross motor), grid walking and climbing
Wang et al. (2015)	Rat	T9–Contusive SC	Quadrupedal treadmill training (exercise/gross motor)	Open-field locomotion Gross motor) and grid walking (gross motor)

Study	Model	Injury	Training	Negative Transfer to
Girgis et al. (2007)	Rat	C2/C3–Dorsolateral quadrant lesion	Reaching training (fine motor)	Horizontal ladder (gross motor)
De Leon et al. (1999)	Cat	T12/13–Completely transection	Standing (gross motor)	Stepping (gross motor)
De Leon et al. (1999)	Cat	T12/13–Completely transection	Stepping (gross motor)	Stepping (gross motor)
García-Alías et al. (2009)	Rat	C4–Dorsal funiculus transection	Enriched environment (gross motor)	Staircase reaching task (fine motor)

Study	Model	Injury	Training	No Effect
Singh et al. (2011)	Rat	T9/10–Moderate contusion	Staircase climbing (gross motor)	Open-field locomotion (gross motor) and Grid walk (gross motor)
Sandrow-Feinberg et al. (2009)	Rat	C4–Unilateral contusion	Motorized running wheel	Grid walk (Gross motor) and Open field (gross motor)
Goldshmit et al. (2008)	Mouse	T12–Hemisection	Quadrupedal treadmill training (exercise/gross motor)	Grasp test (fine motor)
Smith et al. (2006)	Rat	T9–Contusion	Swimming (exercise)	Over-ground locomotion (gross motor)
Krajacic et al. (2009)	Rat	C2/C3–Dorsolateral quadrant lesion	Delayed grasping (fine motor)	Horizontal ladder (gross motor)
Dai et al. (2009)	Rat	C4-C5–Hemisection with bilaterally dorsal columns injury	Reaching training (fine motor), grid walking (gross motor) and enriched environment gross motor)/running wheel (exercise)	Novel cylinder test (gross motor) and open-field locomotion (gross motor)

was improved by having daily access to a running wheel rather than only having access 3 days a week (Engesser-Cesar et al., 2007). However, the optimal amount of training after an SCI that has a beneficial effect on motor recovery and quality-of-life, compared to the recovery that occurs spontaneously as a result of self-training, is currently undefined (Starkey and Schwab, 2012). De Leon et al. (1998) showed that untrained spinalized cats had some spontaneous recovery, although less than their trained counterparts. In addition, rats with moderate incomplete SCI demonstrated no significant functional improvements in locomotion after 5 weeks of treadmill training when compared to an untrained group (Fouad et al., 2000). Unsurprisingly, the size, type, and location of the SCI have all been identified as factors that affect the amount of possible spontaneous recovery (van Hedel and Dietz, 2010). Currently, it is not known whether increasing the duration and frequency of rehabilitation sessions in human SCI patients impacts on recovery (Starkey and Schwab, 2012).

Variations in frequency and duration training are clearly key factors that have been shown to influence recovery of motor function. However, research to date has focussed mainly on how these parameters alter the efficacy of exercise and gross motor skill training. Currently, no study has attempted to evaluate how changing these parameters in fine motor skill training impacts on functional outcome of rehabilitation in SCI. Considering that recovery of hand function has been identified as a priority for quadriplegics, investigating how to optimize fine motor skill training is clearly a vital question that needs to be investigated (Anderson, 2004).

Onset

Another rehabilitation parameter that has been shown to affect motor recovery is the timing of its onset. For example, Smith et al. (2006) showed that SCI rats had significantly better motor performance when swimming training was initiated 3 days postinjury rather than 2 weeks. Similarly in rats with a T-shaped lesion to T8, initiating motor training 3–4 days after injury resulted in significantly better motor performance than when training was started 3 months after injury (Norrie et al., 2005). Furthermore, Gonzenbach et al. (2010) showed that locomotor training can reduce muscle spasms in a rat model of SCI, but its effectiveness depended on the time of onset; locomotor training starting 1 week after SCI permanently reduced muscle spasms by up to 25%, whereas when it was initiated in the later chronic stage its effect on muscle spasms was only transient.

As previously stated, Girgis et al. (2007) reported that training (4 days after injury) rats with cervical dorsolateral quadrant lesions in a reaching task, negatively affected motor performance on a horizontal ladder. However, Krajacic et al. (2009), using the same rat model and apparatus, reported that when the initiation of reaching training was delayed (12 days after injury) there was no impairment of performance. Furthermore, unlike early onset training, delayed reaching training did not result in an increased motor cortical representation of wrist extensor. Interestingly, delayed onset reaching training (14 days after injury) restored cortical levels of protein kinase A (downstream effect of growth factors), whereas early onset training (4 days after injury) did not.

Overall, it appears that onset of training can influence functional outcome after either continuous exercise or motor skill training. Although the current dogma within the field of SCI is that there is an optimal window where onset of physical rehabilitation would result in maximum motor recovery, Houle and Côté (2013) reported that the capacity for considerable neuroplasticity remained long after the initial SCI; in completely transected rats the onset (5 vs. 28 days) of exercise (passive bicycling) did not affect lumbar spinal cord levels of BDNF or frequency-dependent depression of the H-reflex. Furthermore, the optimal onset of rehabilitation has been shown to alter when used in combination with other treatments; for example, when weight supported treadmill training in a rat model of SCI was combined with the pharmacological agent anti-Nogo-A antibody, the motor outcome was inferior to when either was used in isolation (Maier et al., 2009). By contrast, preliminary evidence suggests that motor recovery is enhanced when weight supported treadmill-training is initiated 2 weeks after the end of anti-Nogo-A antibody treatment (Marsh et al., 2011).

CONCLUSIONS

As reviewed, both continuous exercise and motor skill training may have beneficial effects on functional recovery following an SCI. However, the underlying mechanisms are still not completely understood. While the evidence is increasing, and understanding of the effects of exercise and motor skill training on functional recovery following SCI are accumulating, much remains unknown. For example, while the evidence regarding upregulation of plasticity enhancing factors, such as growth factors, seems robust, the effects of exercise and rehabilitation on plasticity inhibiting factors are much less well understood. Ghiani et al. (2007) demonstrated that access to running wheels in intact rats downregulated expression of myelin associated glycoprotein in the spinal cord. Similarly, we have recently shown that exercise in intact rats results in increased expression of the plastic inhibitory structures, perineuronal nets; the number of perineuronal nets in the dorsal horn, as well of the thickness of the perineuronal nets around the motor neuron in the lumbar spinal cord increasing in rats that were given access to a running wheel (Smith et al., 2015). Clearly, such inhibitory factors play a crucial role in plasticity mechanisms and warrant further investigation.

It is important to realize that in addition to the effects on the CNS after SCI, numerous studies have demonstrated the benefit of exercise on other body systems, which could also contribute to the general recovery of function. For example, bicycle training has been shown to reduce atrophy of the soleus muscle in a rat SCI models (Dupont-Versteegden et al., 2004). Furthermore, cycling has been combined with functional electrical stimulation to improve both muscle mass SC patients and bone density (Mohr et al., 1997; Sadowsky et al., 2013). In clinical studies of patients with SCIs, exercise has been shown to reduce levels of depression and self-reported stress, and to improve physical self-confidence and perceived quality-of-life (Hicks et al., 2003). Numerous studies have also reported increased VO_2 peaks after exercise training in SCI patients (Jacobs and Nash, 2004).

A complete understanding of how activity-based therapies modulate functional recovery is essential for the development of effective treatment strategies. In the future, it is likely that stratified approaches will be adopted; different types of injury and individual circumstances resulting in tailored intervention programs which, for the foreseeable future, are likely to include rehabilitation.

References

Adkins, D.L., Boychuk, J., Remple, M.S., Kleim, J.A., 2006. Motor training induces experience-specific patterns of plasticity across motor cortex and spinal cord. Journal of Applied Physiology 101 (6), 1776–1782. http://dx.doi.org/10.1152/japplphysiol.00515.2006.

Allred, R.P., Jones, T.A., 2004. Unilateral ischemic sensorimotor cortical damage in female rats: forelimb behavioral effects and dendritic structural plasticity in the contralateral homotopic cortex. Experimental Neurology 190 (2), 433–445. http://dx.doi.org/10.1016/j.expneurol.2004.08.005.

Anderson, K.D., 2004. Targeting recovery: priorities of the spinal cord-injured population. Journal of Neurotrauma 21 (10), 1371–1383. http://dx.doi.org/10.1089/neu.2004.21.1371.

Barrière, G., Leblond, H., Provencher, J., Rossignol, S., 2008. Prominent role of the spinal central pattern generator in the recovery of locomotion after partial spinal cord injuries. The Journal of Neuroscience: The Official Journal of the Society for Neuroscience 28 (15), 3976–3987. http://dx.doi.org/10.1523/JNEUROSCI.5692-07.2008.

Behrman, A.L., Harkema, S.J., 2000. Locomotor training after human spinal cord injury: a series of case studies. Physical Therapy 80 (7), 688–700.

Boulenguez, P., Liabeuf, S., Bos, R., Bras, H., Jean-Xavier, C., Brocard, C., Stil, A., Darbon, P., Cattaert, D., Delpire, E., Marsala, M., Vinay, L., 2010. Down-regulation of the potassium-chloride cotransporter KCC2 contributes to spasticity after spinal cord injury. Nature Medicine 16 (3), 302–307. http://dx.doi.org/10.1038/nm.2107.

Boussana, A., Matecki, S., Galy, O., Hue, O., Ramonatxo, M., Le Gallais, D., 2001. The effect of exercise modality on respiratory muscle performance in triathletes. Medicine and Science in Sports and Exercise 33 (12), 2036–2043.

Boyce, V.S., Park, J., Gage, F.H., Mendell, L.M., 2012. Differential effects of brain-derived neurotrophic factor and neurotrophin-3 on hindlimb function in paraplegic rats. The European Journal of Neuroscience 35 (2), 221–232. http://dx.doi.org/10.1111/j.1460-9568.2011.07950.x.

Boyce, V.S., Tumolo, M., Fischer, I., Murray, M., Lemay, M.A., 2007. Neurotrophic factors promote and enhance locomotor recovery in untrained spinalized cats. Journal of Neurophysiology 98 (4), 1988–1996. http://dx.doi.org/10.1152/jn.00391.2007.

Bury, S.D., Jones, T.A., 2002. Unilateral sensorimotor cortex lesions in adult rats facilitate motor skill learning with the 'unaffected' forelimb and training-induced dendritic structural plasticity in the motor cortex. The Journal of Neuroscience: The Official Journal of the Society for Neuroscience 22 (19), 8597–8606.

Cameron, A.A., Smith, G.M., Randall, D.C., Brown, D.R., Rabchevsky, A.G., 2006. Genetic manipulation of intraspinal plasticity after spinal cord injury alters the severity of autonomic dysreflexia. The Journal of Neuroscience: The Official Journal of the Society for Neuroscience 26 (11), 2923–2932. http://dx.doi.org/10.1523/JNEUROSCI.4390-05.2006.

Cha, J., Heng, C., Reinkensmeyer, D.J., Roy, R.R., Edgerton, V.R., De Leon, R.D., 2007. Locomotor ability in spinal rats is dependent on the amount of activity imposed on the hindlimbs during treadmill training. Journal of Neurotrauma 24 (6), 1000–1012. http://dx.doi.org/10.1089/neu.2006.0233.

Cheetham, C., Green, D., Collis, J., Dembo, L., O'Driscoll, G., 2002. Effect of aerobic and resistance exercise on central hemodynamic responses in severe chronic heart failure. Journal of Applied Physiology 93 (1), 175–180. http://dx.doi.org/10.1152/japplphysiol.01240.2001.

Côté, M.-P., Azzam, G.A., Lemay, M.A., Zhukareva, V., Houlé, J.D., 2011. Activity-dependent increase in neurotrophic factors is associated with an enhanced modulation of spinal reflexes after spinal cord injury. Journal of Neurotrauma 28 (2), 299–309. http://dx.doi.org/10.1089/neu.2010.1594.

Côté, M.-P., Gandhi, S., Zambrotta, M., Houlé, J.D., 2014. Exercise modulates chloride homeostasis after spinal cord injury. The Journal of Neuroscience: The Official Journal of the Society for Neuroscience 34 (27), 8976–8987. http://dx.doi.org/10.1523/JNEUROSCI.0678-14.2014.

Courtine, G., Gerasimenko, Y., van den Brand, R., Yew, A., Musienko, P., Zhong, H., Song, B., Ao, Y., Ichiyama, R.M., Lavrov, I., Roy, R.R., Sofroniew, M.V., Edgerton, V.R., 2009. Transformation of nonfunctional spinal circuits into functional states after the loss of brain input. Nature Neuroscience 12 (10), 1333–1342. http://dx.doi.org/10.1038/nn.2401.

Curt, A., Keck, M.E., Dietz, V., 1998. Functional outcome following spinal cord injury: significance of motor-evoked potentials and ASIA scores. Archives of Physical Medicine and Rehabilitation 79 (1), 81–86. http://dx.doi.org/10.1016/S0003-9993(98)90213-1.

Dai, H., MacArthur, L., McAtee, M., Hockenbury, N., Tidwell, J.L., McHugh, B., Mansfield, K., Finn, T., Hamers, F.P., Bregman, B.S., 2009. Activity-based therapies to promote forelimb use after a cervical spinal cord injury. Journal of Neurotrauma 26 (10), 1719–1732. http://dx.doi.org/10.1089/neu.2008.0592.

Davidson, L., Hudson, R., Kilpatrick, K., 2009. Effects of exercise modality on insulin resistance and functional limitation in older adults: a randomized controlled trial. Archives of Internal Medicine 169 (2), 122–131. http://dx.doi.org/10.1001/archinternmed.2008.558.

De Leon, R.D., Hodgson, J.A., Roy, R.R., Edgerton, V.R., 1998. Full weight-bearing hindlimb standing following stand training in the adult spinal cat. Journal of Neurophysiology 80 (1), 83–91.

De Leon, R.D., Hodgson, J.A., Roy, R.R., Edgerton, V.R., 1999. Retention of hindlimb stepping ability in adult spinal cats after the cessation of step training. Journal of Neurophysiology 81 (1), 85–94.

Detloff, M.R., Smith, E.J., Quiros Molina, D., Ganzer, P.D., Houlé, J.D., 2014. Acute exercise prevents the development of neuropathic pain and the sprouting of non-peptidergic (GDNF- and artemin-responsive) c-fibers after spinal cord injury. Experimental Neurology 255, 38–48. http://dx.doi.org/10.1016/j.expneurol.2014.02.013.

Dobkin, B.H., Apple, D., Barbeau, H., Basso, M., Behrman, A., Deforge, D., Ditunno, J., Dudley, G., Elashoff, R., Fugate, L., Harkema, S., Saulino, M., Scott, M., Spinal Cord Injury Locomotor Trial (SCILT) Group, 2003. Methods for a randomized trial of weight-supported treadmill training versus conventional training for walking during inpatient rehabilitation after incomplete traumatic spinal cord injury. Neurorehabilitation and Neural Repair 17 (3), 153–167. http://dx.doi.org/10.1177/0888439003255508.

Dupont-Versteegden, E.E., Houlé, J.D., Dennis, R.A., Zhang, J., Knox, M., Wagoner, G., Peterson, C.A., 2004. Exercise-induced gene expression in soleus muscle is dependent on time after spinal cord injury in rats. Muscle and Nerve 29 (1), 73–81. http://dx.doi.org/10.1002/mus.10511.

Engesser-Cesar, C., Anderson, A.J., Basso, D.M., Edgerton, V.R., Cotman, C.W., 2005. Voluntary wheel running improves recovery from a moderate spinal cord injury. Journal of Neurotrauma 22 (1), 157–171. http://dx.doi.org/10.1089/neu.2005.22.157.

Engesser-Cesar, C., Ichiyama, R.M., Nefas, A.L., Hill, M.A., Edgerton, V.R., Cotman, C.W., Anderson, A.J., 2007. Wheel running following spinal cord injury improves locomotor recovery and stimulates serotonergic fiber growth. The European Journal of Neuroscience 25 (7), 1931–1939. http://dx.doi.org/10.1111/j.1460-9568.2007.05469.x.

Ernfors, P., Lee, K.F., Kucera, J., Jaenisch, R., 1994. Lack of neurotrophin-3 leads to deficiencies in the peripheral nervous system and loss of limb proprioceptive afferents. Cell 77 (4), 503–512.

Fouad, K., Metz, G.A.S., Merkler, D., Dietz, V., Schwab, M.E., 2000. Treadmill training in incomplete spinal cord injured rats. Behavioural Brain Research 115 (1), 107–113. http://dx.doi.org/10.1016/S0166-4328(00)00244-8.

Fouad, K., Tetzlaff, W., 2012. Rehabilitative training and plasticity following spinal cord injury. Experimental Neurology 235 (1), 91–99.

Ganzer, P.D., Manohar, A., Shumsky, J.S., Moxon, K.A., 2016. Therapy induces widespread reorganization of motor cortex after complete spinal transection that supports motor recovery. Experimental Neurology. http://dx.doi.org/10.1016/j.expneurol.2016.01.022.

García-Alías, G., Barkhuysen, S., Buckle, M., Fawcett, J.W., 2009. Chondroitinase ABC treatment opens a window of opportunity for task-specific rehabilitation. Nature Neuroscience 12 (9), 1145–1151. http://dx.doi.org/10.1038/nn.2377.

Ghiani, C.A., Ying, Z., de Vellis, J., Gomez-Pinilla, F., 2007. Exercise decreases myelin-associated glycoprotein expression in the spinal cord and positively modulates neuronal growth. Glia 55 (9), 966–975. http://dx.doi.org/10.1002/glia.20521.

Giehl, K.M., Tetzlaff, W., 1996. BDNF and NT-3, but not NGF, prevent axotomy-induced death of rat corticospinal neurons in vivo. The European Journal of Neuroscience 8 (6), 1167–1175.

Girgis, J., Merrett, D., Kirkland, S., Metz, G.A.S., Verge, V., Fouad, K., 2007. Reaching training in rats with spinal cord injury promotes plasticity and task specific recovery. Brain: A Journal of Neurology 130 (Pt 11), 2993–3003. http://dx.doi.org/10.1093/brain/awm245.

Goldshmit, Y., Lythgo, N., Galea, M.P., Turnley, A.M., 2008. Treadmill training after spinal cord hemisection in mice promotes axonal sprouting and synapse formation and improves motor recovery. Journal of Neurotrauma 25 (5), 449–465. http://dx.doi.org/10.1089/neu.2007.0392.

Gómez-Pinilla, F., Ying, Z., Opazo, P., Roy, R.R., Edgerton, V.R., 2001. Differential regulation by exercise of BDNF and NT-3 in rat spinal cord and skeletal muscle. The European Journal of Neuroscience 13 (6), 1078–1084. http://dx.doi.org/10.1046/j.0953-816x.2001.01484.x.

Gómez-Pinilla, F., Ying, Z., Roy, R., Molteni, R., Edgerton, R., 2002. Voluntary exercise induces a BDNF-mediated mechanism that promotes neuroplasticity. Journal of Neurophysiology 88 (5), 2187–2195. http://dx.doi.org/10.1152/jn.00152.2002.

Gonzenbach, R.R., Gasser, P., Zörner, B., Hochreutener, E., Dietz, V., Schwab, M.E., 2010. Nogo-A antibodies and training reduce muscle spasms in spinal cord-injured rats. Annals of Neurology 68 (1), 48–57. http://dx.doi.org/10.1002/ana.22009.

Grasso, R., Ivanenko, Y.P., Zago, M., Molinari, M., Scivoletto, G., Lacquaniti, F., 2004. Recovery of forward stepping in spinal cord injured patients does not transfer to untrained backward stepping. Experimental Brain Research 157 (3), 377–382. http://dx.doi.org/10.1007/s00221-004-1973-3.

Graziano, A., Foffani, G., Knudsen, E.B., Shumsky, J., Moxon, K.A., 2013. Passive exercise of the hind limbs after complete thoracic transection of the spinal cord promotes cortical reorganization. PLoS One 8 (1), e54350. http://dx.doi.org/10.1371/journal.pone.0054350.

Greenough, W.T., Larson, J.R., Withers, G.S., 1985. Effects of unilateral and bilateral training in a reaching task on dendritic branching of neurons in the rat motor-sensory forelimb cortex. Behavioral and Neural Biology 44 (2), 301–314.

Griesbach, G.S., Hovda, D.A., Gomez-Pinilla, F., 2009. Exercise-induced improvement in cognitive performance after traumatic brain injury in rats is dependent on BDNF activation. Brain Research 1288, 105–115. http://dx.doi.org/10.1016/j.brainres.2009.06.045.

Grill, R., Murai, K., Blesch, A., Gage, F.H., Tuszynski, M.H., 1997. Cellular delivery of neurotrophin-3 promotes corticospinal axonal growth and partial functional recovery after spinal cord injury. The Journal of Neuroscience: The Official Journal of the Society for Neuroscience 17 (14), 5560–5572.

Hicks, A.L., Martin, K.A., Ditor, D.S., Latimer, A.E., Craven, C., Bugaresti, J., McCartney, N., 2003. Long-term exercise training in persons with spinal cord injury: effects on strength, arm ergometry performance and psychological well-being. Spinal Cord 41 (1), 34–43. http://dx.doi.org/10.1038/sj.sc.3101389.

Houle, J.D., Côté, M.-P., 2013. Axon regeneration and exercise-dependent plasticity after spinal cord injury. Annals of the New York Academy of Sciences 1279 (1), 154–163. http://dx.doi.org/10.1111/nyas.12052.

Hutchinson, K.J., Gómez-Pinilla, F., Crowe, M.J., Ying, Z., Basso, D.M., 2004. Three exercise paradigms differentially improve sensory recovery after spinal cord contusion in rats. Brain: A Journal of Neurology 127 (Pt 6), 1403–1414. http://dx.doi.org/10.1093/brain/awh160.

Ichiyama, R., Broman, J., Roy, R., Zhong, H., Edgerton, R., Havton, L., 2011. Locomotor training maintains normal inhibitory influence on both alpha- and gamma-motoneurons after neonatal spinal cord transection. The Journal of Neuroscience: The Official Journal of the Society for Neuroscience 31 (1), 26–33. http://dx.doi.org/10.1523/JNEUROSCI.6433-09.2011.

Ichiyama, R., Courtine, G., Gerasimenko, Y.P., Yang, G.J., van den Brand, R., Lavrov, I.A., Zhong, H., Roy, R.R., Edgerton, V.R., 2008. Step training reinforces specific spinal locomotor circuitry in adult spinal rats. The Journal of Neuroscience: The Official Journal of the Society for Neuroscience 28 (29), 7370–7375. http://dx.doi.org/10.1523/JNEUROSCI.1881-08.2008.

Ichiyama, R., Potuzak, M., Balak, M., Kalderon, N., Edgerton, R., 2009. Enhanced motor function by training in spinal cord contused rats following radiation therapy. PLoS One 4 (8), e6862. http://dx.doi.org/10.1371/journal.pone.0006862.

IV. EXERCISE AS THERAPY FOR NEUROLOGICAL DISEASES

Jacobs, P.L., Nash, M.S., 2004. Exercise recommendations for individuals with spinal cord injury. Sports Medicine (Auckland, N.Z.) 34 (11), 727–751.

Kleim, J.A., Barbay, S., Nudo, R.J., 1998. Functional reorganization of the rat motor cortex following motor skill learning. Journal of Neurophysiology 80 (6), 3321–3325.

Kleim, J.A., Hogg, T.M., VandenBerg, P.M., Cooper, N.R., Bruneau, R., Remple, M., 2004. Cortical synaptogenesis and motor map reorganization occur during late, but not early, phase of motor skill learning. The Journal of Neuroscience: The Official Journal of the Society for Neuroscience 24 (3), 628–633. http://dx.doi.org/10.1523/JNEUROSCI.3440-03.2004.

Krajacic, A., Ghosh, M., Puentes, R., Pearse, D.D., Fouad, K., 2009. Advantages of delaying the onset of rehabilitative reaching training in rats with incomplete spinal cord injury. The European Journal of Neuroscience 29 (3), 641–651. http://dx.doi.org/10.1111/j.1460-9568.2008.06600.x.

Krajacic, A., Weishaupt, N., Girgis, J., Tetzlaff, W., Fouad, K., 2010. Training-induced plasticity in rats with cervical spinal cord injury: effects and side effects. Behavioural Brain Research 214 (2), 323–331. http://dx.doi.org/10.1016/j.bbr.2010.05.053.

Krassioukov, A., Claydon, V.E., 2006. The clinical problems in cardiovascular control following spinal cord injury: an overview. In: Weaver, L.C., Polosa, C. (Eds.), Progress in Brain Research, vol. 152. Elsevier, pp. 223–229. Retrieved from: http://www.sciencedirect.com/science/article/pii/S0079612305520144.

Krenz, N.R., Meakin, S.O., Krassioukov, A.V., Weaver, L.C., 1999. Neutralizing intraspinal nerve growth factor blocks autonomic dysreflexia caused by spinal cord injury. The Journal of Neuroscience: The Official Journal of the Society for Neuroscience 19 (17), 7405–7414.

Krenz, N.R., Weaver, L.C., 1998. Sprouting of primary afferent fibers after spinal cord transection in the rat. Neuroscience 85 (2), 443–458.

Lankhorst, A.J., ter Laak, M.P., van Laar, T.J., van Meeteren, N.L., de Groot, J.C., Schrama, L.H., Hamers, F.P., Gispen, W.-H., 2001. Effects of enriched housing on functional recovery after spinal cord contusive injury in the adult rat. Journal of Neurotrauma 18 (2), 203–215. http://dx.doi.org/10.1089/08977150150502622.

Liebl, D.J., Tessarollo, L., Palko, M.E., Parada, L.F., 1997. Absence of sensory neurons before target innervation in brain-derived neurotrophic factor-, neurotrophin 3-, and TrkC-deficient embryonic mice. The Journal of Neuroscience: The Official Journal of the Society for Neuroscience 17 (23), 9113–9121.

Liu, G., Detloff, M.R., Miller, K.N., Santi, L., Houlé, J.D., 2012. Exercise modulates microRNAs that affect the PTEN/mTOR pathway in rats after spinal cord injury. Experimental Neurology 233 (1), 447–456. http://dx.doi.org/10.1016/j.expneurol.2011.11.018.

Liu, K., Lu, Y., Lee, J.K., Samara, R., Willenberg, R., Sears-Kraxberger, I., Tedeschi, A., Kyungsuk Park, K., Jin, D., Cai, B., Xu, B., Connolly, L., Steward, O., Zheng, B., He, Z., 2010. PTEN deletion enhances the regenerative ability of adult corticospinal neurons. Nature Neuroscience 13 (9), 1075–1081. http://dx.doi.org/10.1038/nn.2603.

Lovely, R.G., Gregor, R.J., Roy, R.R., Edgerton, V.R., 1986. Effects of training on the recovery of full-weight-bearing stepping in the adult spinal cat. Experimental Neurology 92 (2), 421–435.

Macias, M., Nowicka, D., Czupryn, A., Sulejczak, D., Skup, M., Skangiel-Kramska, J., Czarkowska-Bauch, J., 2009. Exercise-induced motor improvement after complete spinal cord transection and its relation to expression of brain-derived neurotrophic factor and presynaptic markers. BMC Neuroscience 10, 144. http://dx.doi.org/10.1186/1471-2202-10-144.

Maier, I.C., Ichiyama, R.M., Courtine, G., Schnell, L., Lavrov, I., Edgerton, V.R., Schwab, M.E., 2009. Differential effects of anti-Nogo-A antibody treatment and treadmill training in rats with incomplete spinal cord injury. Brain: A Journal of Neurology 132 (Pt 6), 1426–1440. http://dx.doi.org/10.1093/brain/awp085.

Maldonado, M.A., Allred, R.P., Felthauser, E.L., Jones, T.A., 2008. Motor skill training, but not voluntary exercise, improves skilled reaching after unilateral ischemic lesions of the sensorimotor cortex in rats. Neurorehabilitation and Neural Repair 22 (3), 250–261. http://dx.doi.org/10.1177/1545968307308551.

Marsh, B.C., Astill, S.L., Utley, A., Ichiyama, R.M., 2011. Movement rehabilitation after spinal cord injuries: emerging concepts and future directions. Brain Research Bulletin 84 (4), 327–336.

Mohr, T., Podenphant, J., Biering-Sorensen, F., Galbo, H., Thamsborg, G., Kjaer, M., 1997. Increased bone mineral density after prolonged electrically induced cycle training of paralyzed limbs in spinal cord injured man. Calcified Tissue International 61 (1), 22–25.

Multon, S., Franzen, R., Poirrier, A.-L., Scholtes, F., Schoenen, J., 2003. The effect of treadmill training on motor recovery after a partial spinal cord compression-injury in the adult rat. Journal of Neurotrauma 20 (8), 699–706. http://dx.doi.org/10.1089/089771503767869935.

Murray, K.C., Nakae, A., Stephens, M.J., Rank, M., D'Amico, J., Harvey, P.J., Li, X., Harris, R.L., Ballou, E.W., Anelli, R., Heckman, C.J., Mashimo, T., Vavrek, R., Sanelli, L., Gorassini, M.A., Bennett, D.J., Fouad, K., 2010. Recovery of motoneuron and locomotor function after spinal cord injury depends on constitutive activity in 5-HT2C receptors. Nature Medicine 16 (6), 694–700. http://dx.doi.org/10.1038/nm.2160.

Norrie, B.A., Nevett-Duchcherer, J.M., Gorassini, M.A., 2005. Reduced functional recovery by delaying motor training after spinal cord injury. Journal of Neurophysiology 94 (1), 255–264. http://dx.doi.org/10.1152/jn.00970.2004.

Nudo, R.J., Milliken, G.W., Jenkins, W.M., Merzenich, M.M., 1996. Use-dependent alterations of movement representations in primary motor cortex of adult squirrel monkeys. The Journal of Neuroscience: The Official Journal of the Society for Neuroscience 16 (2), 785–807.

Ollivier-Lanvin, K., Keeler, B.E., Siegfried, R., Houlé, J.D., Lemay, M.A., 2010. Proprioceptive neuropathy affects normalization of the H-reflex by exercise after spinal cord injury. Experimental Neurology 221 (1), 198–205. http://dx.doi.org/10.1016/j.expneurol.2009.10.023.

Park, K.K., Liu, K., Hu, Y., Smith, P.D., Wang, C., Cai, B., Xu, B., Connolly, L., Kramvis, I., Sahin, M., He, Z., 2008. Promoting axon regeneration in the adult CNS by modulation of the PTEN/mTOR pathway. Science (New York, N.Y.) 322 (5903), 963–966. http://dx.doi.org/10.1126/science.1161566.

Petruska, J.C., Ichiyama, R.M., Jindrich, D.L., Crown, E.D., Tansey, K.E., Roy, R.R., Edgerton, V.R., Mendell, L.M., 2007. Changes in motoneuron properties and synaptic inputs related to step training after spinal cord transection in rats. The Journal of Neuroscience: The Official Journal of the Society for Neuroscience 27 (16), 4460–4471. http://dx.doi.org/10.1523/JNEUROSCI.2302-06.2007.

Phadke, C.P., Flynn, S.M., Thompson, F.J., Behrman, A.L., Trimble, M.H., Kukulka, C.G., 2009. Comparison of single bout effects of bicycle training versus locomotor training on paired reflex depression of the soleus H-reflex after motor incomplete spinal cord injury. Archives of Physical Medicine and Rehabilitation 90 (7), 1218–1228. http://dx.doi.org/10.1016/j.apmr.2009.01.022.

Ploughman, M., Windle, V., MacLellan, C.L., White, N., Doré, J.J., Corbett, D., 2009. Brain-derived neurotrophic factor contributes to recovery of skilled reaching after focal ischemia in rats. Stroke 40 (4), 1490–1495. http://dx.doi.org/10.1161/STROKEAHA.108.531806.

Sadowsky, C.L., Hammond, E.R., Strohl, A.B., Commean, P.K., Eby, S.A., Damiano, D.L., Wingert, J.R., Bae, K.T., McDonald, J.W., 2013. Lower extremity functional electrical stimulation cycling promotes physical and functional recovery in chronic spinal cord injury. The Journal of Spinal Cord Medicine 36 (6), 623–631. http://dx.doi.org/10.1179/2045772313Y.0000000101.

Sandrow-Feinberg, H.R., Houlé, J.D., 2015. Exercise after spinal cord injury as an agent for neuroprotection, regeneration and rehabilitation. Brain Research 1619, 12–21. http://dx.doi.org/10.1016/j.brainres.2015.03.052.

Sandrow-Feinberg, H.R., Izzi, J., Shumsky, J.S., Zhukareva, V., Houle, J.D., 2009. Forced exercise as a rehabilitation strategy after unilateral cervical spinal cord contusion injury. Journal of Neurotrauma 26 (5), 721–731. http://dx.doi.org/10.1089/neu.2008.0750.

Sanes, J.N., Donoghue, J.P., 2000. Plasticity and primary motor cortex. Annual Review of Neuroscience 23, 393–415. http://dx.doi.org/10.1146/annurev.neuro.23.1.393.

Shephard, R.J., 1968. Intensity, duration and frequency of exercise as determinants of the response to a training regime. Internationale Zeitschrift fu¨r Angewandte Physiologie, Einschliesslich Arbeitsphysiologie 26 (3), 272–278.

Singh, A., Murray, M., Houle, J.D., 2011. A training paradigm to enhance motor recovery in contused rats: effects of staircase training. Neurorehabilitation and Neural Repair 25 (1), 24–34. http://dx.doi.org/10.1177/1545968310378510.

Skinner, R.D., Houle, J.D., Reese, N.B., Berry, C.L., Garcia-Rill, E., 1996. Effects of exercise and fetal spinal cord implants on the H-reflex in chronically spinalized adult rats. Brain Research 729 (1), 127–131. http://dx.doi.org/10.1016/0006-8993(96)00556-2.

Smith, C., Mauricio, R., Nobre, L., Marsh, B., Wüst, R.C., Rossiter, H.B., Ichiyama, R.M., 2015. Differential regulation of perineuronal nets in the brain and spinal cord with exercise training. Brain Research Bulletin 111, 20–26. http://dx.doi.org/10.1016/j.brainresbull.2014.12.005.

Smith, R., Shum-Siu, A., Baltzley, R., Bunger, M., Baldini, A., Burke, D.A., Magnuson, D.S.K., 2006. Effects of swimming on functional recovery after incomplete spinal cord injury in rats. Journal of Neurotrauma 23 (6), 908–919. http://dx.doi.org/10.1089/neu.2006.23.908.

Starkey, M.L., Schwab, M.E., 2012. Anti-Nogo-A and training: can one plus one equal three? Experimental Neurology 235 (1), 53–61. http://dx.doi.org/10.1016/j.expneurol.2011.04.008.

Swain, R.A., Harris, A.B., Wiener, E.C., Dutka, M.V., Morris, H.D., Theien, B.E., Konda, S., Engberg, K., Lauterbur, P.C., Greenough, W.T., 2003. Prolonged exercise induces angiogenesis and increases cerebral blood volume in primary motor cortex of the rat. Neuroscience 117 (4), 1037–1046. http://dx.doi.org/10.1016/S0306-4522(02)00664-4.

Tashiro, S., Shinozaki, M., Mukaino, M., Renault-Mihara, F., Toyama, Y., Liu, M., Nakamura, M., Okano, H., 2015. BDNF induced by treadmill training contributes to the suppression of spasticity and allodynia after spinal cord injury via upregulation of KCC2. Neurorehabilitation and Neural Repair 29 (7), 677–689. http://dx.doi.org/10.1177/1545968314562110.

Tessarollo, L., Vogel, K.S., Palko, M.E., Reid, S.W., Parada, L.F., 1994. Targeted mutation in the neurotrophin-3 gene results in loss of muscle sensory neurons. Proceedings of the National Academy of Sciences of the United States of America 91 (25), 11844–11848.

Tiidus, P., Ianuzzo, C., 1982. Effects of intensity and duration of muscular exercise on delayed soreness and serum enzyme activities. Medicine and Science in Sports and Exercise 15 (6), 461–465.

van Hedel, H.J.A., Dietz, V., 2010. Rehabilitation of locomotion after spinal cord injury. Restorative Neurology and Neuroscience 28 (1), 123–134. http://dx.doi.org/10.3233/RNN-2010-0508.

Wainberg, M., Barbeau, H., Gauthier, S., 1990. The effects of cyproheptadine on locomotion and on spasticity in patients with spinal cord injuries. Journal of Neurology, Neurosurgery and Psychiatry 53 (9), 754–763. http://dx.doi.org/10.1136/jnnp.53.9.754.

Wang, H., Liu, N.-K., Zhang, Y.P., Deng, L., Lu, Q.B., Shields, C.B., Walker, M.J., Li, J., Xu, X.-M., 2015. Treadmill training induced lumbar motoneuron dendritic plasticity and behavior recovery in adult rats after a thoracic contusive spinal cord injury. Experimental Neurology 271, 368–378. http://dx.doi.org/10.1016/j.expneurol.2015.07.004.

Weishaupt, N., Blesch, A., Fouad, K., 2012. BDNF: the career of a multifaceted neurotrophin in spinal cord injury. Experimental Neurology 238 (2), 254–264. http://dx.doi.org/10.1016/j.expneurol.2012.09.001.

Wenger, H.A., Bell, G.J., 1986. The interactions of intensity, frequency and duration of exercise training in altering cardiorespiratory fitness. Sports Medicine (Auckland, N.Z.) 3 (5), 346–356.

Wessels, M., Lucas, C., Eriks, I., de Groot, S., 2010. Body weight-supported gait training for restoration of walking in people with an incomplete spinal cord injury: a systematic review. Journal of Rehabilitation Medicine 42 (6), 513–519. http://dx.doi.org/10.2340/16501977-0525.

West, C.R., Crawford, M.A., Laher, I., Ramer, M.S., Krassioukov, A.V., 2015. Passive hind-limb cycling reduces the severity of autonomic dysreflexia after experimental spinal cord injury. Neurorehabilitation and Neural Repair. http://dx.doi.org/10.1177/1545968315593807.

Withers, G.S., Greenough, W.T., 1989. Reach training selectively alters dendritic branching in subpopulations of layer II-III pyramids in rat motor-somatosensory forelimb cortex. Neuropsychologia 27 (1), 61–69.

Ying, Z., Roy, R.R., Edgerton, V.R., Gómez-Pinilla, F., 2005. Exercise restores levels of neurotrophins and synaptic plasticity following spinal cord injury. Experimental Neurology 193 (2), 411–419. http://dx.doi.org/10.1016/j.expneurol.2005.01.015.

Ying, Z., Roy, R.R., Zhong, H., Zdunowski, S., Edgerton, V.R., Gomez-Pinilla, F., 2008. BDNF-exercise interactions in the recovery of symmetrical stepping after a cervical hemisection in rats. Neuroscience 155 (4), 1070–1078. http://dx.doi.org/10.1016/j.neuroscience.2008.06.057.

12

Neural Structure, Connectivity, and Cognition Changes Associated to Physical Exercise

S. Bonavita, G. Tedeschi

1st Clinic of Neurology, Second University of Naples, Naples, Italy

Abstract

Cognition is affected by aging with attention and memory being the most affected domains. A significant contribution to age-related declines is represented by impairment of executive functions (EF) that depend on prefrontal cortex, indeed age-related decline in cortical thickness is greatest in the frontal, and prefrontal areas. Variability in cognitive performances among elderly people may find explanation in several factors; among these, lifestyle differences have been associated with different cognitive features. Better cognitive performances have been associated with active lifestyles, with aerobic exercise benefitting especially EF. Neuroimaging studies, indeed, have shown that increased cardiorespiratory fitness and active aerobic exercise positively impact brain structure and function in particular in cortical areas and neural circuits involved in EF.

INTRODUCTION

Cognition, as well as brain structure and function, is affected by aging in a variable way across people. Age-related changes are not uniform through the cognitive domains or across individual elderly subjects. The cognitive domains most affected by age are attention and memory, however, language processing and decision making may also be impaired. Moreover, a significant contribution to age-related declines is represented by impairment of executive function (EF). Declines in attention may deeply impact everyday life; elderly people, are slower than younger adults in performing selective attention tasks (i.e., Stroop color test), and even more in the divided attention.

Memory complaints are often reported by elderly people; episodic memory (personal experiences occurred in a specific place and at a particular time) seems susceptible to age-related brain damage, particularly in the prefrontal regions, as well as the retrieval of information depending on the hippocampus and prefrontal cortex function. An aspect of episodic memory that may be impaired in aging people is the storage and consolidation of information that depend on the integrity of medial temporal lobe (MTL) structures, particularly the hippocampus. On the other hand, semantic and autobiographical memory, as well as procedural, perspective, and implicit memory are largely preserved with age. Working memory, which implies the active manipulation of information and the involvement of attention capabilities, is also impaired in older adults as a result of the reduction of divided attention performances (for all the previously reported data, see Glisky, 2007).

Neuroimaging studies (Wager and Smith, 2003) demonstrated a significant involvement of dorsolateral prefrontal cortex (PFC) in the manipulation of information in working memory task, with the left PFC involved more in verbal tasks and the right PFC in visuospatial tasks.

A simplistic interpretation of age-related cognitive declines confers a causal role to executive control deficits. EF consists of working memory, task flexibility, and problem solving, as well as planning and execution of tasks; it depends critically on PFC, via extensive reciprocal connections with posterior cortical regions. The hypothesis that the deficit of EF may be the main responsibility for age-related cognitive decline finds support in structural and functional magnetic resonance imaging (fMRI) studies revealing in older adults the almost specific reduction in volume and function in prefrontal brain regions (West, 1996).

Variability in cognitive performances among elderly people may find some explanation in biological and psychological factors, as well as environmental and lifestyle differences. In terms of biological factors, a possible explanation may rely on the different implementation of compensatory mechanisms. Indeed, fMRI studies have found different patterns of brain activation in older and younger adults while performing identical memory tasks: older adults, particularly if "high-performing," showed a bilateral activation of brain areas that in young subjects were activated only unilaterally (Cabeza et al., 2002). This increased activation has been interpreted as a compensatory mechanism, operated by a reorganization of the aging brain. Recently, particular attention has been focused on lifestyle variables as a source of variance in differential cognitive aging. Better cognitive performances are associated with active lifestyles, and furthermore aerobic exercise has been shown to benefit especially EF (Colcombe and Kramer, 2003).

Indeed, physical exercise can preserve brain health and cognitive function under normal or disease conditions, and protects against cognitive decline and neurodegenerative diseases (Meeusen, 2005).

Physiological Mechanisms Underlying Cognitive Improvement After Physical Exercise

The mechanisms to explain the effects of physical exercise on cognition are far to be completely known, however, there may be some possible interpretation either at a cellular or at a behavioral level.

At a cellular level, it has been shown that the mammalian brain exhibits persistent plasticity throughout all stages of life (Leuner and Gould, 2010). Neuronal plasticity allows to learn new skills, to consolidate and retrieve memories, to reorganize neuronal networks, particularly in response to environmental stimuli (Knaepen et al., 2010). In particular, the hippocampus is a highly plastic region associated with spatial memory (Knaepen et al., 2010), and declarative memory consolidation (Leahey and Harris, 2001) that is formed by two areas, the cornus ammonis and the dentate gyrus (DG). The DG seems to be involved in the capacity of discriminating between stimuli (Marr, 1971), is able, in rodents, to generate new neurons, and can double or triple in size after physical exercise (van Praag, 2008). Indeed, in rodents, physical exercise may induce hippocampal neurogenesis, cell proliferation, and dendritic branching (Eadie et al., 2005); moreover, voluntary exercise on the activity wheel for 7 days could enhance brain-derived neurotrophic factor (BDNF) gene expression in the hippocampus and in the caudal region of the neocortex (Neeper et al., 1995). In this regard, it is worthwhile to pinpoint that peripheral levels of this neurotrophin have been proposed to be associated with cognition in mice (Pang et al., 2004). It is well-known that physical exercise is a compelling stimulant of angiogenesis during development or in the adult brain (Bloor, 2005) and that these effects seem to be mediated by insulin growth factors (IGF-1) and BDNF. In particular, it has been shown that resistance training increases blood levels of IGF-1 in humans (Vale et al., 2009) and positive correlations have been reported between increased blood IGF-1 levels and cognitive function improvement (Kalmijn et al., 2000). Other trophic factors, such as nerve growth factor, vascular endothelial growth factor, and fibroblast growth factor 2, may be influenced by physical exercise (Neeper et al., 1996; Gomez-Pinilla et al., 1997) and have been proposed to promote exercise-induced neurogenesis; the increase of these neurotrophins, indeed, may result in angiogenesis and ultimately in neurogenesis (Trejo et al., 2008).

At a behavioral level, it is possible that, with practice, tasks become automatic, and less demanding in terms of attention. Alternatively, continuous physical training may facilitate the development of less attention demanding strategies.

The amelioration of task performances after aerobic exercise concerns tasks involving executive control of attention, largely controlled by PFC.

It has been hypothesized that cardiovascular fitness may improve the efficiency of neural processes or may provide increased metabolic resources for task performance.

Effective Connectivity and Functional Connectivity

Neuroimaging studies showed that aerobic exercise impacts on neural circuitries either during the performance of cognitive tasks or during a resting condition. To better understand the studies (reported in the following) on the effect of physical exercise on cognition and brain structure/function, it is worth to explain the concept of brain connectivity, including differences between effective connectivity (EC) and functional connectivity (FC).

EC refers to the influence of a neuronal system upon another and to the interactions between activated brain areas. The founding concept is that connectivity links together different brain areas involved in a certain processing of information; strictly linked to the concept of connectivity is the pivotal role of brain networks. These are different functionally interacting brain regions, that may be distant in anatomical space but linked via long-range connections. FC refers to the temporal coherence between the oscillatory firing rate of neuronal groups (Friston, 1994). fMRI, that relies on blood-oxygen-level-dependent (BOLD) signal, by detecting the temporal correlation between fluctuations in the BOLD signal of discrete anatomical regions (Fox and Raichle, 2007) is capable of identifying correlated activities within brain networks.

It is now recognized that the brain is constantly active, even if the subjects are in a resting state condition, without performing a cognitive task or being exposed to external stimuli. These self-referential states are thought to arise from neuronal activity coherently organized in the so-called default mode network (DMN), a network of brain regions, including precuneus/posterior cingulate cortex (PCC), medial PFC (MPFC), and medial, lateral, and inferior parietal cortex. The DMN is active in the resting state with a high degree of FC between brain areas, particularly PCC and ventral anterior cingulate cortex (ACC), while it is attenuated immediately before and during task performance (Greicius et al., 2003). The DMN has received much attention for its capacity to predict individual cognitive differences in diseases such as Alzheimer's disease (AD) and mild cognitive impairment (MCI), as well as cognitive performance in healthy college-age and elderly adults. Beside the DMN, there are other networks at rest (Damoiseaux et al., 2006) that adaptively reorganize themselves in a task-related and goal-oriented manner. During cognitive tasks requiring self-referential thought or working memory only specific DMN regions are specifically deactivated (Broyd et al., 2009). For this peculiarity, several studies indicated that FC changes in DMN have potential utility in distinguishing between AD and healthy controls (Greicius et al., 2004). Resting state fMRI thus seems to provide connectivity-related biomarkers that distinguish AD patients from normal controls; therefore, the study of DMN connectivity is particularly useful to identify functional changes associated to cognitive impairment. However, it is still unclear whether functional abnormalities of the DMN are causal rather than the result of the pathology. The structural substrate of the DMN has been identified by diffusion tensor imaging tractography combined with resting state fMRI. Beside the MPFC, PCC, and ACC, the DMN includes MTLs. These regions are thought to be engaged in episodic memory processing. The fMRI connectivity maps combined with DTI analysis showed structural connections between the MTLs and the retrosplenial cortex (RSC), while MPFC is connected with the PCC, and indicate that FC (deduced from resting state fMRI) indeed reflects structural connections. Therefore, we anticipate that fMRI changes induced by physical exercise depend mainly and/or primarily on FC changes and more profoundly by structural changes.

Neuroimaging studies investigating associations between fitness levels, cognitive performances, and the pattern of brain FC on one side, and the potential changes induced by active physical training intervention (either at a behavioral level or structural/functional) on the other, are particularly interesting to better understand the neural correlates of cardiorespiratory fitness (CRF) level and cognition in the normal brain.

Neuroimaging Studies in Healthy People

Structural Studies

In terms of structural changes, in older adults, increased aerobic fitness levels were associated with increased volume in the right and left hippocampi, and this correlation sustains the relationship between aerobic fitness and spatial memory performance (Erickson et al., 2009).

A number of evidences from the current literature strongly suggest that active physical exercise impacts on brain structure. An interesting study by Hamzei et al. (2012) investigated the time course of gray matter (GM) changes and the association between GM changes and the parallel, dynamic course of the functional modulation during the time duration of a short motor skill training. Healthy subjects were trained to perform a specific motor skill (writing their signature with the nondominant left hand) during four sessions of 30 min per day over a 5-day-period (this duration is the shortest reported time period necessary to induce GM changes (May et al., 2007)) The subjects were scanned on a daily basis to capture the initial stages and temporal dynamics of the structural and functional task-related changes and to investigate the association between the functional and structural changes in the motor network.

Structural changes were evaluated by voxel-based morphometry and functional changes by fMRI acquired during task performance. The performance improvement over the motor skill training period was associated with an increase of GM volume in distinct secondary cortical motor areas. A very early significant GM increase occurred after 3 days of training in the right ventral striatum; this early GM change within ventral striatum was functionally linked to the training associated GM changes within several cortical regions. Consequently, the authors suggested that motor skill training promotes structural change that is based on a dynamic functional integrative network processing between striatum and secondary cortical motor areas.

If we equalize motor learning (i.e., learning of motor sequences) to physical exercise we may hypothesize that similar structural changes may occur early after physical training and may thus influence cortical networks involved in different tasks (likely including cognitive ones). Probably, different patterns of plastic changes apply for different types of tasks.

Taubert et al. (2010) reported structural GM and white matter (WM) changes in response to balance training and demonstrated (Taubert et al., 2011) a tight positive correlation between training-induced functional and structural brain plasticity. They trained subjects in a dynamic balance task for 45 min once a week over 6 consecutive weeks and acquired resting-state fMRI prior to training, and later in the 1, 3, 5, and 7 weeks after training. By using a sophisticated network analysis technique (the eigenvector centrality mapping), they identified regions in which FC increased as a result of training; moreover, by multimodal correlation analyses they investigated whether functional and structural changes occurring in the same brain networks within the same participants had comparable temporal dynamics across the 6 weeks of training. Increased fronto-parietal network connectivity was evident 1 week after two brief motor training sessions. Repeated training sessions over 6 consecutive weeks progressively modulated these changes in accordance with individual performance improvements. These coincident changes were most prominent in the first 3 weeks of training. In contrast, changes in fronto-parietal FC and the underlying WM fibers structure developed gradually during the 6 weeks. These resting state fMRI highlighted the persistence of balance training-induced functional changes.

FC Studies on Relationship Between CRF Levels and Cognitive Performances

Age-related differences in neural connectivity and brain structure exist between young and elderly adults; indeed, age-related decline in cortical thickness is greatest in the frontal, prefrontal, and parietal cortices (Raz, 2000), regions that are also thought to support EF, which show the greatest behavioral improvement with CRF training in aging humans (Colcombe et al., 2004). EF can be investigated by fMRI studies while patients perform an executive task requiring to inhibit or filter misleading information provided by incongruent (Inc) stimuli. Indeed, neuroimaging studies showed that regions implicated in selective attention and resolution of response conflict are electively the frontal and parietal cortices, particularly the middle frontal gyrus (MFG), superior frontal gyrus (SFG), and the superior and inferior parietal lobules (SPL and IPL). Successful task completion in the presence of Inc stimuli would require older adults to invoke selective spatial attention through the frontal and parietal circuitry; if this circuitry is properly working, the information provided by the peripheral stimuli is reduced, which then leads to reduction in conflict at the response stage, and facilitation of the correct response. As a result, the successful involvement of the attentional network in the presence of conflicting response cues should result in a relative decrease in reaction time to Inc trials, as well as a reduction of task-related activity in the ACC, a region of the DMN known to be sensitive to response conflict (Casey et al., 2000).

With respect to resting state FC changes induced by exercise or associated to CRF, many neuroimaging studies focused on the DMN because of its reported disruption in healthy cognitive aging (Andrews-Hanna et al., 2007; Damoiseaux et al., 2008), and its association with diagnosis of AD (Greicius et al., 2004). In the context of healthy aging, specific network disruptions between the PCC/RSC and the frontal medial cortex (FMC) and the medial temporal and hippocampal/parahippocampal cortices are preferentially associated with age-related cognitive decline (Andrews-Hanna et al., 2007). Moreover, a disrupted connectivity is most apparent along an anterior–posterior anatomical dimension and is a source of variance in cognitive performance.

Healthy lifestyle factors are associated with increased cognitive and cortical function. So far, it has been demonstrated that increased aerobic fitness is structurally and functionally neuroprotective in healthy older adults, and may even delay the onset, or reduce the rate of decline of AD and vascular dementias (Colcombe et al., 2006).

Voss et al. (2010) examined whether increased FC of the DMN, as a function of aerobic fitness level, reflects a mechanism by which increased fitness is associated with better cognitive performance on tests of EF and memory. They studied two groups of individuals, college-age and elderly participants, by a seed-based FC analysis, to find areas most characteristic of age-related dysfunctional connectivity with the PCC/RSC. They also examined whether in the group of elderly adults aerobic fitness was associated with increased FC in the same areas that showed the largest age-related differences in connectivity, and whether increased connectivity, as a function of increased fitness, was associated with better cognitive performance on tests of EF and spatial memory. They studied 32 young adults (YA) and 120 elderly participants cognitively preserved, who were evaluated for aerobic fitness level and underwent a switching task, the Wisconsin Card Sorting Task (WCST) (assessing working memory, inhibition, and switching processes), and a spatial memory paradigm previously associated with aerobic fitness and hippocampal volume (Erickson et al., 2009). fMRI scans were acquired during three passive viewing tasks for FC seeding analysis. Age-related differences in FC with the PCC/RSC showed five ROIs of interest, derived from the age-group analysis, including the left MFG, FMC, bilateral medial temporal gyri (MTG), PCC, and bilateral parahippocampal gyri (PHG). The analysis on the direct effects of aerobic fitness on cognition in the elderly adults showed that increased aerobic fitness was associated with fewer perseverative errors on the WCST; with better average accuracy and mean response time across all levels of the spatial memory task. In elderly adults, the connection between the PCC and

MFG showed a statistically significant positive association with aerobic fitness; the connection between the PCC and FMC was associated with better performances in the switching task; and faster response speed in the spatial memory task was associated with greater connectivity in MFG/FMC. With a Multiple Mediator Model analysis, the authors examined the extent to which increased connectivity, as positively associated with aerobic fitness, was correlated with individual differences in cognitive function. With respect to perseverative errors in the WCST, the 18.8% of the total effect was attributable to PCC–FMC connectivity; while for the local switch cost (attentional set reconfiguration and inhibition) at the switching task, the 14.7% of the total effect was attributable to MTG–MFG connectivity. These results show that long-range connectivity between the PCC/RSC and the FMC is associated with better cognitive performance in elderly and particularly that FC along the same direction (anterior–posterior) mediates the association between aerobic fitness and performance on a classic test of EF, the WCST. Therefore aerobic fitness training may lead to increased DMN connectivity and in turn provide a pathway for improved EF.

A growing body of literature illustrates that higher levels of aerobic fitness also relate to higher academic achievement, superior cognitive abilities, larger brain structures, and elevated brain function in children (Castelli et al., 2007; Chaddock et al., 2010; Hillman and Kramer, 2012). To examine the association between aerobic fitness and brain function in children, Chaddock et al. (2012) used fMRI focusing on differences in brain activity of high fit (HF) and low fit (LF) children during a cognitive control task. They studied 14 HF and 18 LF children who underwent an fMRI scan during an event related modified Eriksen flanker task (Eriksen and Eriksen, 1974). The task consisted in responding differently to different (congruent (Con) and Inc) stimuli: array of arrows presented on an MRI back projection (a Con trial consisted of >>>>> and <<<<< arrow displays in which the target arrow was flanked by arrows of the same direction. An Inc trial consisted of >><>> and <<><< arrow displays in which the target arrow was flanked by the opposing arrow response). Changes in accuracy across the experiment varied as a function of both aerobic fitness, group and task condition; indeed, it decreased during Inc task in both groups but HF participants maintained their accuracy on Inc trials across both early and late task blocks, while LF participants showed decreased performance during the late task block relative to the early task block. fMRI brain activation measured during the flanker paradigm helped providing a neural substrate for differences in performance as a function of aerobic fitness. During the Con condition, all children, regardless of aerobic fitness level, had greater activation in the prefrontal and parietal cortex (i.e., LMFG, supplementary motor area (SMA), ACC, LSPL) early in task performance, followed by a significant reduction in activity in these regions later in the task. When increased cognitive demands were required during the Inc condition, HF children showed greater activation than LF children in the prefrontal and parietal cortex (i.e., LMFG, RMFG, SMA, ACC, LSPL) during the early task block, and only HF children demonstrated a decrease in brain activity in these regions across time, while maintaining a high level of accuracy. LF children, on the other hand, demonstrated a decrease in accuracy in Inc trials between the first and second halves of the task block, coupled with no change in fMRI activity in most regions of the attentional network. This pattern of results suggested that changes in brain activity across a flanker task vary as a function of childhood aerobic fitness and cognitive control demands. The authors interpreted the overall task accuracy decline in terms of fatigue, and suggested that the maintenance of performance across the experiment during increased cognitive demands in HF children may be due to the increased recruitment of prefrontal and parietal areas early in task performance, which is to say that these changes may have served to offset some of the fatigue effects later in the block. The authors also suggested that HF children modulate cognitive control resources more flexibly than their less fit peers, therefore they postulate that aerobic fitness is involved in the ability to adapt neural processes to meet and maintain task goals. Furthermore, by having a superior ability to activate frontal and parietal brain regions (important for the monitoring, maintenance, and strategizing of higher level cognitive control abilities), they may have better academic performances.

The same research group (Voss et al., 2011) investigated whether, as compared to YA, preadolescent children had different pattern of brain activity during a challenging cognitive task and how it related to aerobic fitness level.

During fMRI scanning, participants performed a flanker paradigm. From a behavioral point of view, children performed poorer than YA on the task condition requiring greater cognitive control (Inc condition), and showed generally slower response speed. HF children showed greater overall accuracy and less interference cost than LF children; in particular, accuracy cost was not significantly different between HF children and YA, and LF children showed significantly more cost than both HF and YA. For the previous results, the authors suggested that in children accuracy may be more sensitive to individual differences in fitness. While performing a task that modulated cognitive control requirements, after matching LF and HF children for performance level, LF children had greater activation of a network associated with cognitive control compared with HF children. According to the different task condition (Con or Inc), LF and HF children activated different brain areas: in the HF group, greater activation in the left central opercular and dorsal ACCs during the Inc condition was associated with greater Inc accuracy. Interestingly, in both of these regions, HF children had greater activation during the Con condition and showed either significantly less (opercular) or the same (ACC) activation than LF children during the Inc condition. Since groups were matched for performance, the authors interpreted the results in the context of different task strategies made possible by differences in brain function between LF and HF children. Overall, HF showed a pattern of greater activation in the Con condition than Inc, whereas LF activated more in the Inc than the Con condition. Therefore, they invoked the theory of Pontifex et al. (2011) where LF children are hypothesized to engage in reactive control strategies compared with HF children, who are more likely to engage in proactive cognitive control. Reactive control is transiently engaged following stimulus selection but preceding response execution, whereas proactive control engages the cognitive control system based on task context, involving maintenance of a flexible task set that biases attention to relevant stimuli before selection and response.

Effect of Training Intervention on Brain Structure

Training intervention studies demonstrated that aerobic exercise significantly impacts on brain structure. Colcombe et al. (2006) found increased volume of the ACC, SMA, right inferior frontal gyrus, left superior temporal gyrus, and anterior corpus callosum in the aerobic training group relative to a nonaerobic stretching control group.

Ruscheweyh et al. (2011) demonstrated that improvements in physical activity (assessed with a questionnaire) after a 6-month exercise training period were associated with GM volume increase in the cingulate gyrus (including the ACC and PCC), the left SFG, the left medial parietal cortex and regions of the occipital cortex. Likewise in a study focusing on the MTLs (Erickson et al., 2011), aerobically trained older adults demonstrated an ~2% increase in hippocampal volume, whereas a 1.4% decrease was observed in the stretching control group. Improvements in CRF were positively associated with hippocampal volume. These data are particularly striking given that the volumetric increase greatly offsets the annualized age-related MTL volume loss of 1–2% in this age group (Raz et al., 2004).

In cardiovascular disease (CVD), exercise training is a key component of cardiac rehabilitation. In a study by Anazodo et al. (2013) it has been demonstrated that, prior to the exercise intervention, CVD patients, relative to controls, exhibited smaller GM volume of the SFG, MFG and IFG, SPG and IPG, MTG and STG, and the posterior cerebellum. After completion of a 6-month cardiovascular rehabilitation intervention, CVD patients exhibited GM recovery of the SFG, STG, and posterior cerebellum, in addition to GM increase in SMAs.

Effect of Training Intervention on Cerebral Blood Flow and FC

Chapman et al. (2013) demonstrated that even a short-term aerobic exercise intervention impacts on cognitive performances and on brain FC. They examined changes in CBF, cognition, and fitness level in 37 cognitively healthy sedentary adults (57–75 years of age) who were randomized into physical training or a wait-list control group. The physical training group received supervised aerobic exercise for 3 sessions per week (1 h each) for 12 weeks. Cognitive evaluation and fMRI studies were acquired at baseline, after 6 weeks and at the end of the training (12 weeks). After 3 months training, higher resting CBF was found in the physical training group, as compared to the control group, in the ACC. The improved immediate and delayed memory performances were manifested in the exercise group; these improvements also showed a significant positive association with increases in both left and right hippocampal CBF. In detail, increased CBF and behavioral gains were not simultaneous; the temporal mismatch between the positive correlation between increased CBF in left and right hippocampi at 6 weeks and the improved immediate and delayed memory at 12 weeks, suggested that the brain-behavior relationship is a meaningful gain. The authors, therefore, proposed that exercise training initially increased the CBF and then led to memory performance improvement. These data suggest that even shorter-term aerobic exercise can facilitate neuroplasticity and eventually reduce both the biological and cognitive consequences of aging in sedentary adults.

Several studies (Colcombe et al., 2006; Voss et al., 2010, 2011; Erickson et al., 2011) investigated the effects of aerobic exercise intervention in older adults by pre- and postintervention MRI.

Walking (with varying duration and intensity levels) was the primary type of exercise training in at least one of the studied groups, targeting enhanced CRF as the main training effect. Sedentary subjects (e.g., not more than two bouts of physical activity >30 min in the previous 6 months) were recruited on the assumption that improvements in CRF associated with aerobic exercise intervention would be most prominent in respect to baseline sedentary behaviors and presumably in respect to the most prominent neurologic changes as well.

In this perspective, Colcombe et al. (2004) provided glimpses into the neural bases of cognitive enhancement through CRF in aging humans. They investigated highly functioning older adults to depict relationship between CRF level, behavioral performance on a modified version of the Eriksen flanker task (Eriksen and Eriksen, 1974) (as indication of EF efficiency), and fMRI activated brain areas. Their study consisted of two phases: a cross-sectional and a longitudinal one. In the cross-sectional one, patients were tested for CRF level and executed the flanker paradigm during the fMRI study; in the longitudinal phase a subgroup of patients was randomly assigned to participate in either a CRF aerobic group, or a stretching and toning control group. The exercise training was planned with three sessions per week for 6 months and consisted of walking for 40–45 min/session in the aerobic group and a program of stretching, limbering, and toning for the whole body for the control group. Participants underwent the same cognitive testing and fMRI scanning as in the cross-sectional study, 1 week before beginning the 6-month intervention, and again 1 week after completion of the intervention. Patients participating in the cross-sectional study were separated by a median split on a measure of their maximal oxygen uptake in HF and LF. Comparing the HF and LF participants, HF older adults were reliably more efficient in dealing with the conflicting cues than the LF older adults, and demonstrated significantly greater activation in several cortical regions associated with effective attentional control (right MFG, SFG, and SPL), and significantly less activity in the ACC. After the 6-month intervention, participants in the aerobic group demonstrated a significant improvement in the task performance with an 11% reduction of behavioral conflict and, compared with nonaerobic control participants, showed a significantly greater level of task-related activity in attentional control areas (MFG, SFG, and SPL), and a significantly reduced level of activity in the ACC. It is worth to remark that these regions overlap, in both spatial and directional terms, with those identified as differing between HF and LF participants in the cross-sectional study.

The authors suggest two possible explanations for these results. One is that, the increase in cardiovascular fitness may augment the number of interconnections (synapses) in frontal and parietal GM, allowing for greater systematic recruitment of these areas under higher cognitive load. Another possibility is that the increase in fitness leads to increases in blood (capillary) supply in these regions, which, in turn, provides the metabolic resources necessary to coherently respond during task performance.

Voss et al. (2010) explored aerobic exercise-related changes in FC in several brain networks: that is, the DMN and the frontal-insular and frontal-parietal networks that are associated with EF. YA and elderly sedentary subjects underwent baseline structural and functional MRI scans; elderly participants were further randomized to either an aerobic walking group or a control group that participated in a stretching and toning program.

Elderly adults underwent the fMRI study during passive viewing tasks also at 6 and 12 months after aerobic exercise training (walking) or flexibility, toning, and balance training. In the aerobic training group, as compared to the nonaerobic training one, 12 months of aerobic training produced increased connectivity in MTL, parietal, and frontal regions and enhanced FC between PHG and MTG, the PHG and bilateral inferior parietal cortex, and the left MFG and MTG. Therefore, aerobic training improved the aging brain's resting functional efficiency in higher-level cognitive networks; 1 year of walking increased FC between aspects of the frontal, posterior, and temporal cortices within the DMN and the frontal executive network, two brain networks central to age-related cognitive dysfunction.

Length of training was an important factor: effects in favor of the walking group were observed only after 12 months of training, compared to nonsignificant trends after 6 months. The nonaerobic stretching and toning group also showed increased FC in the DMN after 6 months and in the frontal parietal network after 12 months, possibly reflecting experience-dependent plasticity. Finally, increased FC was associated with greater improvement in EF. Therefore, the authors suggested that exercise may induce functional plasticity in large-scale brain systems in the aging brain.

Rosano et al. (2010) investigated whether the effect of a physical activity intervention on brain FC and cognitive performances persisted after its termination.

Participants of the lifestyle interventions and independence for elders—pilot study (Pahor et al., 2006) were examined 2 years after completing a 1-year treatment, consisting of either physical activity or education in successful aging (control group). Twenty subjects of the physical activity arm who did not completely stop their training and 10 subjects of the sedentary control group who kept being sedentary, underwent a fMRI study and a Digit symbol substitution test (DSST, evaluating EF). The group of previously sedentary older adults who began and kept having a moderate physical activity program showed distinct patterns of brain activation and higher performance on DSST, compared with those who remained sedentary over the same period. Specifically, differences in brain activation during task performance were localized within regions important for EF. Greater physical activity levels were also directly associated with greater fMRI signal restricted to the inferior frontal gyrus, 2 years after the intervention ended.

If physical activity affects the brain through increased cardiovascular conditioning, then it is likely that the watershed region, such as the dorsolateral PFC, would be the most sensitive to cerebrovascular and oxygenation levels' changes after physical activity. If physical activity has a stronger effect on these regions than on others, then this could explain why the effect of physical activity on cognitive function is stronger for the EF.

In conclusion, all the previous studies have shown that basal CRF is positively associated with better cognitive performance (in particular EFs) either in older adults or in children, with HF subjects outperforming LF ones.

CRF Level, Training Intervention, and Cognition in Central Nervous System Diseases

The effect of CRF on cognitive performances has been demonstrated also in some CNS diseases.

In multiple sclerosis (MS) cognitive deficits are frequently seen in working memory, EF, attention and concentration, and speed of information processing. They progress with declines in WM and GM volume and brain function (Bobholz and Rao, 2003), impacting on quality of life and leading to disease-related unemployment. Consequently, development of strategies to maintain or enhance cognitive function in MS is an important public health goal. In this perspective, Prakash et al. (2007) examined whether higher CRF levels enhanced cognitive and neural plasticity in MS patients. They studied 24 relapsing-remitting MS patients by 3T fMRI while performing a task of working memory: the visual version of the paced auditory serial addition test (PVSAT). With respect to behavioral results, they showed that the reaction time were significantly correlated to CRF level, with higher levels associated with faster responding on the PVSAT. Moreover, higher levels of fitness were associated with a greater recruitment of right inferior FG/MFG during task performance along with a reduction in activity in the ACC. Furthermore, by splitting patients in HF and LF, HF participants showed a greater percent signal change than the LF participants in the right inferior FG/MFG, whereas the LF participants recruited more of the ACC. Greater recruitment of ACC by LF participants was attributed to a greater need for executive control due to higher interference from the preprogrammed response. Inferior FG/MFG is a cortical region known to be recruited by MS patients during performance of PVSAT, presumably to compensate for the decline in information processing speed owing to compromised neuronal function. The authors suggested that the associations between lower levels of aerobic fitness with enhanced ACC activity may be due to the fact that the PVSAT task requires to inhibit conflict and engage the contents of working memory. Thus additional ACC activity in LF participants may be indicative of the presence of a larger amount of conflict and a greater need to engage in top–down attentional control to resolve such conflict; alternatively, it may be due to increased effort being devoted towards the task. The possibility that CRF may be related to cognitive function and brain structure in MS is exciting and opening new perspective of patients' management.

Although AD is typically associated with memory loss, executive dysfunction is common and may be one of the earliest manifestations of the disease (Bisiacchi et al., 2008). In people with AD, higher CRF levels are associated with increased whole brain volume (Burns et al., 2008) and hippocampal volume (Honea et al., 2009), while lower CRF levels are associated with faster dementia progression over 2 years (Vidoni et al., 2012).

The available evidences suggest that individuals with cognitive impairment activate additional frontoparietal regions during executive tasks in comparison with their peers without dementia. Vidoni et al. (2013) recently described the relationship between regional brain activity during cognitive tasks and CRF level in people with and without AD. In details, in people without dementia, they found increased MFG and SPL and decreased ACC activity, that was associated with CRF, during the executive task. The same CRF and brain activity associations were not evident in the AD group. The authors suggested that AD alters or overrides the relationship of CRF with brain function. On the other hand, the possible positive role of exercise training has also been suggested in these patients based on preliminary evidences showing that exercise may support functional plastic change in the earliest stages of AD (Nagamatsu et al., 2012).

Smith et al. (2013) demonstrated that a 12-week walking exercise intervention positively affects semantic memory, fMRI activation, and neuropsychological outcomes in individuals diagnosed with MCI, compared to cognitively intact older adults. Patients underwent an extensive neuropsychological test battery and a fMRI famous name recognition task at baseline and after the 12 weeks of treadmill walking intervention. The exercise intervention led to a 10% increase in maximal aerobic capacity and an associated decrease in semantic memory retrieval-related fMRI activation in MCI participants, and cognitively intact older adults. Learning task improved both in the MCI participants and in cognitively intact elders. While these cognitive improvements did not differ statistically between the groups, the quality of the cognitive improvement in MCI participants was remarkable given their history of cognitive impairment and likelihood for future cognitive decline. The cognitive improvement in the MCI participants was supported by the changes in task-activated fMRI. The authors suggested that exercise training may enhance cognitive and neural reserve in MCI through a reduced neural workload during successful engagement of semantic memory networks. Particularly interesting are the results concerning the PCC that, in an exploratory post hoc analysis, showed that the decrease over time was significant in the control group, but not in the MCI group. Because a valued hypothesis is that in MCI precuneus/PCC hyperactivation is a compensatory response to hippocampal neurodegeneration, the authors suggested that the effects of exercise training on precuneus/PCC activation were blunted in the MCI participants to preserve compensatory activation in presence of early hippocampal neurodegenerative processes. Moreover, MCI participants also showed new areas of activation after the intervention, particularly in left SFG, MFG, and left lateral occipital and fusiform gyri. These results are consistent with the findings of Belleville et al. (2011) and partly support theories that cognitive improvement or compensation will result in the recruitment of new neural circuits (Reuter-Lorenz and Lustig, 2005).

All together the previous studies are in favor of a meaningful effect of CRF levels and aerobic exercise training on cognitive function. The positive effects have been shown either on healthy (both young and elderly) people or in neurological diseases. With this evidence, physical exercise should be encouraged in all individuals since early childhood to build up an efficient brain reserve and should be included in the management of cognitive impairment in healthy aging and brain diseases involving cognition.

References

Anazodo, U.C., Shoemaker, J.K., Suskin, N., St Lawrence, K.S., 2013. An investigation of changes in regional gray matter volume in cardiovascular disease patients, pre and post cardiovascular rehabilitation. NeuroImage Clinical 3, 388–395.

Andrews-Hanna, J.R., Snyder, A.Z., Vincent, J.L., Lustig, C., Head, D., Raichle, M.E., Buckner, R.L., 2007. Disruption of large-scale brain systems in advanced aging. Neuron 56, 924–935.

Belleville, S., Clement, F., Mellah, S., Gilbert, B., Fontaine, F., Gauthier, S., 2011. Training-related brain plasticity in subjects at risk of developing Alzheimer's disease. Brain 134, 1623–1634.

Bisiacchi, P.S., Borella, E., Bergamaschi, S., Carretti, B., Mondini, S., 2008. Interplay between memory and executive functions in normal and pathological aging. Journal of Clinical and Experimental Neuropsychology 30, 723–733.

Bloor, C.M., 2005. Angiogenesis during exercise and training. Angiogenesis 8, 263–271.

Bobholz, J.A., Rao, S.M., 2003. Cognitive dysfunction in multiple sclerosis: a review of recent developments. Current Opinion in Neurology 16, 283–288.

Broyd, S.J., Demanuele, C., Debener, S., Helps, S.K., James, C.J., Sonuga-Barke, E.J.S., 2009. Default-mode brain dysfunction in mental disorders: a systematic review. Neuroscience & Biobehavioral Reviews 33, 279–296.

Burns, J.M., Cronk, B.B., Anderson, H.S., Donnelly, J.E., Thomas, G.P., Harsha, A., Brooks, W.M., Swerdlow, R.H., 2008. Cardiorespiratory fitness and brain atrophy in early Alzheimer disease. Neurology 71, 210–216.

Cabeza, R., Anderson, N.D., Locantore, J.K., McIntosh, A.R., 2002. Aging gracefully: compensatory brain activity in high-performing older adults. Neuroimage 17, 1394–1402.

Casey, B.J., Thomas, K.M., Welsh, T.F., Badgaiyan, R.D., Eccard, C.H., Jennings, J.R., Crone, E.A., 2000. Dissociation of response conflict, attentional selection, and expectancy with functional magnetic resonance imaging. Proceedings of the National Academy of Sciences of the United States of America 97, 8728–8733.

Castelli, D.M., Hillman, C.H., Buck, S.M., Erwin, H.E., 2007. Physical fitness and academic achievement in third- and fifth-grade students. Journal of Sport & Exercise Psychology 29, 239–252.

Chaddock, L., Erickson, K.I., Prakash, R.S., Kim, J.S., Voss, M.W., VanPatter, M., Pontifex, M.B., Raine, L.B., Konkel, A., Hillman, C.H., Cohen, N.J., Kramer, A.F., 2010. A neuroimaging investigation of the association between aerobic fitness, hippocampal volume and memory performance in preadolescent children. Brain Research 1358, 172–183.

Chaddock, L., Erickson, K.I., Prakash, R.S., Voss, M.W., VanPatter, M., Pontifex, M.B., Hillman, C.H., Kramer, A.F., 2012. A functional MRI investigation of the association between childhood aerobic fitness and neurocognitive control. Biological Psychology 89, 260–268.

Chapman, S.B., Aslan, S., Spence, J.S., Defina, L.F., Keebler, M.W., Didehbani, N., Lu, H., 2013. Shorter term aerobic exercise improves brain, cognition, and cardiovascular fitness in aging. Frontiers in Aging Neuroscience 12 (5), 75.

Colcombe, S., Kramer, A.F., 2003. Fitness effects on the cognitive function of older adults: a meta-analytic study. Psychological Science 14, 125.

Colcombe, S.J., Kramer, A.F., Erickson, K.I., Scalf, P., McAuley, E., Cohen, N.J., Webb, A., Jerome, G.J., Marquez, D.X., Elavsky, S., 2004. Cardiovascular fitness, cortical plasticity, and aging. Proceedings of the National Academy of Sciences of the United States of America 101, 3316–3321.

Colcombe, S.J., Kramer, A.F., Erickson, K.I., Scalf, P., Kim, J.S., Prakash, R., McAuley, E., Elavsky, S., Marquez, D.X., Hu, L., Kramer, A.F., 2006. Aerobic exercise training increases brain volume in aging humans. Journals of Gerontology Series A: Biological Sciences and Medical Sciences 61, 1166–1170.

Damoiseaux, J.S., Rombouts, S.A., Barkhof, F., Scheltens, P., Stam, C.J., Smith, S.M., Beckmann, C.F., 2006. Consistent resting-state networks across healthy subjects. Proceedings of the National Academy of Sciences of the United States of America 103, 13848–13853.

Damoiseaux, J.S., Beckmann, C.F., Arigita, E.J., Barkhof, F., Scheltens, P., Stam, C.J., Smith, S.M., Rombouts, S.A., 2008. Reduced resting-state brain activity in the "default network" in normal aging. Cerebral Cortex 18, 1856–1864.

Eadie, B.D., Redila, V.A., Christie, B.R., 2005. Voluntary exercise alters the cytoarchitecture of the adult dentate gyrus by increasing cellular proliferation, dendritic complexity, and spine density. Journal of Comparative Neurology 486, 39–47.

Erickson, K.I., Prakash, R.S., Voss, M.W., Chaddock, L., Hu, L., Morris, K.S., White, S.M., Wojcicki, T.R., McAuley, E., Kramer, A.F., 2009. Aerobic fitness is associated with hippocampal volume in elderly humans. Hippocampus 19, 1030–1039.

Erickson, K.I., Voss, M.W., Prakash, R.S., Basak, C., Szabo, A., Chaddock, L., Kim, J.S., Heo, S., Alves, H., White, S.M., Wojcicki, T.R., Mailey, E., Vieira, V.J., Martin, S.A., Pence, B.D., Woods, J.A., McAuley, E., Kramer, A.F., 2011. Exercise training increases size of hippocampus and improves memory. Proceedings of the National Academy of Sciences of the United States of America 108, 3017–3022.

Eriksen, B.A., Eriksen, C.W., 1974. Effects of noise letters on the identification of a target letter in a nonsearch task. Perception & Psychophysics 16, 143–149.

Fox, M.D., Raichle, M.E., 2007. Spontaneous fluctuations in brain activity observed with functional magnetic resonance imaging. Nature Reviews Neuroscience 8, 700–711.

Friston, K.J., 1994. Functional and effective connectivity in neuroimaging: a synthesis. Human Brain Mapping 2, 56–78.

Glisky, E.L., 2007. Changes in cognitive function in human aging. In: Brain Aging: Models, Methods, and Mechanisms. CRC Press/Taylor & Francis, Boca Raton (FL) (Chapter 1).

Gomez-Pinilla, F., Dao, L., So, V., 1997. Physical exercise induces FGF-2 and its mRNA in the hippocampus. Brain Research 764, 1–8.

Greicius, M.D., Krasnow, B., Reiss, A.L., Menon, V., 2003. Functional connectivity in the resting brain: a network analysis of the default mode hypothesis. Proceedings of the National Academy of Sciences of the United States of America 100, 253–258.

Greicius, M.D., Srivastava, G., Reiss, A.L., Menon, V., 2004. Default-mode network activity distinguishes Alzheimer's disease from healthy aging: evidence from functional MRI. Proceedings of the National Academy of Sciences of the United States of America 101, 4637–4642.

Hamzei, F., Glauche, V., Schwarzwald, R., May, A., 2012. Dynamic gray matter changes within cortex and striatum after short motor skill training are associated with their increased functional interaction. NeuroImage 59, 3364–3372.

Hillman, C.H., Kramer, A.F., 2012. A functional MRI investigation of the association between childhood aerobic fitness and neurocognitive control. Biological Psychology 89, 260–268.

Honea, R.A., Thomas, G.P., Harsha, A., Anderson, H.S., Donnelly, J.E., Brooks, W.M., Burns, J.M., 2009. Cardiorespiratory fitness and preserved medial temporal lobe volume in Alzheimer disease. Alzheimer Disease and Associated Disorders 23, 188–197.

Kalmijn, S., Janssen, J.A., Pols, H.A., Lamberts, S.W., Breteler, M.M., 2000. A prospective study on circulating insulin-like growth factor I (IGF-I), IGF-binding proteins, and cognitive function in the elderly. Journal of Clinical Endocrinology & Metabolism 85, 4551–4555.

Knaepen, K., Goekint, M., Heyman, E.M., Meeusen, R., 2010. Neuroplasticity-exercise-induced response of peripheral brain derived neurotrophic factor: a systematic review of experimental studies in human subjects. Sports Medicine 40, 765–801.

Leahey, T.H., Harris, R.J., 2001. Neurophysiology of learning and cognition. In: Leahey, T.H., Harris, R.J. (Eds.), Learning and Cognition. Prentice-Hall, New Jersey, pp. 353–377.

Leuner, B., Gould, E., 2010. Structural plasticity and hippocampal function. Annual Review of Psychology 61, 111–113.

Marr, D., 1971. Simple memory: a theory for archicortex. Philosophical Transactions of the Royal Society of London. Series B, Biological Sciences 262, 23–81.

May, A., Hajak, G., Ganssbauer, S., Steffens, T., Langguth, B., Kleinjung, T., Eichhammer, P., 2007. Structural brain alterations following 5 days of intervention: dynamic aspects of neuroplasticity. Cerebral Cortex 17, 205–210.

Meeusen, R., 2005. Exercise and the brain: insight in new therapeutic modalities. Annals of Transplantation 10, 49–51.

Nagamatsu, L.S., Handy, T.C., Hsu, C.L., Voss, M., Liu-Ambrose, T., 2012. Resistance training promotes cognitive and functional brain plasticity in seniors with probable mild cognitive impairment. Archives of Internal Medicine 172, 666–668.

Neeper, S.A., Gomez-Pinilla, F., Choi, J., Cotman, C., 1995. Exercise and brain neurotrophins. Nature 373, 109.

Neeper, S.A., Gomez-Pinilla, F., Choi, J., Cotman, C.W., 1996. Physical activity increases mRNA for brain-derived neurotrophic factor and nerve growth factor in rat brain. Brain Research 726, 49–56.

Pahor, M., Blair, S., Espeland, M., 2006. Effects of a physical activity intervention on measures of physical performance: results of the lifestyle interventions and independence for elders pilot (LIFE-P) study. Journals of Gerontology Series A: Biological Sciences and Medical Sciences 61, 1157–1165.

Pang, P.T., Teng, H.K., Zaitsev, E., Woo, N.T., Sakata, K., Zhen, S., Teng, K.K., Yung, W.H., Hempstead, B.L., Lu, B., 2004. Cleavage of proBDNF by tPA/plasmin is essential for long-term hippocampal plasticity. Science 306, 487–491.

Pontifex, M.B., Raine, L.B., Johnson, C.R., Chaddock, L., Voss, M.W., Cohen, N.J., Kramer, A.F., Hillman, C.H., 2011. Cardiorespiratory fitness and the flexible modulation of cognitive control in preadolescent children. Journal of Cognitive Neuroscience 23, 1332–1345.

Prakash, R.S., Snook, E.M., Erickson, K.I., Colcombe, S.J., Voss, M.W., Motl, R.W., Kramer, A.F., 2007. Cardiorespiratory fitness: a predictor of cortical plasticity in multiple sclerosis. Neuroimage 34 (3), 1238–1244.

Raz, N., 2000. In: Craik, F.I.M., Salthouse, T.A. (Eds.), The Handbook of Aging and Cognition. Lawrence Erlbaum Associates, Mahwah, NJ, pp. 1–90.

Raz, N., Rodrigue, K.M., Head, D., Kennedy, K.M., Acker, J.D., 2004. Differential aging of the medial temporal lobe – a study of a five-year change. Neurology 62, 433–438.

Reuter-Lorenz, P.A., Lustig, C., 2005. Brain aging: reorganizing discoveries about the aging mind. Current Opinion in Neurobiology 15, 245–251.

Rosano, C., Venkatraman, V.K., Guralnik, J., Newman, A.B., Glynn, N.W., Launer, L., Taylor, C.A., Williamson, J., Studenski, S., Pahor, M., Aizenstein, H., 2010. Psychomotor speed and functional brain MRI 2 years after completing a physical activity treatment. Journals of Gerontology Series A: Biological Sciences and Medical Sciences 65, 639–647.

Ruscheweyh, R., Willemer, C., Kruger, K., Duning, T., Warnecke, T., Sommer, J., Völker, K., Ho, H.V., Mooren, F., Knecht, S., Flöel, A., 2011. Physical activity and memory functions: an interventional study. Neurobiology of Aging 32, 1304–1319.

Smith, J.C., Nielson, K.A., Antuono, P., Lyons, J.A., Hanson, R.J., Butts, A.M., Hantke, N.C., Verber, M.D., 2013. Semantic memory functional MRI and cognitive function after exercise intervention in mild cognitive impairment. Journal of Alzheimer's Disease 37, 197–215.

Taubert, M., Draganski, B., Anwander, A., Müller, K., Horstmann, A., Villringer, A., Ragert, P., 2010. Dynamic properties of human brain structure: learning-related changes in cortical areas and associated fiber connections. Journal of Neuroscience 30 (35), 11670–11677.

Taubert, M., Lohmann, G., Margulies, D.S., Villringer, A., Ragert, P., 2011. Long-term effects of motor training on resting-state networks and underlying brain structure. NeuroImage 57, 1492–1498.

Trejo, J.L., Llorens-Martin, M.V., Torres-Aleman, I., 2008. The effects of exercise on spatial learning and anxiety-like behavior are mediated by an IGF-I-dependent mechanism related to hippocampal neurogenesis. Molecular and Cellular Neuroscience 37, 402–411.

Vale, R.G., de Oliveira, R.D., Pernambuco, C.S., de Meneses, Y.P., Novaes, J.S., de Andrade, A.F., 2009. Effects of muscle strength and aerobic training on basal serum levels of IGF-1 and cortisol in elderly women. Archives of Gerontology and Geriatrics 49, 343–347.

van Praag, H., 2008. Neurogenesis and exercise: past and future directions. NeuroMolecular Medicine 10, 128–140.

Vidoni, E.D., Honea, R.A., Billinger, S.A., Swerdlow, R.H., Burns, J.M., 2012. Cardiorespiratory fitness is associated with atrophy in Alzheimer's and aging over 2 years. Neurobiology of Aging 33, 1624–1632.

Vidoni, E.D., Gayed, M.R., Honea, R.A., Savage, C.R., Hobbs, D., Burns, J.M., 2013. Alzheimer disease alters the relationship of cardiorespiratory fitness with brain activity during the stroop task. Physical Therapy 93, 993–1002.

Voss, M.W., Prakash, R.S., Erickson, K.I., Basak, C., Chaddock, L., Kim, J.S., Alves, H., Heo, S., Szabo, A.N., White, S.M., Wójcicki, T.R., Mailey, E.L., Gothe, N., Olson, E.A., McAuley, E., Kramer, A.F., 2010. Plasticity of brain networks in a randomized intervention trial of exercise training in older adults. Frontiers in Aging Neuroscience 2.

Voss, M.W., Chaddock, L., Kim, J.S., Vanpatter, M., Pontifex, M.B., Raine, L.B., Cohen, N.J., Hillman, C.H., Kramer, A.F., 2011. Aerobic fitness is associated with greater efficiency of the network underlying cognitive control in preadolescent children. Neuroscience 199, 166–176.

Wager, T.D., Smith, E.E., 2003. Neuroimaging studies of working memory: a meta-analysis. Cognitive, Affective, & Behavioral Neuroscience 3, 255.

West, R.L., 1996. An application of prefrontal cortex function theory to cognitive aging. Psychological Bulletin 120, 272.

13

The Effect of Exercise on Motor Function and Neuroplasticity in Parkinson's Disease

J. Watson[1], *K.E. Welman*[1], *B. Sehm*[2,3]

[1]Stellenbosch University, Stellenbosch, South Africa; [2]Max Planck Institute for Human Cognitive and Brain Sciences, Leipzig, Germany; [3]University of Leipzig, Leipzig, Germany

Abstract

Every second millions of neural cells in the human brain fire together, creating and maintaining intricate networks that allows us to move our bodies, recall our memories, and experience our surroundings. The discovery that these neural networks are adaptive well into adulthood and even aging has sparked great interest in multiple levels of scientific analyses, specifically in neurorehabilitative inquiries. Indeed, there is increasing evidence that neuroplastic mechanisms might beneficially influence the course of neurodegenerative diseases. We here focus on idiopathic Parkinson's disease (PD), one of the major age-related neurodegenerative diseases. While there is increasing research on the behavioral effects of exercise in PD on neurological functioning, only a few studies have investigated effects of exercise and physical activity on potential underlying brain changes. This chapter provides an overview of the current scientific evidence of how physical activity and exercise influence both motor function and associated brain changes in the parkinsonian brain. We incorporate different levels of neuroscientific evidence, both including investigations on molecular and systems level in animal models and human studies.

INTRODUCTION

Every second millions of neural cells in the human brain fire together, creating and maintaining intricate networks that allows us to move our bodies, recall our memories, and experience our surroundings. The discovery that these neural networks are adaptive well into adulthood and even aging has sparked great interest in multiple levels of scientific analyses, specifically in neurorehabilitative inquiries. Indeed, there is increasing evidence that neuroplastic mechanisms might beneficially influence the course of neurodegenerative diseases. We here focus on idiopathic Parkinson's disease (PD), one of the major age-related neurodegenerative diseases. Although there is increasing research on the behavioral effects of exercise in PD on neurological functioning, only a few studies have investigated effects of exercise and physical activity on potential underlying brain changes. This chapter provides an overview of the current scientific evidence of how physical activity and exercise influence both motor function and associated brain changes in the parkinsonian brain. We incorporate different levels of neuroscientific evidence, both including investigations on molecular and systems level in animal models and human studies.

PARKINSON'S DISEASE

Parkinson's disease (PD) is a progressive neurological disease which affects, predominantly, the basal ganglia function of the human brain and leads to neurological symptoms that affect both motor and nonmotor function (Abbruzzese et al., 2016). Typical motor symptoms include bradykinesia, rigidity, tremor, gait-impairment, and postural instability. In order to understand the changes induced by exercise and physical activity on motor function in PD, a short overview about the predominantly affected brain regions and their connectivity patterns will be provided: The basal lie deep in the center of the brain, composed of the striatum (subdivided into the caudate and putamen), the globus pallidus [subdivided into internal (GPi) and external pallidus (GPe)], the substantia

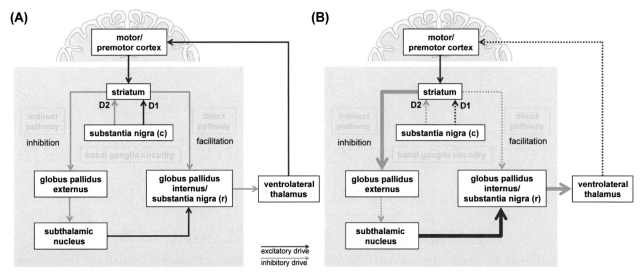

FIGURE 13.1   Schematic illustration of the major structures and pathways of the basal ganglia circuitry, based on the model by Mink (1996). (A) Model of excitatory (*red arrows*) and inhibitory (*blue arrows*) influences within the basal ganglia circuitry under physiological conditions. (B) Changes within the basal ganglia circuitry in the Parkinsonian brain (*bold arrows*, increase in excitation/inhibition; *dotted arrows*, decrease in excitation/inhibition).

nigra [pars reticulate (SNr) and pars compacta (SNc)], and the subthalamic nucleus. The neuronal degeneration affects predominantly, but not exclusively, dopamine-producing cells in the SNc of the substantia nigra and results in a lack of dopamine within the cortico-basal ganglia-thalamo-cortical loop, a network involved in modulating motor cortical excitability (see Fig. 13.1 for a schematic illustration of the basal ganglia substructures and connectivity).

The basal ganglia are largely responsible to regulate motor and nonmotor behavior. These structures form a loop, that receives glutamatergic (excitatory) projections and send inhibitory projections back to the cortex via the thalamus (see Fig. 13.1A). The neural pathways within this loop can further be divided into direct, indirect, and nigrostriatal dopaminergic pathways (for the sake of simplicity we will not go in detail about the fourth pathway, the hyperdirect pathway). Importantly, within these single pathways, differences in the main neurotransmitters provide for the synergistic action of these structures on thalamus and cortex. Conceptualized by the model of Mink (1996), the striatum [i.e., the medium spiny neurons (MSN) within this structure] receives excitatory glutamatergic input from the cortex. In the striatum, MSN sends projections via direct and indirect pathways. The direct pathway acts straight from the striatum on the GPi, whereas the indirect pathway acts on the GPi via the GPe and STN (see Fig. 13.1A). Hence, the direct pathway acts on the main output nucleus of the basal ganglia, the GPi, inhibitory, whereas the indirect pathway has an overall facilitatory influence on the GPi. Therefore, the inhibitory tone ("the brake") of the GPi on thalamus and cortex is "released" by the direct pathway and "applied" by the indirect. Both pathways are equally important in motor control as they modulate the facilitation of intended motor programs and the inhibition of unintended motor programs via this model, also coined as "brake/release model" (Mink, 1996). On the basis of this concept, an imbalance between these pathways may lead to what is known as hyperkinetic (hemiballism) or hypokinetic (PD) movement disorders. The neurotransmitter dopamine is expressed within the nigrostriatal pathway and differentially modulates the glutamatergic cortical input on MSN based on the dopamine receptor type (D1- or D2-receptors): while D2-receptors enhance the cortical glutamatergic input on the MSN, D2-receptors dampen the cortical input. Importantly, both receptor types are differentially expressed in the direct and indirect pathways. While in the direct pathway, mainly D1-receptors are expressed, in the indirect pathways, there are mainly D2 receptors. Hence, dopamine has an overall synergistical facilitatory effect on the basal ganglia loop, by either enhancing the facilitatory effect of the direct pathway or dampening the inhibitory effect of the indirect pathway (Fig. 13.1B).

In PD, the progressive decline in dopamine levels due to cell death in the subtantia nigra affects both direct and indirect pathways. This decrease in dopamine results in an increase in the inhibitory drive of the basal ganglia loop on the motor cortex (Fig. 13.1B). Furthermore, this brain network is particularly important in different phases of motor learning (Shumway-Cook and Woollacott, 2012), underlining the importance to better understand interactions between the parkinsonian brain and neurorehabilitative interventions, such as exercise and physical activity.

EXERCISE INTERVENTIONS IN PARKINSON'S DISEASE PATIENTS

Exercise therapies are considered as complimentary to pharmacological and surgical treatments, to improve motor function and secondary complications (Abbruzzese et al., 2016; Picelli et al., 2015; Fox et al., 2011). A growing number of randomized controlled trials suggest the efficacy of exercise, physical therapy, and motor skill training on motor and nonmotor PD symptoms. This is supported by recent metaanalyses suggesting that, in general, physiotherapy interventions (including general physiotherapy, exercise, treadmill training, cueing, dance, and martial arts) are beneficial and improve movement parameters such as speed, gait, and balance, as well as clinical scores in PD (Tomlinson et al., 2013). However, it remains elusive, whether one therapy modality has superior effects on PD symptoms than another. This is partly due to methodological issues of the studies performed thus far (such as small sample sizes, problems in study design etc.). Hence, high-level evidence, generated by randomized controlled trials, is needed to better understand effectiveness of different interventions and to allow therapists to chose one exercise modality over another (Tomlinson et al., 2014).

Despite the multitude of different approaches, exercise therapy in general is a customized exercise prescription (taking into account the existing medical condition) aiming to restore health and prevent further disease or impairment. Exercise therapy therefore includes physical activity that is planned, structured, and repetitive for the purpose of physical conditioning and typically provides advice regarding exercise frequency, intensity, time, and type (FITT principles) (Uhrbrand et al., 2015).

Evidence-based practices for PD to date that combine goal-based motor skill training with cognitive engagement include treadmill training, amplitude training, forced cycling, yoga, balance, dance, martial arts, and combat activities such as Tai Chi and boxing (Petzinger et al., 2013; Uhrbrand et al., 2015; Abbruzzese et al., 2016). These exercises generally deliver modest and short-lived but significant and clinically important benefits for motor functioning by improving balance, mobility, and gait parameters in PD (Gallo and Garber, 2011). There are other benefits from exercise, in particular endurance and resistance training, such as improved cardiorespiratory fitness, muscle strength, quality of life (Uhrbrand et al., 2015; Gallo and Garber, 2011), disease severity, executive functioning, (Tanaka et al., 2009) as well as enjoyable and social aspects (Abbruzzese et al., 2016) which may indirectly improve motor function (Uhrbrand et al., 2015).

Promising innovative approaches in PD to improve motor function include motor imagery, action observation therapy, virtual reality, and robotic rehabilitation. These exercise therapies show potential benefit, however clinical effectiveness must still be determined (Abbruzzese et al., 2016).

Exercise therapy is complicated due to the heterogeneity of PD, and as a result various different exercise approaches are used by rehabilitation specialists (i.e., physiotherapist, occupational, and exercise therapist). Consequently, the question still remains what the best practices for exercise interventions are at different stages of the disease (King et al., 2015). Therapist should take into account that research on exercise interventions mostly include early PD (mild to moderate clinical stage), hence more evidence-based practices is needed for advance stages of PD (Petzinger et al., 2013; Hirsch et al., 2016). Multidisciplinary approaches have been proposed in PD, but the debate between isolated and more integrated intervention is still ongoing. Favorable exercise approaches do share a number of "practice variables," that is, intensity, repetition, specificity, difficulty, and complexity (Abbruzzese et al., 2016), and include cognitive engagement via feedback (verbal or proprioceptive), cueing and dual tasking, (attentional demand) and motivation (Petzinger et al., 2013).

Exercise guidelines for optimal benefits are still needed. Hirsch et al. (2016) reviewed PD patient exercise studies and reported that 20–24 treadmill or cycling sessions, for 45–60 min, over 4–8 weeks, respectively, at an age predicted heart rate max of 60–75% resulted in exercise-dependent neuroplasticity. Klamroth et al. (2016) instead evaluated the effective dose for balance interventions (in isolation and in combination with other activities) and reported postural stability benefits for balance interventions in PD, by training 2–3 days per week between 40–60 min over 4–12 weeks.

Phenotypic variability and progressive nature of disease severity contributes to the heterogeneity in PD, thus different individualized approaches are suggested, since the different clinical subtypes as well as disease stages may respond differently to various interventions. Consequently, evidence-based training approaches and practice variables are still needed and established by means of high-quality research, taking into account the variability of the disease type and stage.

THE EFFECTS OF EXERCISE ON THE PARKINSONIAN BRAIN—ANIMAL MODELS

Exercise-induced neuroplasticity has become an operative word in clinical neuroscience, as it is known that experiences may alter the structure and functioning of the brain. The major part of scientific evidence, how exercise may alter the function of the brain in PD, is derived from mice models. These studies, which investigated neural as well as behavioral changes, have largely focused on aerobic treadmill training (Hirsch et al., 2016). It is an important step to understand the relationship between exercise and neural correlates in animal models as they may provide important insights into the mammalian brain, and thus ultimately, human PD research and rehabilitation.

Dopamine Metabolism, Dopamine Receptor Functions and Neurotrophic Factors

The most identifiable pathogenetic marker in PD is the insufficient production, and uptake, of the neurotransmitter dopamine. Dopaminergic D1- and D2-receptors and dopamine are involved in the initial phases of motor learning, while the D2 receptor and dopamine may play an important role in the subsequent phases of learning (Petzinger et al., 2010; Shumway-Cook and Woollacott, 2012). Thus, researchers have investigated what, if any, effects exercise may have changes on receptor function in PD.

In a high intensity treadmill training study over 30 days, in a mice model of PD (i.e., 1-methyl-4-phenyl-1,2,3, 6-tetrahydropuridine (MPTP)–lesioned mice) it was found that exercise led to significantly increased D2 mRNA expression in the dorsolateral striatum of the exercised MPTP-mice, compared to MPTP-mice who received no training (Fisher et al., 2004). In addition, the authors found changes in striatal postsynaptic dopamine transporter proteins (DAT) in MPTP–lesioned mice, with all groups showing reduced DAT activity to the training (groups included: saline-only; saline-exercise; MPTP-only, and MPTP-exercise). Particularly, the saline group showed significant reductions, compared to nonexercised groups, suggesting that training alone affected DAT metabolism and induced positive behavioral changes in the mouse-model PD brain (Fisher et al., 2004). These results are particularly interesting because DAT is predominantly involved in the clearance of dopamine. The reduction of DAT activity may lead to an increased dopamine receptor binding potential within the striatum, thus, ultimately leading to a possible improvement in dopamine uptake as a result of exercise.

Similarly, Petzinger et al. (2007) proposed that intensive aerobic exercise led to a downregulation of DAT as well as Tyrosine Hydroxylase (TH)—proteins observed in MPTP-exercise mice, compared to MPTP only. This may also have led to increased synaptic availability of dopamine, since TH acts as a rate-limiting enzyme to dopamine, catalyzing the hydroxylation of tyrosine to L-DOPA, a precursor to dopamine.

Other studies have observed an effect of exercise on the glutamatergic system. It has been reported that high intensity treadmill exercise may lead to changes in postsynaptic glutamatergic neurotransmission in MSN of the dorsolateral striatum via an increase in GLuR2 transcript and protein in mice (VanLeeuwen et al., 2009). These changes were stated to reverse hyper-excitability of the synapses due to dopamine depletion and therefore, lead to improvements in motor performance of MPTP mice (VanLeeuwen et al., 2009).

Neurotrophic factors, such as brain-derived neurotrophic factor (BDNF) have been shown to be a driver of neuroplastic changes in healthy humans (Vaynman et al., 2004) and be impaired in PD (Howells et al., 2000). The downregulation of the BDNF in the substantia nigra and striatum has been reported in animal models of PD (Hirsch et al., 2016). But what are the potential effects of exercise on neurotrophic factors in PD animal models?

Real et al. (2013) used a PD animal model that makes use of the neurotoxic effects of 6-hydroxydopamine (6-OHDA) in rats. They proposed that exercise had an influence on the reduction of the damage induced by 6-OHDA in adult male Wistar rats, and that this was mediated by the BDNF. Another neurotrophic factor with a potential protective effect is the glial cell derived neurotrophic factor (GDNF) (Cohen et al., 2003). Increased levels of GDNF due to prior limb-use was shown to attenuate the damage caused by 6–OHDA infusion, suggesting a possible mechanism behind physical activity as a protective factor in PD related to disease onset and progression.

Taken together, exercise may induce improvements in motor symptoms via different neuroplastic mechanisms including changes in dopamine (mainly D2 receptors) and glutamate receptor function, changes in dopamine clearance as well as an increase in neurotrophic factors.

Functional Changes in Brain Networks

While in previously mentioned studies, the effect of exercise was investigated on molecular changes, recent studies used neuroimaging techniques in PD animal models to investigate changes in brain structure and function from a network perspective.

In this line, a neuroimaging study of the whole brain detected functional network changes in response to 4 weeks of aerobic training in parkinsonian (6-OHDA) rats (Wang et al., 2013). Changes in the functional reorganization of both motor and limbic circuits were reported in both saline and lesioned groups following aerobic exercise, suggestive of functional reorganization in regions connected to the cerebellar-thalamocortical circuit. In comparison to the lesioned-only group, the 6-OHDA-exercise group showed increase in regional cerebral blood flow-related activity in both basal ganglia, brain stem, and cortical brain structures: the striatum, globus pallidus, thalamus, pedunculopontine nucleus, and rostral secondary motor cortex. Although these effects were significantly lower compared to the nonlesioned exercise group, these results suggest that also the PD animals demonstrated functional changes in a brain network that was induced by exercise interventions (Wang et al., 2013).

A more recent study investigated the effects of exercise on functional connectivity using resting-state functional neuroimaging and found that exercise induced not only a reintegration of the lesioned dorsolateral striatum into a functional network, but also increased functional connectivity in regions beyond the localization of the lesion, such as motor cortex, thalamus, and cerebellum (Wang et al., 2015a). Similarly, an increase in recruitment of the prefrontal cortex as well as the cerebellum was found in a study that looked at task-specific exercise in 6-OHDA rats (Wang et al., 2015b). These results are interesting in the light of recent hypotheses that assign the cerebellum a potential compensatory role for basal ganglia dysfunction in PD. Interestingly, this result is convergent with recent human neuroimaging studies on exercise-induced structural brain changes (see the following section).

Taken together, these animal experiments provide evidence that exercise-induced changes in functional activation and connectivity also occur beyond the lesioned brain area, within the functional circuitry of motor control and include cortical, subcortical, and brain stem structures.

THE EFFECTS OF EXERCISE ON THE PARKINSONIAN BRAIN—HUMAN STUDIES

Clinical human cross-sectional studies in PD patients compared to healthy controls, have provided evidence that not only the neurodegeneration but also compensatory brain mechanisms determine the onset and course of PD. Magnetic resonance imaging (MRI) studies suggest that, at both presymptomatic and symptomatic disease stages, an increase in gray matter volume within putamen and globus pallidus is indicative of long-term adaptation to chronic dopaminergic dysfunction (Binkofski et al., 2007; Reetz et al., 2010). Interestingly, functional MRI studies showed an additional functional recruitment of cortical and cerebellar brain areas in PD patients as compared to healthy controls when successfully learning/exerting a motor task, potentially indicating a compensatory role of these structures (Mentis et al., 2003; Palmer et al., 2009).

Yet, there is only a limited number of longitudinal studies which have investigated molecular and/or brain network effects of exercise, or physical activity, in human PD. Current studies are heterogeneous in the physical training methods implemented and the level of disease progression analyzed. Although these first studies are important and may provide a "proof of principle," more research is needed in order to systemize these neuroplastic effects according to clinical parameters and the respective exercise intervention.

Dopamine Receptor Changes and Neurotrophic Factors

A study by Fisher et al. (2013) used PET imaging to investigate the effect of an 8-week program of continuous treadmill walking on D2 receptor binding potential. As mentioned previously, these receptors are involved in modulating glutamatergic cortical input within the MSN in the striatum (Fisher et al., 2013). The results showed an increase in dopamine D2 receptor density in the putamen of the experimental group following the treadmill exercise in PD patients.

A study by Zoladz et al. (2014) investigated the effects of intermittent aerobic training, by means of a forced-use paradigm, on BDNF serum levels in mild to moderately affected PD patients. The authors found increase in basal serum BDNF levels following the exercise intervention. This is relevant as the exercise intensity was of a moderate level over a period of 8 weeks—suggesting that even moderate levels of exercise could produce increased levels of serum BDNF.

Similar results were found in another recent study: In a more ecological setting, increased levels of BDNF serum levels were found with multidisciplinary training methods (Frazzitta et al., 2013). Here, training methods included intensive physiotherapy sessions that focussed on cardiovascular, mobility, and balance training. In addition, occupational therapy was included that focussed on improving independency in activities of daily living such as hand functionality and bed transfers. The intervention design is noteworthy as multiple training techniques were implemented which led to a general increase in BDNF factors, whether this was due to a combined effect of the training methods used, or a particular intervention in isolation is unclear.

Taken together, these human longitudinal studies at least partly confirm results that have been obtained in animal models, and suggest that both changes in D2 receptor function as well as BDNF might mediate neuroplastic mechanisms underlying the effects of exercise interventions in PD.

Functional and Structural Changes in Brain Networks

Fisher et al. (2008) used transcranial magnetic stimulation (TMS) in order to assess potential changes in motorcortical excitability in PD patients induced by a high intensity body-weight supported treadmill training over 8 weeks. The intervention resulted in an increased motor performance in self-selected walking speed and other gait parameters. These behavioral changes were accompanied by an increase in corticomotor excitability as assessed by TMS. Since attenuated corticomotor excitability is suggested to be present in PD, these changes might reflect a normalization of motor cortex function induced by the exercise intervention (Fisher et al., 2008).

In a recent study, Shah et al. (2016) used resting-state functional magnetic resonance imaging as a measure for functional connectivity between brain regions before and after an 8-week forced-rate cycling exercise intervention compared to a voluntary-rate pedaling intervention. The authors showed an increased thalamo-cortical connectivity in the forced-pedaled PD group, an effect that persisted after a 4-week retention period, compared to the slower pedalling PD control group. These findings provide preliminary evidence that higher intensity forced-rate cycling influences the functional connectivity between motor cortex and thalamus as potential neuroplastic mechanism induced by the exercise intervention.

Athough the aforementioned studies investigated functional brain network changes in response to an exercise intervention, Sehm et al. (2014) investigated learning-related gray-matter structure alterations in PD patients compared to healthy controls. In this study, a 6 week, complex balance-task training was performed and four MRI scans were performed before, during, and after the training. The task itself consisted of time spent in balance on a specially constructed balance-board, enforcing a discovery-learning approach to perform and learn to keep a platform in a horizontal position. The results suggest that, even in the PD brain, structural brain changes occur while patients learn to master the task. Gray matter changes that correlated with balance learning in the PD patient group were found in different cortical areas (involving the right anterior precuneus, left parietal cortex, left ventral premotor cortex, bilateral anterior cingulate cortex, and left middle temporal gyrus). Furthermore, and more important, as evidenced by a significant time by group interaction analysis, PD patients showed an increase in structural brain changes over time as compared to the control group in the cerebellum. This result is especially interesting in the light of other studies (see previous paragraph on animal models) and assign the cerebellum a potential role for exercise-induced compensatory neuroplastic mechanisms in PD.

Taken together, these first studies provide evidence that exercise interventions may induce both functional and even structural changes in the brain of PD patients. Potential localizations of such exercise-induced neuroplastic changes involve not only the network affected by the disease pathology (i.e., areas within the cortico-basal ganglia-thalamo-cortical loop) but also alternative networks that modulate motor function such as the cerebellum.

CONCLUSION

The knowledge regarding exercise-induced neuroplastic changes in the parkinsonian brain is still scarce. However, first studies provide the "proof of principle" that functional and structural brain changes underlie beneficial effects of different exercise modalities on clinical symptoms. Potential mechanisms observed so far include changes in dopamine and glutamate transmission in the basal ganglia pathways, increase in neurotrophic factors as well as changes in function ad structure within and beyond the brain network affected by the disease pathology. These changes represent intrinsic regenerative processes that counteract the symptom-inducing pathogenetic processes, that is, the neurodegeneration of dopamine producing cells in the substantia nigra. In future, these markers may be used to monitor and assess the effectiveness of exercise, thereby helping to guide effective interventions. Furthermore, knowledge regarding the neuroanatomical substrates of neuroplastic changes may guide new innovative approaches that aim at enhancing these processes such as plasticity-inducing noninvasive brain stimulation protocols. This could open a new avenue of therapeutic approaches, in addition to the established pharmacological substitution therapy and deep brain stimulation.

References

Abbruzzese, G., Marchese, R., Avanzino, L., Pelosin, E., 2016. Rehabilitation for Parkinson's disease: current outlook and future challenges. Parkinsonism & Related Disorders 22, S60–S64.

Binkofski, F., Reetz, K., Gaser, C., Hilker, R., Hagenah, J., Hedrich, K., van Eimeren, T., Thiel, A., Buchel, C., Pramstaller, P.P., Siebner, H.R., Klein, C., 2007. Morphometric fingerprint of asymptomatic Parkin and PINK1 mutation carriers in the basal ganglia. Neurology 69, 842–850.

Cohen, A., Tillerson, J., Smith, A., Schallert, T., Zigmond, M., 2003. Neuroprotective effects of prior limb use in 6-hydroxydopamine-treated rats: possible role of GDNF. Journal of Neurochemistry 85 (2), 299–305.

Fisher, B., Petzinger, G., Nixon, K., Hogg, E., Bremmer, S., Meshul, C., Jakowec, M., 2004. Exercise-induced behavioral recovery and neuroplasticity in the 1-methyl-4-phenyl-1,2,3,6-tetrahydropyridine-lesioned mouse basal ganglia. Journal of Neuroscience Research 77 (3), 378–390.

Fisher, B., Wu, A., Salem, G., Song, J., Lin, C., Yip, J., 2008. The effect of exercise training in improving motor performance and corticomotor excitability in people with early Parkinson's disease. Archives of Physical Medicine and Rehabilitation 89 (7), 1221–1229.

Fisher, B.E., Li, Q., Nacca, A., Salem, G.J., Song, J., Yip, J., Hui, J.S., Jakowec, M.W., Petzinger, G.M., 2013. Treadmill exercise elevates striatal dopamine D2 receptor binding potential in patients with early Parkinson's disease. Neuroreport 24 (10), 509–514.

Fox, S.H., Katzenschlager, R., Lim, S.Y., Ravina, B., Seppi, K., Coelho, M., Poewe, W., Rascol, O., Goetz, C.G., Sampaio, C., 2011. The movement disorder society evidence-based medicine review update: treatments for the motor symptoms of Parkinson's disease. Movement Disorders 26 (S3), S2–S41.

Frazzitta, G., Maestri, R., Ghilardi, M., Riboldazzi, G., Perini, M., Bertotti, G., 2013. Intensive rehabilitation increases BDNF serum levels in parkinsonian patients: a randomized study. Neurorehabilitation and Neural Repair 28 (2), 163–168.

Gallo, P.M., Garber, C.E., 2011. Parkinson's disease: a comprehensive approach to exercise prescription for the health fitness professional. ACSM's Health & Fitness Journal 15 (4), 8–17.

Hirsch, M., Iyer, S., Sanjak, M., 2016. Exercise-induced neuroplasticity in human Parkinson's disease: what is the evidence telling us? Parkinsonism & Related Disorders 22, S78–S81.

Howells, D.W., Porritt, M.J., Wong, J.Y., Batchelor, P.E., Kalnins, R., Hughes, A.J., Donnan, G.A., 2000. Reduced BDNF mRNA expression in the Parkinson's disease substantia nigra. Experimental Neurology 166, 127–135.

King, L.A., Wilhelm, J., Chen, Y., Blehm, R., Nutt, J., Chen, Z., Serdar, A., Horak, F.B., 2015. Effects of group, individual, and home exercise in persons with Parkinson disease: a randomized clinical trial. Journal of Neurologic Physical Therapy 39 (4), 204–212.

Klamroth, S., Steib, S., Devan, S., Pfeifer, K., 2016. Effects of exercise therapy on postural instability in Parkinson disease: a meta-analysis. Journal of Neurologic Physical Therapy 40 (1), 3–14.

Mentis, M.J., Dhawan, V., Nakamura, T., Ghilardi, M.F., Feigin, A., Edwards, C., Ghez, C., Eidelberg, D., 2003. Enhancement of brain activation during trial-and-error sequence learning in early PD. Neurology 60, 612–619.

Mink, J.W., 1996. The basal ganglia: focused selection and inhibition of competing motor programs. Progress in Neurobiology 50 (4), 381–425.

Palmer, S.J., Ng, B., Abugharbieh, R., Eigenraam, L., McKeown, M.J., 2009. Motor reserve and novel area recruitment: amplitude and spatial characteristics of compensation in Parkinson's disease. European Journal of Neuroscience 29, 2187–2196.

Petzinger, G.M., Walsh, J.P., Akopian, G., Hogg, E., Abernathy, A., Arevalo, P., Turnquist, P., Vuckovic, M., Fisher, B.E., Togasaki, D.M., Jakowec, M.W., 2007. Effects of treadmill exercise on dopaminergic transmission in the MPTP-lesioned mouse model of basal ganglia injury. Journal of Neuroscience 27 (20), 5291–5300.

Petzinger, G.M., Fisher, B.E., Van Leeuwen, J.E., Vukovic, M., Akopian, G., Meshul, C.K., Holschneider, D.P., Nacca, A., Walsh, J.P., Jakowec, M.W., 2010. Enhancing neuroplasticity in the basal ganglia: the role of exercise in Parkinson's disease. Movement Disorders 25 (S1), S141–S145.

Petzinger, G.M., Fisher, B., McEwen, S., Beeler, J., Walsh, J., Jakowec, M., 2013. Exercise-enhanced neuroplasticity targeting motor and cognitive circuitry in Parkinson's disease. The Lancet Neurology 12 (7), 716–726.

Picelli, A., Herman, T., Paul, S.S., King, L.A., 2015. Rehabilitation procedures in the management of Parkinson's disease. Parkinson's Disease 2015.

Real, C.C., Ferreira, A.F., Chaves-Kirsten, G.P., Torrao, A.S., Pires, R.S., Britto, L.R., 2013. BDNF receptor blockade hinders the beneficial effects of exercise in a rat model of Parkinson's disease. Neuroscience 237, 118–129.

Reetz, K., Tadic, V., Kasten, M., Bruggemann, N., Schmidt, A., Hagenah, J., Pramstaller, P.P., Ramirez, A., Behrens, M.I., Siebner, H.R., Klein, C., Binkofski, F., 2010. Structural imaging in the presymptomatic stage of genetically determined parkinsonism. Neurobiology of Disease 39, 402–408.

Sehm, B., Taubert, M., Conde, V., Weise, D., Classen, J., Dukart, J., Draganski, B., Villringer, A., Ragert, P., 2014. Structural brain plasticity in Parkinson's disease induced by balance training. Neurobiology of Aging 35 (1), 232–239.

Shah, C., Beall, E.B., Frankemolle, A.M.M., Penko, A., Phillips, M.D., Lowe, M.J., Alberts, J.L., 2016. Brain Connectivity 6 (1), 25–36.

Shumway-Cook, A., Woollacott, M., 2012. Motor Control. Wolters Kluwer Health, Lippincott Williams & Wilkins, Philadelphia. [u.a.].

Tanaka, K., de Quadros, A.C., Santos, R.F., Stella, F., Gobbi, L.T.B., Gobbi, S., 2009. Benefits of physical exercise on executive functions in older people with Parkinson's disease. Brain and Cognition 69 (2), 435–441.

Tomlinson, C.L., Patel, S., Meek, C., Herd, C.P., Clarke, C.E., Stowe, R., Shah, L., Sackley, C., Deane, K.H., Wheatley, K., Ives, N., 2013. Physiotherapy versus placebo or no intervention in Parkinson's disease. Cochrane Database of Systematic Reviews 8, CD002817.

Tomlinson, C.L., Herd, C.P., Clarke, C.E., Meek, C., Patel, S., Stowe, R., Deane, K.H., Shah, L., Sackley, C., Wheatley, K., Ives, N., 2014. Physiotherapy for Parkinson's disease: a comparison of techniques. Cochrane Database of Systematic Reviews 6, CD002815.

Uhrbrand, A., Stenager, E., Pedersen, M.S., Dalgas, U., 2015. Parkinson's disease and intensive exercise therapy–a systematic review and meta-analysis of randomized controlled trials. Journal of the Neurological Sciences 353 (1), 9–19.

VanLeeuwen, J., Petzinger, G., Walsh, J., Akopian, G., Vuckovic, M., Jakowec, M., 2009. Altered AMPA receptor expression with treadmill exercise in the 1-methyl-4-phenyl-1,2,3,6-tetrahydropyridine-lesioned mouse model of basal ganglia injury. Journal of Neuroscience Research 88 (3), 650–668.

Vaynman, S., Ying, Z., Gomez-Pinilla, F., 2004. Hippocampal BDNF mediates the efficacy of exercise on synaptic plasticity and cognition. European Journal of Neuroscience 20 (10), 2580–2590.

Wang, Z., Myers, K.G., Guo, Y., Ocampo, M.A., Pang, R.D., Jakowec, M.W., Holschneider, D.P., 2013. Functional reorganization of motor and limbic circuits after exercise training in a rat model of bilateral parkinsonism. PLoS One 8 (11), e80058 21.

Wang, Z., Guo, Y., Myers, K.G., Heintz, R., Peng, Y.H., Maarek, J.M., Holschneider, D.P., 2015a. Exercise alters resting-state functional connectivity of motor circuits in parkinsonian rats. Neurobiology of Aging 36 (1), 536–544.

Wang, Z., Guo, Y., Myers, K.G., Heintz, R., Holschneider, D.P., 2015b. Recruitment of the prefrontal cortex and cerebellum in Parkinsonian rats following skilled aerobic exercise. Neurobiology of Disease 77, 71–87.

Zoladz, J.A., Majerczak, J., Zeligowska, E., Mencel, J., Jaskolski, A., Jaskolska, A., Marusiak, J., 2014. Moderate-intensity interval training increases serum brain-derived neurotrophic factor level and decreases inflammation in Parkinson's disease patients. Journal of Physiology and Pharmacology 65 (3), 441–448.

IV. EXERCISE AS THERAPY FOR NEUROLOGICAL DISEASES

Physical Exercise and Its Effects on Alzheimer's Disease

A.M. Stein, R.V. Pedroso
Univ Estadual Paulista, Rio Claro, São Paulo, Brazil

Abstract

Physical exercise has frequently been the target of research studies related to the treatment of Alzheimer's disease. The level and routine of physical exercise can influence the progression of the disease, as well as influence the intensity of the deleterious effects from Alzheimer's disease. The objective of this article is to introduce the reader to this subject and point out the main findings in scientific literature related to physical exercise and its effects on Alzheimer's disease. This article will identify the general characteristics of the disease, the exercise programs currently used, and the main effects for each of these topics. It will also address a very current topic related to this issue, blood markers, and other techniques for future studies with this population.

INTRODUCTION

In the last few decades, physical education has been studied as part of the treatment for Alzheimer's disease (AD). The evidence is very interesting for researchers and the public health industry, since the disease has become increasingly prevalent and 60–80% of all cases of dementia in the world are AD, in accordance with the current report from the Alzheimer's Association (2013).

This article aims to increase knowledge about the effects that exercise has on AD, and is divided into six topics which address the general aspects of AD and the effects that different levels of physical activity have on the progression of the disease.

ALZHEIMER'S DISEASE AND LEVEL OF PHYSICAL ACTIVITY

Physical activity is defined as any body movement produced as a result of a muscular contraction with a caloric expenditure (Caspersen et al., 1985). The association between physical activity and good health is noteworthy in AD. There are studies showing the possible relationship between having an active lifestyle and being less at risk of developing the disease (Barnesand and Yaffe, 2011; Rolland et al., 2008).

Barnes and Yaffe (2011) identified the lack of physical activity as one of the six risks factors for the disease's development and estimated that around 13% (almost 4.3 million) of the AD cases could be attributed to physical inactivity. They also noted that a 10% reduction in the prevalence of physical inactivity could help avoid over 380,000 new cases, while a 25% decrease would cause a reduction of over 1 million new cases around the world. These results become more important, due to the fact that almost one fifth of the population (~17.3%) is considered inactive (Dumith et al., 2011).

Therefore, it is very important for people to embrace a healthy lifestyle, considering the importance of it on the aging process. In the relationship between physical conditioning and cognitive reserve in the elderly, studies have shown that better conditioned individuals show more cognitive reserve, that they have acquired during life, which could be a defense mechanism against cognitive impairment (Deary et al., 2006).

Besides the relationship between physical activity and AD genesis, studies have also verified the relationship between the level of activity and AD progression. Although scarce, studies have shown low levels of physical activities in this population (Lima et al., 2010; Vital et al., 2012a; Stein et al., 2012; Andrade et al., 2013; Garuffi et al., 2013).

Lima et al. (2010) studies quantified the level of physical activity of older people through a questionnaire and pedometer. The authors verified that, no matter the method used, the level of physical activity was considered low; there was an average of 4400 steps per day. They suggested that 6000–6500 steps per day would be a reasonable recommendation for this population. Holthoff et al. (2015) also used a pedometer and suggested a range from 5818 to 6662 steps, which means some of the group Lima studied can still be considered to be at a low level, if the suggested recommendation is taken into consideration.

Vital et al. (2012a), Stein et al. (2012), Andrade et al. (2013), and Garuffi et al. (2013) all evaluated elderly people with AD in the low and moderate phases of the disease through the modified Baecke questionnaire for older adults and identified a low level of physical activity was common. The average points vary among the studies from 1.7 to 5.4 points. Vital et al. (2012a) also found that the lower scores are mainly due to the lack of leisure activity and lack of systematic physical activity.

Although there are some barriers to overcome to be able to engage in regular physical activity, when systematic, the physical activity can promote many benefits to cognitive functions, in behavioral disorders and in functionality of elderly people with dementia (Pedroso et al., 2012a; Coelho et al., 2009; Vital et al., 2012a,b; Hernandez et al., 2010). All of which will be addressed in the following topics "Alzheimer's Disease, Physical Exercise, and Cognitive Functions," "Alzheimer's Disease, Physical Exercise, and Neuropsychiatric Symptoms," and "Alzheimer's Disease, Physical Exercise, and Functional Capacity."

Therefore, considering that old people with AD present low levels of physical activity and benefits shown for slowing the progression of the disease, it becomes even more important to practice regular and systematic physical activity. Some of the exercise programs already used with this population can be analyzed in the next section.

ALZHEIMER'S DISEASE AND PHYSICAL ACTIVITY PROGRAMS

As seen in the previous topic, the physical activity level has been associated with AD progression and is one of the strategies used to try to increase the activity levels of the elderly, which can help prevent or slow the effects of the disease. Physical exercise is defined as any planned, structured, and repetitive activity that aims to improve or to maintain the components of physical fitness (Caspersen et al., 1985).

The current theme in literature is that physical exercise programs have been employed aiming to analyze the effects on the disease, either in animal examination or in patients with AD (Phillips et al., 2015). It is known that different kinds of exercises, as well as the intensity and frequency of those exercises, all result in different results. Besides that, because the studies are with patients at different stages of the disease, ages, amount of time with the disease, and the presence or not of AD symptoms, this limits some affirmations on the topic of exercise and AD until more research studies are done. Therefore, the goal is to provide the reader with an overview of the studies already presently made and indicate programs, in chronological order, regarding the training principles, and the findings in each of the programs. Such information can be seen on Table 14.1.

ALZHEIMER'S DISEASE, PHYSICAL EXERCISE, AND COGNITIVE FUNCTIONS

The cognitive impairment can be considered as one of the first clinical manifestation in AD patients, which is affected gradually according to the evolution of the disease. At first, the patient has greater impairment of recent memory and, with clinical course, changes occur in semantic memory, language disorder, attention deficits, deficits in visual-spatial skills, and executive functions. Those cognitive changes damage ability to perform daily activities and affect family, social, and occupational living (Yaari and Bloom, 2007).

Regular physical activity has been shown to be effective for nonpharmacological treatment of AD by showing benefits of controlling cognitive changes. A systematic review done by Coelho et al. (2009) included eight studies that verified the effects of systematic physical activities on cognitive functions in older people with AD. In all studies, they all contributed to improving, even if just temporarily, their attention, executive functions, and language.

Recently, another metaanalysis study by Farina et al. (2014) also verified the effects of physical activities, including programs that used only physical exercise with no extra stimulus on cognitive function in people with AD. The study concluded that it had a positive result in controlling the rate of cognitive decline and global cognitive function.

TABLE 14.1 Characteristics of Studies That Analyzed the Effects of Physical Exercise in the Elderly With Alzheimer's Disease

Reference	Protocol	Time/Session; Frequency/Week; Duration	Intensity	Overload	Results
Namazi et al. (1994)	Resistance, flexibility, respiration, and ADL exercises	40 min; daily; 4 weeks	Mild	No overload	Decrease of depressive symptoms
Palleschi et al. (1996)	Aerobic training (treadmill)	20 min; 3; 12 weeks	70% PRF	No overload	Improvement of attention and global cognitive functions
Arkin and Howell (1999)	Aerobic training (treadmill and stationary bicycle), stretching, balance, and resistance exercises	At least 20 min; 2; 6–12 weeks	NR	Increase of total training volume	Improvement of physical fitness, mood, and socialization
Cott et al. (2002)	Walk with conversation	30 min; 5; 16 weeks	NR	NR	Maintenance of communication
Heyn (2003)	Multisensory exercise program: aerobic, stretching, and resistance exercises, relaxation, dance	15–70 min; 3; 8 weeks	NR	Increase of total training volume (15–70 min)	Maintenance of global cognitive functions. Improvement of resting heart rate, mood and in engagement of physical activity
Teri et al. (2003)	Home-exercise program: aerobic, stretching, balance, and resistance exercises	At least 30 min; daily; 12 weeks	Moderate	NR	Decrease of depressive symptoms increased of level of physical activity, health and motor function
Rolland et al. (2007)	Aerobic, stretching, balance, and resistance exercises	60 min; 2; 12 months	Moderate	NR	Improvement in ADL
Arkin (2007)	Aerobic training (stationary bicycle), stretching, and balance exercises, resistance training	NR; 2; 10 weeks	NR	Increase of total training volume	Maintenance of global cognitive functions
Williams and Tappen (2008)	Comprehensive individual exercise: stretching, balance, and resistance exercises and walk. Supervised individual walking: Walk	20–30 min, respectively; 5; 15 weeks	NR	Increase of total training volume	Decrease of depressive symptoms
Santana-Sosa et al. (2008)	Resistance, motor co-ordination, and mobility exercises	75 min; 3; 12 weeks	NR	NR	Improvement of muscular resistance, flexibility, agility, balance and in ADL
Aman and Thomas (2009)	Aerobic, stretching, and resistance exercises	30 min; 3; 3 weeks	Mild	No overload	Improvement of physical fitness. Decreased of anxiety
Steinberg et al. (2009)	Home-based protocol: walk, stretching, balance, and resistance exercises	NR; 3; 12 weeks	NR	NR	Improvement of functional performance
Christofoletti et al. (2009)	Agility, balance, and resistance exercises Spatial orientation, proprioception, and cognitive stimulation	50 min; 3; 12 weeks	80% HRmax	Increase of the training stimulus	Decrease of depressive symptoms. Improvement of flexibility, motor coordination, balance and aerobic capacity
Hernandez et al. (2010)	Multimodal exercises: stretching and resistance exercises, circuits, sports games, dance, and relaxation	60 min; 3; 24 weeks	60–80% HRmax	NR	Maintenance of global cognitive functions. Improvement of mobility and balance

Continued

TABLE 14.1   Characteristics of Studies That Analyzed the Effects of Physical Exercise in the Elderly With Alzheimer's Disease—cont'd

Reference	Protocol	Time/Session; Frequency/Week; Duration	Intensity	Overload	Results
Yaguez et al. (2011)	Brain Gym	60 min; 1; 6 weeks	NR	NR	Improvement of attention, visuospatial memory, and working memory
Stella et al. (2011)	Multimodal exercises: walk, dance, stretching, agility, motor coordination, and resistance exercises	60 min; 3; 24 weeks	Moderate	Every 5 weeks	Attenuation of neuropsychiatric disorders
Venturelli et al. (2011)	Program of walk	30 min; 4; 24 weeks	Moderate	NR	Maintenance of global cognitive functions and improvement in ADL
Vreugdenhil et al. (2012)	Home-based exercise: home-based exercises and walking under the supervision of their caregiver	NR; 1; 16 weeks	NR	Increase of the training stimulus	Improvement of global cognitive functions, muscular resistance, balance, mobility and in ADL
Nascimento et al. (2012)	Multimodal exercises: Resistance, motor coordination, stretching, and balance exercises and cognitive exercises	60 min; 3; 24 weeks	70% HRmax	Every 4 weeks	Attenuation of neuropsychiatric disorders and improvement in ADL
Pedroso et al. (2012a)	Physical activity with dual task: aerobic, resistance, flexibility, agility, and balance exercises encompassed cognitive component	60 min; 3; 16 weeks	NR	NR	Improvement of executive functions, balance. Reduction in the number of falls
Garuffi et al. (2013)	Resistance training: peck deck, the pull down, leg press, supported barbell curls performed with free weights and triceps pulley	60 min; 3; 16 weeks	85% of 20 RM	Every 15 days	Improvement of muscular resistance, balance, flexibility and in ADL
Groppo et al. (2012)	Multimodal exercises: aerobic, resistance, agility, and balance exercises and cognitive exercises	60 min; 3; 24 weeks	60–80% HRmax	Every 4 weeks	Decrease of depressive symptoms
Vital et al. (2012b)	Resistance training: peck deck, the pull down, leg press, supported barbell curls performed with free weights and triceps pulley	60 min; 3; 16 weeks	85% of 20 RM	Every 15 days	No difference after the intervention
Coelho et al. (2013)	Physical activity with dual task: aerobic, resistance, flexibility, agility, and balance exercises encompassed cognitive components	60 min; 3; 16 weeks	65–75% HRmax	Increase of the training stimulus	Improvement of global cognitive functions
Andrade et al. (2013)	Physical activity with dual task: aerobic, stretching, flexibility, and balance exercises encompassed cognitive components (executive function, attention, and language)	60 min; 3; 16 weeks	65–75% HRmax	Every 4 weeks	Improvement of postural control, muscular resistance, gait and flexibility
Coelho et al. (2014)	Aerobic training (treadmill)	17 min; NR; 1 day (acute exercise)	Moderate	NA	Increase of BDNF concentration
Arcoverde et al. (2014)	Aerobic training (treadmill)	30 min; 2; 12 weeks	60% VO$_{2máx}$	NR	Improvement of global cognitive functions, balance, and mobility
Nascimento et al. (2014)	Multimodal exercise: flexibility, resistance, motor coordination, and balance exercises	60 min; 3; 24 weeks	60–80% HRmax	Every 4 weeks	Decrease of depressive symptoms. Improvement in ADL
Hulshof et al. (2015)	Movement trainer—ReckMOTOmed	30 min; 3; 12 weeks	Level 2–4 of movement trainer	No overload	Improvement of global cognitive functions, functional capacity and in ADL

ADL, activities of daily living; *BDNF*, brain-derived neurotrophic factor; *HRmax*, maximum heart rate; *Min*, minutes; *NA*, not applicable; *NR*, not related; *PRF*, pulse repetition frequency; *RM*, repetition maximum.

However, not only Coelho et al. (2009) but also Farina et al. (2014) agree that there is still no consensus or sufficient theoretical basis to define what the ideal intervention program is to produce results such as cognitive benefits in this population. That difficulty is a result of the articles, wide variation between the different designs of each study. However, there is a positive initial indication that the effectiveness of regular physical activity is evident.

Other studies also show improvements in global cognitive functions (Hernandez et al., 2010; Venturelli et al., 2011; Vreugdenhil et al., 2012; Arcoverde et al., 2014), advancements in sustained attention and visual-spatial memory (Yaguez et al., 2011), and improvements in executive and frontal functions (Pedroso et al., 2012a; Coelho et al., 2013). The intervention programs were different in each study and can be reviewed in the topic "Alzheimer's Disease and Physical Activity Programs."

The mechanisms by which exercise can generate such cognitive benefits are not yet fully understood, but there are some theories. Many authors have pointed out that physical exercise can induce molecular cascades and cellular processes that promote angiogenesis, neurogenesis, and synaptogenesis; increase cerebral blood flow; and increase the supply of neurotransmitters (Deslandes et al., 2009).

Ratey and Loehr (2011) divided these possible mechanisms in three groups: neural system (cognitive: attention, learning, and memory), molecular (growth factors), and cellular (angiogenesis, neurogenesis, and synaptic plasticity). Also note that the authors point out that these mechanisms would all be interconnected. But beyond the neurological mechanisms, one cannot omit the benefits derived from the social interaction surrounding the physical exercise group.

ALZHEIMER'S DISEASE, PHYSICAL EXERCISE, AND NEUROPSYCHIATRIC SYMPTOMS

Although AD is commonly known by the cognitive alterations, there are other manifestations of the disease known as neuropsychiatric, behavioral and psychological symptoms of dementia or neuropsychiatric symptoms (NPS). NPS reach between 60% and 80% of AD patients, and the most prevalent are apathy, depression, anxiety, aggression, agitation, and psychosis. These factors contribute to increased patient suffering and heightened care giver burden, which may represent one of the factors to premature institutionalization and they also accelerate disease progression (Jalbert et al., 2008). Given this context, studies of exercises have been proposed in an attempt to figure out if this type of intervention could be effective for the control of NPS.

In a study by Hernandez et al. (2011), there were positive results regarding the effects of physical activity on depression symptoms, sleep disturbances, and restlessness. In this review, of the eight analyzed articles, six showed benefits related to NPS.

In another review by Vital et al. (2010), it was found that there is no definite answer to the effectiveness of physical exercise on the symptoms of depression. Of the four studies analyzed in this review, two pointed out benefits and two did not show any significant changes.

Regarding the programs described in the previous section, that were not analyzed by Hernandez et al. (2011) and Vital et al. (2010), we can see that five studies reinforce the findings, such as reducing depressing symptoms (Christofoletti et al., 2009; Groppo et al., 2012); mitigation and reduction of NPS (Stella et al., 2011; Nascimento et al., 2012) and a decrease in sleep disorders (Nascimento et al., 2014).

Nascimento et al. (2014) adds that the sleeping disturbances can be related to changes in neurotransmitters, signaling hormones, and neurotrophic factors. Also, an explanation about the effects of exercise on brain health could be the greatest contribution of afferent neurotransmitters to the hippocampus, such as norepinephrine and serotonin and also the brain-derived neurotrophic factor (BDNF).

In general, most studies analyzed in this topic showed that an exercise program lowers and weakens the NPS. Therefore, exercise seems to play an important role in the control of this manifestation.

ALZHEIMER'S DISEASE, PHYSICAL EXERCISE, AND FUNCTIONAL CAPACITY

Besides the cognitive changes and NPS, the AD patients show functional changes that are relative to the levels of decreased functional capacity that may be present in the early stages of the disease (Perry and Hodges, 2000; Eggermont et al., 2010; Cedervall et al., 2015).

Eggermont et al. (2010) found that elderly people in the mild stage of AD showed decreases in balance and functional mobility compared to cognitively preserved elderly. The same difference between groups was found in several studies based on other components of functional capacity, such as strength, agility, and aerobic capacity (Cedervall et al., 2015; Coelho et al., 2014).

Cedervall et al. (2015) identified that over 2 years, elderly in the mild stage of AD declined in all functional capacity components, with the aerobic capacity the least affected. Besides that, the cognitive impairment seems to contribute to such damage. Therefore, the practice of the physical activity aimed to improve functional capacity as it becomes important, because besides contributing to attenuate cognitive decline and NPS, one can also avoid the sharp decline in functional capacity.

Blankevoort et al. (2010) reviewed 16 studies that investigated the effects of physical activity in strength, balance, mobility, and performance, on the activities of daily living in elderly patients with dementia. The authors found that, in every stage of the disease, the practice of physical activities have benefits. Furthermore, they concluded that interventions such as "multimodal," which are group activities that encourage all components of functional capacity, are the ones that promote greater benefits in walking speed, mobility, and balance, in comparison to interventions such as resistance training, that prioritize only one component of functional capacity. However, for the resistance strength of the lower limbs, both types of intervention result in improvement.

After 2009, more studies were done and the findings are described in the following. Hernandez et al. (2010) developed a multimodal intervention program and found improvements in mobility and balance. Pedroso et al. (2012a) and Andrade et al. (2013) conducted a multimodal intervention program with double task, and in addition to the improvements reported by Hernandez et al. (2010), there were improved postural control, pace of walking, flexibility, and strength in the legs.

Although Blankevoort et al. (2010) indicates greater benefits from multimodal interventions, Garuffi et al. (2013) found some improvements after a resistance training program. Those advancements included increased strength endurance of the lower limbs and improved balance and flexibility. Arcoverde et al. (2014) also applied an individualized aerobic training, performed on a treadmill, and found increases in balance and mobility. Also Vreugdenhil et al. (2012)'s study which consisted of a domiciliary of supervised walks that provided improvements in balance, mobility, and strength in the legs. Therefore, it can be seen that several programs were sufficient in generating benefits in physical components of functional capacity. Details about the programs can be seen in the topic "Alzheimer's Disease and Physical Activity Programs" in this chapter.

Also note, because there is no specific recommendation for physical activities for the elderly with Alzheimer's disease there is difficulty defining exactly what would be the best kind of program for this population. However, in the case of the benefits of physical activity for the health of older people in general, you can follow the guidelines from the American College of Medicine and Sports for the Elderly (2009). They recommend that exercise for the elderly should include aerobic exercises, muscle strengthening, and flexibility and balance exercises, specifically when they are at risk of falling or having mobility impairment, as is the case of older people with dementia.

Therefore, in accordance with the guidelines and the results discussed here, multimodal interventions seem to be important for the improvement of functional capacity, but remember that other programs also found interesting results.

ALZHEIMER'S DISEASE, PHYSICAL EXERCISE, AND BIOMARKERS

In an attempt to clarify what would be the best possible mechanisms by which physical exercise leads to benefits in AD, several studies have proposed different and complementary hypotheses. In this context, Deslandes et al. (2009), in a review article, suggests some neurophysiological hypotheses as to why exercise can promote improvements in mental health, such as regulation of reactive oxygen species, release of growth factors, neurotransmitter synthesis, oxygenation increase in the brain, and glucose uptake and changes in cerebral blood flow.

Therefore, one of the possible putative mechanisms for cognitive improvement induced by exercise is the growth factors. Among these, the BDNF growth factor similar to −1 (IGF-1) and the vascular endothelial growth factor (VEGF), have been identified as the main mechanisms that work together to produce functional effects related to plasticity, functionality, and brain health (Cotman et al., 2007).

The BDNF, among other functions, is the main regulator of synaptic transmission and plasticity in various regions of the central nervous system. Furthermore, the BDNF may act as a modulator of neuroplasticity in cognitive processes and some studies have found that there is an association between the BDNF levels and cognitive performance (Komulainen et al., 2008), reinforcing the idea that the BDNF may be an indicator of cognitive impairment.

Regarding AD, a study by Coelho et al. (2014) pointed out that there is a relationship between physical activity and the BDNF levels. The AD patients have low levels in both variables, therefore strengthening the role of physical activity and neurotrophic factors in this disease. In the same study, it was found that aerobic exercise of moderate intensity can increase the BDNF levels in AD patients, which would be interesting because of the deficiency of this factor related to the disease. Given these observations, the authors point out that physical exercise could contribute to and prevent neurodegeneration from arising in AD (Coelho et al., 2014).

Besides the BDNF, another factor associated is the VEGF, which is produced by endothelial cells and plays a key role in the processes of angiogenesis, a process related to increased blood flow and increased perfusion of oxygen (Bloor, 2005). In regard to the nervous system, VEGF may act on migration and neuronal survival, improvement in synaptic transmission, axon growth and orientation, denditrogenege, glial cell migration and survival, and oligo-dentrocytes migration. Also, it can aid in neurogenesis and synaptic plasticity regulation (Carmeliet and Ruiz de Almodovar, 2013).

Studies have indicated that AD patients have a lower concentration of VEGF when compared to older people without cognitive impairment (Huang et al., 2013). On the other hand, exercises appear to stimulate increased levels of the VEGF contributing to increased capillary (Prior et al., 2003).

In AD, IGF-1 appears to exert a neuroprotective effect, neurogenesis, development, differentiation, synapse formation, and utilization of glucose in the brain (Gasparini and Xu, 2003). Regarding cognitive functions, IGF-I can benefit them as it has neurotrophic property and opposes the processes of beta-amyloid and tau hyperphosphorylation (Duron et al., 2012). In healthy elderly, there is a positive association between serum levels, IGF-I and working memory, selective attention, and executive functions (Bellar et al., 2011).

In a study by Trejo et al. (2001), it was reported that blocking IGF-1 entry into the brain results in preventing the proliferation of neurons in the dentade gyrus of the hippocampus, strengthening the role of this factor in neurogenesis and cognitive performance. Also, another study has demonstrated that blocking IGF-1 receptors in the choroid plexus triggers a series of disorders such as amyloidosis, cognitive impairment, loss of synaptic vesicle protein, glucose, and abnormal forms of tau protein, similar to the disturbances in AD (Carro et al., 2006).

Other studies in animal models have demonstrated that IGF-1 is also a mediator of angiogenesis induced by exercise, besides being a stimulus to increase the central level BDNF and increase production of VEGF (Lopez-Lopez et al., 2004; Ding et al., 2006). Thus, IGF-1 appears to exert a neural and vascular response induced by exercise, since the growth factors BDNF and VEGF are also linked to the processes of neurogenesis, synaptogenesis, and angiogenesis.

Trueba-Sáiz et al. (2013) defend the IGF-1 insert as a biomarker to be included in the early diagnosis of AD, as well as the inclusion of this in the development of new exercises. Moreover, the authors advocate the insertion of electroencephalogram (EEG) in the AD diagnosis. Routine EEG visual analysis has been considered an interesting method in the differential diagnosis aid in different types of dementia (Caramelli et al., 2011). EEG records are easy to use, common in clinics, are not expensive, as well as being a type of noninvasive method (Trueba-Sáiz et al., 2013). The use of EEG has also been used to verify the effect of exercise on the brains of the elderly (Moraes et al., 2007).

Exercises can cause changes in the brain activity, as pointed out by Moraes et al. (2007), and electrophysiological alterations could indicate reorganization of several systems. Among them are the metabolic system, physiological, biochemical, as well as, emotional, and cognitive functions. Studies suggest that after physical exercise there is an increase in the alpha wave activity that can be related to decrease in cortical activation, level of fatigue, relaxation, or reduction of anxiety (Petruzzello et al., 1991; Moraes et al., 2007). Moreover, Moraes et al. (2007) pointed out a series of evidence in relation to increased beta activity induced by exercise, indicating greater cortical activation, changes in cerebral blood flow, and hypothalamic modulation increasing temperature.

Another EEG component that has been used to understand how physical activity can modulate neural circuits is the P300 (Hillman et al., 2002, 2006). The P300 is a positive curve of large amplitude generated from 250 to 500 ms after the presence of an uncommon target stimulus, which is being presented through an eccentric paradigm in which the subjects are instructed to identify the infrequent stimulus while other irrelevant stimuli are also presented (Johnson, 1993).

There are two most relevant aspects of P300: latency, the information processing time, and amplitude, which is associated with the attention span and working memory (Polich, 1996). With the process of aging and the development of AD, studies indicate an increased latency, which is a slower cognitive processing speed and decreased amplitude, lower attention span and working memory, of P300 (Pedroso et al., 2012b; Polich, 1996).

In healthy elderly, physical activity appears to modulate these values in a positive way. Several studies have found more intense exercise programs are effective in generating these changes, such as swimming programs, Tai Chi, running, dancing, and resistance training (Ozkaya et al., 2005; Zhang et al., 2014).

Besides P300 being altered in AD, and studies show that physical activity could be associated with their values, there are no studies that investigate the effects of exercise on P300 elderly with AD. So having future studies, specific to this population, becomes necessary to clarify the effects of exercise on EEG and P300 as well as the neurotrophic factors.

IV. EXERCISE AS THERAPY FOR NEUROLOGICAL DISEASES

FINAL CONSIDERATIONS

It can be seen that there is an ample amount of scientific research investigating the positive effects of physical exercise on the characteristic changes of Alzheimer's disease, such as easing the rate of cognitive decline, improving the physical components of the functional capacity, and reduction of neuropsychiatric disorders. Despite the evidence, there are gaps related to physical activity programs that do not allow more conclusive recommendations; such as, what the ideal type is, frequency, and intensity of the physical activity to have greater benefits. Other doubts remain. Is there a dose–response relation between the activity and the benefits arising from it, with regard to the health of the elderly with Alzheimer's disease?

In addition to the cognitive, functional, and behavioral benefits, studies suggest that physical activity could also alter biomarkers of the disease, but there are more recent studies which are not fully consolidated. Therefore, it is necessary to develop further research in this area that can contribute to the knowledge covered in this article.

References

Alzheimer's Association, 2013. Alzheimer's disease facts and figures. Alzheimer's & Dementia 8 (2), 1–72.

Aman, E., Thomas, D.R., 2009. Supervised exercise to reduce agitation in severely cognitively impaired persons. Journal of the American Medical Directors Association 10, 271–276.

Andrade, L.P., Gobbi, L.T., Coelho, F.G., Christofoletti, G., Costa, J.L., Stella, F., 2013. Benefits of multimodal exercise intervention for postural control and frontal cognitive functions in individuals with Alzheimer's disease: a controlled trial. Journal of the American Geriatrics Society 61 (11), 1919–1926.

Arcoverde, C., Deslandes, A., Moraes, H., Almeida, C., Araujo, N.B., de Vasques, P.E., et al., 2014. Treadmill training as an augmentation treatment for Alzheimer's disease: a pilot randomized controlled study. Arquivos de Neuropsiquiatria 72, 190–610.

Arkin, S.M., Howell, N.M., 1999. Elder rehab: a student-supervised exercise program for Alzheimer's patients. The Gerontologist 39 (6), 279–775.

Arkin, S., 2007. Language-enriched plus socialization slows cognitive decline in Alzheimer's disease. American Journal of Alzheimer's Diseases and Other Dementias 22 (1), 62–77.

Barnes, D.E., Yaffe, K., 2011. The projected effect of risk factor reduction on Alzheimer's disease prevalence. The Lancet Neurology 10, 819–828.

Bellar, D., Glickman, E.L., Juvancic-Heltzel, J., Gunstad, J., 2011. Serum insulin like growth factor-1 is associated with working memory, executive function and selective attention in a sample of healthy, fit older adults. Neuroscience 178, 133–137.

Blankevoort, C.G., van Heuvelen, M.J.G., Boersma, F., Luning, H., de Jong, J., Scherder, E.J.A., 2010. Review of effects of physical activity on strength, balance, mobility and ADL performance in elderly subjects with dementia. Dementia and Geriatric Cognitive Disorders 30, 392–402.

Bloor, C.M., 2005. Angiogenesis during exercise and training. Angiogenesis 83, 263–271.

Caramelli, P., Teixeira, A.L., Buchpiguel, C.A., Lee, H.W., Livramento, J.A., Fernandes, L.L., et al., 2011. Diagnóstico da Doença de Alzheimer no Brasil: exames complementares. Dementia & Neuropsychologia 5 (1), 10–11.

Carmeliet, P., Ruiz de Almodovar, C., 2013. VEGF ligands and receptors: implications in neurodevelopment and neurodegeneration. Cellular and Molecular Life Sciences 70, 1763–1778.

Carro, E., Trejo, J.L., Spuch, C., Bohl, D., Heard, J.M., Torres-Aleman, I., 2006. Blockade of the insulin-like growth factor I receptor in the choroid plexus originates Alzheimer's-like neuropathology in rodents: new cues into the human disease? Neurobiology of Aging 27, 1618–1631.

Caspersen, C.J., Powell, K.E., Christenson, G.M., 1985. Physical activity, exercise and physical fitness. Public Health Reports 100 (2), 126–131.

Cedervall, Y., Kilander, L., Aberg, A.C., 2015. Declining physical capacity but maintained aerobic activity in early Alzheimer's disease. American Journal of Alzheimer's Diseases and Other Dementias 27 (3), 180–187.

Christofoletti, G., Oliani, M.M., Corazza, D.I., Stella, F., Gobbi, S., Gobbi, L.T.B., et al., 2009. Influencia de la actividad física en la enfermedad de Alzheimer: un caso clínico. RIFK 12 (2), 96–100.

Coelho, F.G.M., Galduróz-Santos, R.F., Gobbi, S., Stella, F., 2009. Atividade física sistematizada e desempenho cognitivo com demência de Alzheimer: uma revisão sistemática. Revista Brasileira de Psiquiatria 31, 163–170.

Coelho, F.G., Andrade, L.P., Pedroso, R.V., Santos-Galduróz, R.F., Gobbi, S., Costa, J.L.R., et al., 2013. Multimodal exercise intervention improves frontal cognitive functions and gait in Alzheimer's disease: a controlled trial. Geriatrics & Gerontology International 13 (1), 198–203.

Coelho, F.G., Vital, T.M., Stein, A.M., Arantes, F.J., Rueda, A.V., Camarini, R., Teodorov, et al., 2014. Acute aerobic exercise increases brain-derived neurotrophic factor levels in elderly with Alzheimer's disease. Journal of Alzheimer's Disease 39 (2), 401–408.

Cotman, C.W., Berchtold, N.C., Christie, L., 2007. Exercise builds brain health: key roles of growth factor cascades and inflammation. Trends in Neurosciences 20 (9), 464–472.

Cott, C.A., Dawson, P., Sidani, S., Wells, D., 2002. The effects of a walking/talking program on communication, ambulation, and functional status in residents with Alzheimer. Alzheimer Disease and Associated Disorders 16 (2), 81–87.

Deary, I.J., Whalley, L.J., Batty, G.D., Starr, J.M., 2006. Physical fitness and lifetime cognitive change. Neurology 67, 1195–1200.

Deslandes, A., Moraes, H., Ferreira, C., Veiga, H., Silveira, H., Mouta, R., et al., 2009. Exercise and mental health: many reasons to move. Neuropsychobiology 59, 191–198.

Ding, Q., Akhavan, M., Ying, Z., Gomez-Pinilla, F., 2006. Insulin-like growth factor I interfaces with brain-derived neurotrophic factor-mediated synaptic plasticity to modulate aspects of exercise-induced cognitive function. Neuroscience 40 (3), 823–833.

Dumith, S.C., Hallal, P.C., Reis, R.S., Kohl III, H.W., 2011. Worldwide prevalence of physical inactivity and its association with human development index in 76 countries. Preventive Medicine 53, 24–28.

Duron, E., Funalot, B., Brunel, N., Coste, J., Quinquis, L., Viollet, C., et al., 2012. Insulin-like growth factor-I and insulin-like growth factor binding protein-3 in Alzheimer's disease. The Journal of Clinical Endocrinology and Metabolism 97, 4673–4681.

Eggermont, L.H., Gavett, B.E., Volkers, K.M., Blankevoort, C.G., Scherder, E.J., Jefferson, A.L., et al., 2010. Lower-extremity function in cognitively healthy aging, mild cognitive impairment, and Alzheimer's disease. Archives of Physical Medicine and Rehabilitation 91, 584–588.

Farina, F., Rusted, J., Tabet, N., 2014. The effect of exercise interventions on cognitive outcome in Alzheimer's disease: a systematic review. International Psychogeriatrics 26 (1), 9–18.

Garuffi, M., Costa, J.L.R., Hernández, S.S.S., Vital, T.M., Stein, A.M., Santos, J.G., Stella, F., 2013. Effects of resistance training on the performance of activities of daily living in patients with Alzheimer's disease. Geriatrics & Gerontology International 13, 322–328.

Gasparini, L., Xu, H., 2003. Potential roles of insulin and IGF-1 in Alzheimer's disease. Trends in Neurosciences 26 (8), 404–406.

Groppo, H.S., Nascimento, C.M.C., Stella, F., Gobbi, S., Oliani, M.M., 2012. Efeitos de um programa de atividade física sobre os sintomas depressivos e a qualidade de vida de idosos com demência de Alzheimer. Revista Brasileria de Educação Física e Esporte 26 (4), 543–551.

Hernandez, S.S.S., Coelho, F.G.M., Gobbi, S., Stella, F., 2010. Efeitos de um programa de atividade física nas funções cognitivas, equilíbrio e risco de quedas em idosos com demência de Alzheimer. Brazilian Journal of Physical Therapy 14 (1), 68–74.

Hernandez, S.S., Vital, T.M., Gobbi, S., Stella, F., 2011. Atividade física e sintomas neuropsiquiátricos em pacientes com demência de Alzheimer. Motriz 17 (3), 533–543.

Heyn, P., 2003. The effect of a multisensory exercise program on engagement, behavior, and selected physiological indexes in persons with dementia. American Journal of Alzheimer's Diseases and Other Dementias 1 (4), 247–251.

Hillman, C.H., Weiss, E.P., Hagberg, J.M., Hatfield, B.D., 2002. The relationship to age and cardiovascular fitness to cognitive and motor processes. Psychophysiology 39, 1–10.

Hillman, C.H., Motl, R.W., Pontifex, M.B., Posthuma, D., Stubbe, J.H., Boomsma, D.I., et al., 2006. Physical activity and cognitive function in a cross-section of younger and older community-dwelling individuals. Health Psychology 25, 678–687.

Holthoff, V.A., Marschner, K., Scharf, M., Steding, J., Meyer, S., Koch, R., Donix, M., 2015. Effects of physical activity training in patients with Alzheimer's dementia: results of a pilot RCT study. PLoS One 10 (4).

Huang, L., Jia, J., Liu, R., 2013. Decreased serum levels of the angiogenic factors VEGF and TGF-β1 in Alzheimer's disease and amnestic mild cognitive impairment. Neuroscience Letters 550, 60–63.

Jalbert, J.J., Daiello, L.A., Lapane, K.L., 2008. Dementia of the Alzheimer type. Epidemiologic Reviews 30, 15–34.

Johnson, R., 1993. On the neural generators of the P300 component of the event-related potential. Psychophysiology 30, 90–97.

Komulainen, P., Pedersen, M., Hänninen, T., Bruunsgaard, H., Lakka, T.A., Kivipelto, M., et al., 2008. BDNF is a novel marker of cognitive function in ageing women: the DR's EXTRA study. Neurobiology of Learning and Memory 90, 596–603.

Lima, R.A., Freitas, C.M.S.M., Smethurst, W.S., William, S., Santos, C.M., Barros, M.V.G., 2010. Nível de atividade física em idosos com doença de Alzheimer mediante aplicação do IPAQ e de pedômetros. Revista Brasileria de Atividade Física & Saúde 15, 180–185.

Lopez-Lopez, C., Leroith, D., Torres-Aleman, I., 2004. Insulin-like growth factor I is required for vessel remodeling in the adult brain. Proceedings of the National Academy of Sciences of the United States of America 101 (26), 9833–9838.

Moraes, H., Ferreira, C., Deslandes, A., Cagy, M., Pompeu, F., Ribeiro, P., et al., 2007. Beta and alpha electroencephalographic activity changes after acute exercise. Arquivos de Neuropsiquiatria 65, 637–641.

Namazi, K.H., Paulletta, B.G., Zadorozny, C.A., 1994. A low intensity exercise/movement program for patients with Alzheimer's disease: the TEMP-AD protocol. Journal of Aging and Physical Activity 2, 80–92.

Nascimento, C.M.C., Teixeira, C.V.L., Gobbi, L.T.B., Gobbi, S., Stella, F., 2012. A controlled clinical trial on the effects of exercise on neuropsychiatric disorders and instrumental activities in women with Alzheimer's disease. Geriatrics & Gerontology International 14, 259–266.

Nascimento, C.M., Ayan, C., Cancela, J.M., Gobbi, L.T., Gobbi, S., Stella, F., 2014. Effect of a multimodal exercise program on sleep disturbances and instrumental activities of daily living performance on Parkinson's and Alzheimer's disease patients. Geriatrics & Gerontology International 14 (2), 259–266.

Ozkaya, G.Y., Aydin, H., Toraman, N.F., Kizilay, F., Ozdemir, O., Cetinkaya, V., 2005. Effect of strength and endurance training on cognition in older people. Journal of Sports Science & Medicine 4, 300–313.

Palleschi, L., Vetta, F., Genaro, E., Idone, G., Sottosanti, G., Gianni, W., Marigliano, V., 1996. Effect of aerobic training on the cognitive performance of elderly patients with senile dementia of Alzheimer type. Archives of Gerontology and Geriatrics (Suppl. 5), 47–50.

Pedroso, R.V., Coelho, F.G.M., Santos-Galduróz, R.F., Costa, J.L.R., Gobbi, S., Stella, F., 2012a. Balance, executive functions and falls in elderly with Alzheimer's disease (AD): a longitudinal study. Archives of Gerontology and Geriatrics 54, 348–351.

Pedroso, R.V., Fraga, F.J., Corazza, D.I., Andreatto, C.A.A., Coelho, F.G.M., Costa, J.L.R., et al., 2012b. P300 latency and amplitude in Alzheimer's disease: a systematic review. Brazilian Journal of Otorhinolaryngology 78, 126–132.

Perry, R.J., Hodges, J.R., 2000. Relationship between functional and neuropsychological performance in early Alzheimer disease. Alzheimer Disease and Associated Disorders 14 (1), 1–10.

Petruzzello, S.J., Landers, D.M., Hatfield, B.D., Kubitz, K.A., Salazar, W., 1991. A meta-analysis on the anxiety-reducing effects of acute and chronic exercise. Outcomes and mechanisms. Sports Medicine 11, 143–182.

Phillips, C., Baktir, M.A., Das, D., Lin, B., Salehi, A., 2015. The link between physical activity and cognitive dysfunction in Alzheimer disease. Physical Therapy 95, 1046–1060.

Polich, J., 1996. Meta analysis of P300 normative aging studies. Psychophysiology 33, 334–335.

Prior, B.M., Lloyd, P.G., Yang, H.T., Terjung, R.L., 2003. Exercise-induced vascular remodeling. Exercise and Sport Sciences Reviews 31, 26–33.

Ratey, J.J., Loehr, J.E., 2011. The positive impact of physical activity on cognition during adulthood: a review of underlying mechanisms, evidence and recommendations. Reviews in Neuroscience 22 (2), 171–185.

Rolland, Y., Pillard, F., Klapouszczak, A., Reynish, E., Thomas, D., Andrieu, S., Rivière, D., Vellas, B., 2007. Exercise program for nursing home residents with Alzheimer's disease: a 1-year randomized, controlled trial. Journal of the American Geriatrics Society 55, 158–165.

Rolland, Y., Abellan van Kan, G., Vellas, B., 2008. Physical activity and Alzheimer's disease: from prevention to therapeutic perspectives. Journal of the American Medical Directors Association 9, 390–405.

Santana-Sosa, E., Barriopedro, M.I., Lopez-Mojares, L.M., Perez, M., Lucia, A., 2008. Exercise training is beneficial for Alzheimer's patients. International Journal of Sports Medicine 29 (10), 845–850.

Stein, A.M., Costa, J.L.R., Vital, T.M., Hernandez, S.S.S., Garuffi, M., Teixeira, C.V.L., Stella, F., 2012. Level of physical activity, sleep and quality of life of patients with Alzheimer's disease. Revista Brasileria de Atividade Física & Saúde 17 (3), 200–205.

Steinberg, M., Leoutsakos, J.M., Podewils, L.J., Lyketsos, C.G., 2009. Evaluation of a home-based exercise program in the treatment of Alzheimer's disease: the Maximizing Independence in Dementia (MIND) study. International Journal of Geriatric Psychiatry 24 (7), 680–685.

Stella, F., Canonici, A.P., Gobbi, S., Santos-Galduroz, R.F., de Castilho Cação, J., Gobbi, L.T.B., 2011. Attenuation of neuropsychiatric symptoms and caregiver burden in Alzheimer's disease by motor intervention: a controlled trial. Clinics 66 (8), 1353–1360.

Teri, L., Gibbons, L.E., McCurry, S.M., Logsdon, R.G., Buchner, D.M., Barlow, W.E., Kukull, W.A., LaCroix, A.Z., McCormick, W., Larson, E.B., 2003. Exercise plus behavioral management in patients with Alzheimer disease: a randomized controlled trial. The Journal of the American Medical Association 290 (15), 2015–2022.

Trejo, J.L., Carro, E., Torres-Aleman, I., 2001. Circulating insulin-like growth factor I mediates exercise-induced increases in the number of new neurons in the adult hippocampus. The Journal of Neuroscience 21, 1628–1634.

Trueba-Sáiz, A., Cavada, C., Fernandez, A.M., Leon, T., González, D.A., Fortea Ormaechea, J., 2013. Loss of sérum IGF-I input to the brain as an early biomarker of disease onset in Alzheimer mice. Translational Psychiatry 1–6.

Venturelli, M., Scarsini, R., Schena, F., 2011. Six-month walking program changes cognitive and ADL performance in patients with Alzheimer. American Journal of Alzheimer's Diseases and Other Dementias 26 (5), 381–388.

Vital, T.M., Hernández, S.S.S., Gobbi, S., Costa, J.L.R., Stella, F., 2010. Systematized physical activity and depressive symptoms in Alzheimer's dementia: a systematic review. Journal of Brasileiro de Psiquiatria 59 (1), 58–64.

Vital, T.M., Hernandez, S.S.S., Stein, A.M., Garuffi, M., Corazza, D.I., Andrade, L.P., et al., 2012a. Depressive symptoms and level of physical activity in patients with Alzheimer's disease. Geriatrics & Gerontology International 12 (4), 637–642.

Vital, T.M., Hernández, S.S.S., Pedroso, R.V., Teixeira, C.V.L., Garuffi, M., Stein, A.M., et al., 2012b. Effects of weight training on cognitive functions in elderly with Alzheimer's disease. Dementia & Neuropsychologia 6 (4), 253–259.

Vreugdenhil, A., Cannell, J., Davies, A., Razay, G., 2012. A community-based exercise programme to improve functional ability in people with Alzheimer's disease: a randomized controlled trial. Scandinavian Journal of Caring Sciences 26 (1), 12–19.

Williams, C.L., Tappen, R.M., 2008. Exercise for depressed older adults with Alzheimer disease. Aging and Mental Health 12 (1), 72–80.

Yaari, R., Bloom, J.C., 2007. Alzheimer's disease. Seminars in Neurology 27, 32–41.

Yaguez, L., Shaw, K.N., Morris, R., Matthews, D., 2011. The effects on cognitive functions of a movement-based intervention in patients with Alzheimer's type dementia: a pilot study. International Journal of Geriatric Psychiatry 26 (2), 173–181.

Zhang, X., Ni, X., Chen, P., 2014. Study about the effects of different fitness sports on cognitive function and emotion of the aged. Cell Biochemistry and Biophysics 70, 1591–1596.

15

Cortical Reorganization in Response to Exercise

P. Stephane

University of Montpellier, Montpellier, France

Abstract

While there are clear effects of exercise on brain activity measured subsequent to the bout of physical activity, it is also important to elucidate the nature of the changes that occur in the brain during exercise, because these changes may be linked to sensorimotor performance. Characterization of the cortical contribution to motor control in humans is important for a better understanding of the pathophysiology of sensorimotor deficits after an injury to the central nervous system. This chapter addresses (1) how brain activation patterns change in response to various levels of exercise intensity, (2) in what extend the severity of neuromuscular fatigue modulates brain activation patterns in healthy persons, (3) and how the brain networks adapt to cerebrovascular injury (Stroke) and rehabilitation program to relearn movement.

INTRODUCTION

Understanding the brain function is of high interest in physical activity because every activation of motor units and thereby the establishment of sensorimotor task has its seeds in the central nervous system (CNS). Generation and control of force is required to walk, manipulate objects, and play sports. The ability to accurately produce the various ranges in force can be accomplished through modifying the firing properties and recruitment order of motor units. In order to generate force voluntarily, the motor areas of our brains must be able to communicate effectively with the motor neurons in the spinal cord that are responsible for the force generation of our muscles. When injury to sensorimotor areas of the brain occurs there may be impairment in controlling force. Stroke is one example of such a neurological disorder. In healthy subjects, various processes within the CNS may be responsible for a transient decrease in force generation and leads to the so-called central fatigue (referring to a reduction in the net excitatory input to α-motoneurons, Gandevia, 2001). Furthermore, changes in brain activity may occur secondary to the metabolic changes associated with central fatigue during prolonged exercise (Dalsgaard and Secher, 2007). To compensate for the progressive loss of force due to neuromuscular fatigue during exercise, the CNS usually progressively modulates excitatory input to the motoneuron pool. Adaptive neurophysiological processes within different areas of the CNS might also occur. The output neurons of primary motor cortex (M1) are surrounded by extensive networks of intracortical inhibitory and facilitatory interneurons that regulate the execution of exercise. Thereby, inter-hemispheric inhibition is a powerful mechanism responsible for the inhibition of the mirror movements of the passive limb during unilateral human movements (Kicić et al., 2008). Stroke is functionally characterized by alterations in inter-hemispheric inhibition which neuronal activity in the unaffected hemisphere increases while activity in the affected hemisphere decreases (Nowak et al., 2009). This leads to maladaptive neural activation patterns that are mainly caused by imbalance of inter-hemispheric inhibition. Neural compensation refers to the ability to use alternative brain networks when original networks are damaged (Stern, 2009). Given that improvement in sensorimotor function is the main goal of neuro-rehabilitation programs, understanding the adaptability of the brain networks to exercise is of particular interest. And physical interventions that can modulate motor cortical networks are clinically relevant. While stroke rehabilitation manipulates exercise intensity as an important factor of training, brain responses

Physical Activity and the Aging Brain
http://dx.doi.org/10.1016/B978-0-12-805094-1.00015-0

to exercise have not been well established. In healthy brain, the ability to use compensatory resources (i.e., different or additional brain regions/networks) in the face of increasing demands has been also understudied. Methods to challenge this idea are now emerging. Imaging the brain during increased physiological demand induced by exercise with sufficient ecological validity (Perrey, 2015) is a rapidly growing field. For instance, motor tasks involving a high complexity in the sequencing of movements (Verstynen et al., 2005), various submaximal levels of force to control (Derosière et al., 2014) or during the course of muscle fatigue (Shibuya et al., 2008), elicit stronger and less asymmetric activation pattern in brain motor areas. Taken together, inter-hemispheric remapping in the presence of exercise with sufficient physical loading, mimics the challenge created by neurological disorders.

Neuroimaging techniques provide the ability to examine the brain areas recruitment involved in force generation and its control associated with either recovery after CNS damage or exercise-induced fatigue. Advances in functional neuroimaging techniques of the human brain with behavioral outcomes, such as electroencephalography (EEG) and near-infrared spectroscopy (NIRS), helped recently to generate first valuable data in human exercise and sport and clinical sciences (Jung et al., 2015; Perrey, 2008).

This chapter addresses (1) how brain activation patterns change in response to various levels of exercise intensity, (2) in what extend the severity of fatigue modulates brain activation patterns in healthy persons, (3) and how the brain networks adapt to cerebrovascular injury (Stroke) and rehabilitation program to relearn movement. This chapter outlines several methodological approaches suited for the study of the human brain in movement.

THE EXERCISING BRAIN

Besides the positive effects of exercise on the cardiorespiratory and muscular systems, there is a growing interest in the effects of the exercise on the brain. It is now accepted that exercise might influence the brain responses. Whether or not different regions of the brain respond similarly to exercise has received little attention. Further, characterization of the cortical contribution to motor control in humans is important for a better understanding of the pathophysiology of sensorimotor deficits after an injury to the CNS. Studies examining the influence of exercise features on brain cortical responses are still scarce, which is largely due to the difficulties of using brain-imaging methods during whole body exercise. As a result, different approaches were considered to avoid problems associated for instance with walking (e.g., inability to walk in an MRI scanner, and maintaining balance to avoid motion artifacts). These include recording brain activity immediately after walking (Fukuyama et al., 1997), during imagined walking (Bakker et al., 2008), and during pedaling a stationary bicycle (Christensen et al., 2000; Fontes et al., 2013). In human exercise research, methods such as positron emission tomography (PET), functional magnetic resonance imaging (fMRI), NIRS, and EEG, allowed the exploration of regional brain function during exercise, even if their use is still in its beginning (Boecker et al., 2012). One common approach among the aforementioned neuroimaging methods (PET, fMRI, NIRS) is to evaluate brain hemodynamic responses during exercise since an increase in cerebral blood flow during muscular exercise was described more than 100 years ago (Roy and Sherrington, 1890). Cerebral blood flow changes are considered as a key parameter for a functional monitoring of cortical activation. But little evidence exists regarding exercise-related changes in brain regions or distribution of cerebral blood flow during exercise of various mode, intensity and duration either in healthy subjects or with neurological disorders. Broadly, exercise acting at a constant force and rate can be categorized into three to four discrete intensity domains (moderate-, heavy-, severe-, extreme-intensity exercise; Jones and Poole, 2005) while exercise in the face of a continually increasing power output is known as a maximal incremental test where maximal oxygen uptake (VO_2max) is determined.

In the case of PET studies, changes in neuronal activity are indirectly reflected in the associated changes in regional cerebral blood flow (rCBF). Christensen et al. (2000), for example, detected changes in brain activity with the use of oxygen-15-labelled H_2O PET during moderate-intensity cycling. They found increased brain activation recorded in the primary sensory cortex (S1), M1, supplementary motor cortex (SMA) as well as the anterior part of the cerebellum. One of the first published using single photon emission computed tomography study found also increases in rCBF in the SMA, medial primary sensorimotor cortex (SMC), striatum, visual cortex, and cerebellar vermis after walking (Fukuyama et al., 1997). More recently, these findings were confirmed during moderate steady-state cycling exercise, suggesting that rCBF in the M1, S1, SMA, cerebellum, and left insular cortex could be associated with the central command network as well as afferent inputs from the working muscles (Hiura et al., 2014). However, these valuable studies were not able to perform equivalent measurements under high-intensity conditions.

In fMRI, activation is detected because of the blood oxygen level–dependent (BOLD) effect as deoxyhemoglobin concentration changes in regions of increased neuronal activity. T2*-weighted images are used to detect the BOLD effects in fMRI mapping. As in PET studies, increased BOLD signal with fMRI were found in M1 and the cerebellum during pedaling exercise while lying supine enabling the simultaneous use of fMRI (Fontes et al., 2013). Altogether, these PET and fMRI studies confirm the contribution of several brain areas to the control of whole body dynamic exercise task at moderate intensities.

Unfortunately, the previous techniques require strict motion restriction of the head and therefore are unsuitable for measurements during intense exercise bouts. The use of NIRS to evaluate hemodynamic changes in the brain during exercise has increased as NIRS systems have become more available and are robust to motion artefacts (Perrey, 2008), making it suitable for measuring differences in regional cortical activity during exercise. NIRS is a non-invasive method for detecting dynamic changes in the concentrations of oxyhemoglobin (O_2Hb) and deoxyhemoglobin. NIRS is based on the assumption that an increase in O_2Hb concentration represents an increase in rCBF, which in turn reflects neural activation. Vascular response measured using NIRS within cortical layers are comparable to those described for the BOLD effect in fMRI (Muthalib et al., 2013). In NIRS studies, we can separate the typical O_2Hb changes occurring during short severe exercise (<15–20 min) and those occurring during prolonged moderate exercise (Fig. 15.1). During incremental maximal cycling task, a hyper-oxygenation followed by a decrease in the prefrontal cortex (PFC) before exhaustion (Bhambhani et al., 2007; Rupp and Perrey, 2008) indicate the possibility that this brain region is involved in the decision to stop exercising. Different factors like duration, intensity, and fitness level of the subjects affect the O_2Hb responses of the PFC during incremental dynamic exercise (see the review of Rooks et al., 2010).

Interestingly, in healthy trained humans, O_2Hb profile is maintained over the major portion of a self-paced, 5 km running time trial, and only decreased when subjects voluntarily increased their speed towards the end of the trial (Billaut et al., 2010). Note that Kenyan elite distance runners do not experience a decrease of the PFC before the end of a maximal, self-paced 5 km run, although they have a decrease of the PFC during an incremental test (Santos-Concejero et al., 2015). When exercise is self-paced and work rate is free to vary in response to physiological cues, PFC responses are well preserved even during exhaustive dynamic exercise.

Importantly, different responses between M1 and the PFC areas were reported during both prolonged constant submaximal exercise (Rupp et al., 2013) and incremental maximal exercise (Jung et al., 2015). Whether during prolonged submaximal exercise (Rupp et al., 2013) or a graded exercise to exhaustion (Jung et al., 2015), PFC increases

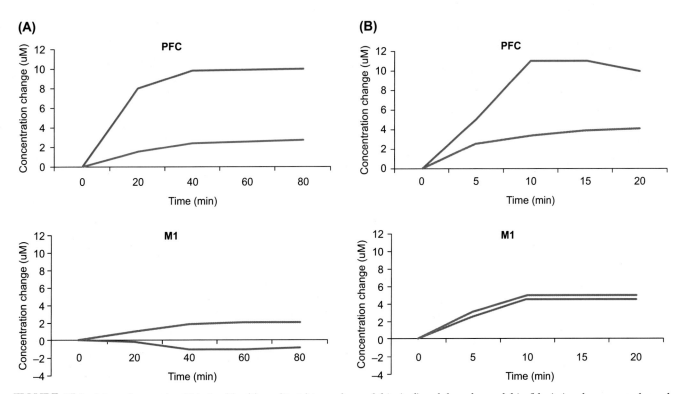

FIGURE 15.1   Mean changes ($n = 10$ trained healthy subjects) in oxyhemoglobin (red) and deoxyhemoglobin (blue) signals across prolonged moderate- (A, 45% of VO_2max, 80 min) and severe- (B, 85% of VO_2max, 20 min) intensity cycling exercise in the prefrontal cortex (PFC) and the primary motor cortex (M1). Personal data.

while M1 significantly decreases simultaneously. In addition, one study (Jung et al., 2015) found that the occipital cortex as a control non-participating brain area was unaffected during an incremental exercise until exhaustion. For prolonged submaximal exercise whatever the exercise intensity (moderate versus intense, constant versus self-paced), there is a constant increase in oxygenation of the PFC during the early phase (3–5 first min), with no marked decrease in PFC before the end of exercise (Fig. 15.1). Activation of the neural circuits involved in the control of gross muscle movements during cycling exercise may draw processing resources away from the frontal lobe networks only in some specific conditions of exercise (i.e., exhaustion) where a decrease of PFC occurs (Dietrich and Sparling, 2004).

EEG belongs to the class of electrophysiological modalities that measure the electrical activity of the brain using scalp electrodes with high temporal resolution (on the order of milliseconds). This is complimentary to other imaging modalities such as fMRI which provide high spatial resolution but relatively low temporal resolution. Since the execution of any sensory or motor activity usually involves fast synchronization of neural processes in different parts of cortical and sub-cortical structures, a high temporal resolution is required to capture these neural events. The source and span of the EEG rhythms can vary from a single neuron to inter-cortical neural structures depending on the motor activity being performed. EEG rhythms are normally associated with five bands: delta (<4 Hz), theta (4–7 Hz), alpha (8–12 Hz), beta (13–30 Hz), and gamma (above 35 Hz). Gamma band is involved in sensory feedback and motor command processing to execute a desired movement (Pfurtscheller, 1981). During initiation and execution of movement, decrease in the power of β frequencies is usually restricted to the electrodes overlying the cortical areas corresponding to the moving limb. An increase in alpha activity is a putative indicator of decreased brain activation. While some studies have described EEG changes immediately after exercise, very few studies have examined EEG during exercise. Numerous EEG studies have consistently shown that exercise is associated with alpha and theta enhancement, particularly in the frontal cortex (Nybo and Nielsen, 2001). Exercise modes (running, cycling, arm cranking) and intensities (moderate vs. heavy) influence differently EEG brain cortical activity measured post exercise (Brümmer et al., 2011a). In the later study, moderate exercise intensity (50% VO$_2$max) evoked an increase in frontal and parietal alpha activity whatever the three exercise modes. Heavy-intensity exercise (80% VO$_2$max) induced a reduced frontal beta activity only in preferred exercise (running) but not in the other exercise modes. These results argue for a dose–response relationship on frontal cortex activity, suggesting that the brain activation patterns are flexible during dynamic exercise resulting in a shift of activity away from brain regions not involved in the task toward regions involved in executing motor commands (SMC).

A handful of studies have acquired EEG data during an acute bout of exercise (Pontifex and Hillman, 2007), and this approach has the potential to offer unique insight into how patterns of neural activity associated with human performance are influenced during exercise. During an incremental exercise test, Robertson and Marino (2015) showed that EEG activity of the PFC increased up to the important metabolic load determined by ventilatory parameters, followed by a significant drop to exhaustion level, while M1 did not change significantly. These EEG responses in agreement with NIRS studies provide further evidence that M1 did maintain its activity with main changes occurring within the PFC. In contrast, others showed that the relative current density of M1 was elevated with increasing exercise intensity, whereas activity of the S1 and that of the PFC were not altered with exercise (Brümmer et al., 2011b). In sum, these studies show that M1 is mainly responsible for movement execution and force output regulation but regions upstream M1 may mediate the decreased cortical output associated with fatigue (see in the following).

Finally, developments of more flexible and robust techniques coupling EEG and NIRS now promise to allow examining changes in electro-cortical and hemodynamic responses within the brain during voluntary movement (Zama and Shimada, 2015). By using both modalities on the same area of cortex, extra information about the observations of neurovascular coupling can be recorded (Muthalib et al., 2013).

Most previous cited human neuroimaging studies identify specialized brain regions associated with the motor control of exercise. This approach basically addresses the magnitude of the brain activation patterns in a set of brain regions involved during exercise. And inferences are made on effects of intensity, duration or modes of exercise on distinct brain regions of interest (Juang et al., 2015) or the brain changes over time (Rupp et al., 2013). With the advent of multi-channel and high-density optical instruments, it also becomes possible to measure dynamic interactions between brain areas through temporal correlations of NIRS signals and therefore deriving a NIRS-based functional connectivity similar to the functional connectivity measured by the fMRI BOLD signal (Anwar et al., 2013). As well, examination of the functional communication between different areas of the brain is allowed with the EEG coherence analysis (Gerloff et al., 2006). Cortical oscillatory drives are also coupled with muscle activation in several different frequency bands as measured by EEG, depending on the functions engaged within the motor system. For example, the oscillation in the beta band (13–30 Hz) is related to strategies for modulating muscle force (Kristeva et al., 2007). Oscillation in the gamma band (30–60 Hz) is related to strategies for controlling stronger muscle force production and dynamic movements (Omlor et al., 2007). Beta band corticomuscular has previously been found to reflect efferent drive from contralateral M1 to the muscle (Gerloff et al., 2006). Therefore, these approaches provide a non-invasive means of assessing how the different brain network regions and the behavioral output are functionally connected, contributing to a better understanding of the changes in brain activity during exercise in fatigue and neurological disorder conditions.

FATIGUE-RELATED BRAIN REORGANIZATION

Central fatigue is defined as a progressive reduction in muscle activation by the CNS (Gandevia, 2001). There are many proposed "models" of muscle fatigue which originate outside of the muscle itself, including psychological/motivational and central governor models (St Clair Gibson et al., 2006). All concepts share some similarities in which the brain has the ability to downregulate the force output of the muscle based on sensory, vicarious or muscle afferent feedback. To date, fatigue is a result of brain function and the CNS is recognized for its pivotal role as the ultimate site where exercise starts and ends (Kayser, 2003). The CNS is thought to play an important role to protect vital organs from injury and damage (Noakes, 2012). Muscle fatigue involving voluntary motor activities is associated with acute adaptations in both the central nervous and muscular systems (van Duinen et al., 2007). Stronger muscle contractions are associated to higher activation of M1, S1, SMA, and PFC (fMRI in Dai et al., 2001; fNIRS in Derosiere et al., 2014; fMRI and PET in Dettmers et al., 1996). Maintaining the performance during a submaximal force task increases brain activation in bilateral S1, M1, cingulate, and PFC (measured by fMRI in Liu et al., 2003). Note that the strongest BOLD signal increased was observed in the PFC. On the basis of the brain activation patterns, several studies by using various neuroimaging methods showed the brain motor network is likely regulated by the PFC during the development of fatigue.

It is thought that the PFC involved in motivational and decision-making processes is an important candidate for acting as relay station in the central fatigue-related network regulating central command (Perrey, 2015). Indeed, the well-recognized PFC disengagement signature during the last stages of incremental exercise (quadratic trend, in Rooks et al., 2010) occurs concomitantly with an increased EMG activity of the active limbs. On the other hand, at a brain level, current evidence supports a network of brain regions that are functionally connected with both the anterior cingulate and orbitofrontal cortices during an ongoing cost-benefit analysis over time (Robertson and Marino, 2016). Overall, these findings suggest that during whole body strenuous exercise PFC plays an important role in regulating force output, by integrating sensory feedback with reinforcement of input signal to M1 to increase the descending command.

Our study of human brain is based on the idea of considering it as a set of correlated variables in a complex network. Within this framework, recent advances in brain functional network analysis provided new tools to study the relationship between different brain areas during movement. As fatigue progress at submaximal intensities, the observed increase of the functional connectivity in cortical regions (SMA, PFC, S1) connected to M1 using fMRI time series (Jiang et al., 2012) suggests a strengthened cortical motor network. Bilateral activation in the primary motor cortices is also a typical brain response as a whole during the course of a muscle fatigue task (Jiang et al., 2012; Liu et al., 2003). Interestingly, the PFC shows the highly significant fatigue-related functional connectivity changes with the M1 (Jiang et al., 2012), suggesting that strength of input from the PFC to lower levels of motor areas such as SMA and M1 likely reinforces the descending command under fatigue condition (Fig. 15.2). These studies indicate that interaction among brain regions is an important factor underpinning the behavioral manifestations of fatigue.

Oscillatory activities are common features of brain signals, as measured by electrophysiological signals. During motor performance the co-activation of different brain regions may occur to varying degrees. Coherence value measured by EEG is one measure of the amplitude of correlation between signals simultaneously recorded from two separate regions on the scalp (Gerloff et al., 2006). EEG coherence analysis is able to examine the cortical networking related to neural adaptation with fatigue or neurological disease states. High EEG coherence indicates communication between particular areas of the cerebral cortex while low coherence displays regional independence. Computing phase synchronization of oscillatory neural activity (insensitive to amplitude) is another measure for testing neurophysiological inter- and intra-hemispheric communication between the time series corresponding to different spatial locations. It appears that the insula additionally plays a key role in central fatigue via CNS connections to the brain M1 and the limbic emotional regulation network. Brain regions, such as the mid/anterior insular cortex, were demonstrated by means of EEG phase synchronization to play an important role in the mediation of motor performance by exerting influence on M1 regions during moderate constant work-load cycling (Hilty et al., 2011). The effect could be to act as a central regulator of motor output to the exercising limbs in keeping with the concept of a central governor mechanism responding to afferent sensory feedback (Noakes, 2012).

FIGURE 15.2 Simplified schematic functional connectivity scenarios among motor regions. The purpose of this figure is to depict schematically some of the many different ways in which functional connectivity in the human cortical network during dynamic motor task can occur in health (fatigue) and neurological disorder (stroke) conditions. The arrow connecting the cortical areas represents the causal relationship. Line thickness indicates connection strength. Patients with subcortical stroke show a significant reduction in intrinsic SMA-M1 coupling in the lesioned hemisphere while fatigue increases the coupling of motor areas. *M1*, primary motor area; *PFC*, prefrontal cortex; *PMC*, premotor cortex; *SMA*, supplementary motor area.

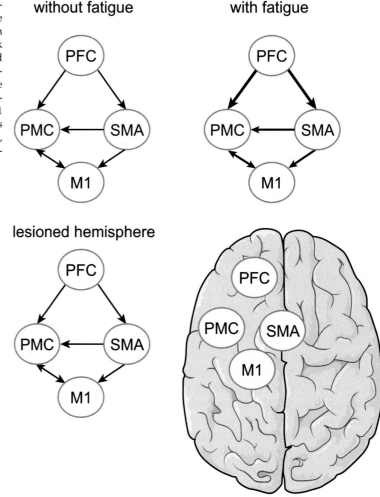

Indications that other regions are also involved in the cortical phenomenon related to muscle fatigue come from alpha and beta power analyses before and after cessation of exhaustive exercise (Brümmer et al., 2011a). These authors found significant increases in alpha and beta power within parietal as well as limbic regions after an incremental cycling exercise. Besides, acute changes in the interaction between the sensorimotor cortex activity (EEG signals) and the muscle activity (EMG signals) revealed a weak coupling during localized muscle fatiguing task to exhaustion (Yang et al., 2009). This weakened corticomuscular coupling may be due to the diminishing motor performance as a result of muscle fatigue. To compensate for diminished force production capability during exercise, brain regions governing the cortical motor control network increase their couplings while brain-muscle coupling decreases. This reorganization of brain function during force production and force modulation can occur after neurological disorder as Stroke.

BRAIN REORGANIZATION AFTER STROKE

Relative to its size, the brain is the most oxygen-dependent organ in the body, but many pathophysiological processes may either cause or result in an interruption to its oxygen supply, as damage to motor areas of the brain caused by disruption of the cerebral blood flow encountered in Stroke. Though it is generally believed that stroke interrupts the neural networks that control movements, little is known regarding the underlying mechanisms of the impairments in the neural connections within the motor cortex network and between cortex and muscle that cause the motor deficits.

After brain injury, the CNS tries to compensate for its loss through plasticity or reorganization of the brain. Neural plasticity after stroke may cause brain functional reorganization during locomotor tasks, such as pedaling (Lin et al.,

2013) and walking (Miyai et al., 2006), suggesting stroke survivors produce different brain activation patterns compared to healthy individuals. Cycling exercise is a common training paradigm for restoring locomotion rhythm in patients. Previous studies reported that impaired locomotion in people post-stroke is associated with bilateral activation of S1 and M1 and reduced brain activities in the same areas when compared to healthy individuals (Luft et al., 2005).

With increasing severity of Stroke and thus poor functional outcome, increased activation in secondary motor areas was often found in compensation for cortical damage (Ward, 2011). This was explained as a result of increased attention (meaning a greater fronto–parietal activity) used by Stroke patients as additional compensation to generate movement. But the latter may induce fatigue which can also influence brain activation, specifically in the SMA and PFC areas (van Duinen et al., 2007). However, there is also evidence for reduced recruitment of secondary motor areas during force production as a function of time recovery since stroke. Alterations in brain activity in people post-stroke are characterized by an excess activation of extra motor areas, abnormally elevated bilateral activation and an abnormal shift of activation between contralateral and ipsilateral hemispheres (Kokotilo et al., 2009). Consistent with these findings is the abnormal corticocortical coherence post-stroke (Gerloff et al., 2006). Abnormal features of corticomuscular coupling have also been reported with the EEG-EMG coherence (i.e., smaller on the affected side, shift anteriorly and/or medially away from ipsilesional M1) measurements in distal muscles for the upper limb (Mima et al., 2001). The observed decrease in the coherence value of gamma in patients performing a reaching task (Fang et al., 2009) is thought to reflect poor communication between the cortex and muscle which may have arisen from cortical changes to the network due to the stroke. Evolution of changes during post-stroke underlines well the cortical reorganization that may contribute to the restoration of motor function.

Rehabilitation programs are able to modify concomitantly brain activation and motor performance in stroke patients. When partial body weight support is applied during treadmill walking in stroke survivors, SMC activation patterns measured with NIRS were found lower and correlated with shifts in gait performance (Miyai et al., 2006). Before rehabilitation, gait is associated with increased SMC activation that is greater in the unaffected versus affected hemisphere, while after rehabilitation, asymmetry in SMC activation tends to be restored and is correlated with improvement of swing phase symmetry during walking (Miyai et al., 2003). Shifting activity of S1 and M1 from bilateral to ipsilesional activity is indicative that a reorganization of the brain regions may contribute to locomotor recovery. Lin et al. (2013) have also demonstrated that increased symmetry between the left and right rectus femoris muscles during pedaling was associated with improved symmetrical brain activation. Recently, reduced brain activation volume during pedaling was found in people post-stroke, as compared to age-matched controls (Promjunyakul et al., 2015). But this was mainly associated with work intensity produced by the paretic leg during pedaling.

As in healthy subjects, a dose effect of whole body exercise intensity on rCBF changes with regards to exercise in Stroke patients needs still to be investigated for optimizing exercise-based stroke rehabilitation. Recently, sensorimotor cortices as measured by rCBF post-exercise in MRI were showed intensity dependent when comparing semi-recumbent cycling at low and moderate intensities in Stroke survivors (Robertson et al., 2015). Interestingly, these authors reported that physical fitness affected the brain in a regionally specific manner. In this framework, the so-called cardiorespiratory fitness hypothesis states that increased level of aerobic fitness (high VO_2max level) would increase rCBF thus allowing better cerebral oxygen supply to the brain (Albinet et al., 2014), and would translate into an improved performance. Cardiorespiratory fitness rather than physical activity is now considered an important factor in moderating the adverse effects of aging on relevant functional brain networks (Voss et al., 2015).

CONCLUSION

While there are clear effects of exercise on brain activity measured subsequent to the bout of physical activity, it is also important to elucidate the nature of the changes that occur in the brain during exercise because these changes may be linked to sensorimotor performance. The investigation of the role of the brain during exercise may aid in the understanding of the central mechanisms involved in the regulation of physical exercise. Over the last few years, many neuroimaging-based techniques have been proposed describing how different brain areas interact with each other under different exercise conditions in healthy persons. Several research areas may benefit, including neurology, psychology, physiotherapy, sports medicine, and sports performance.

References

Albinet, C.T., Mandrick, K., Bernard, P.L., Perrey, S., Blain, H., 2014. Improved cerebral oxygenation response and executive performance as a function of cardiorespiratory fitness in older women: a fNIRS study. Frontiers in Aging Neuroscience 6, 272.

Anwar, A.R., Muthalib, M., Perrey, S., Galka, A., Granert, O., Wolff, S., Deuschl, G., Raethjen, J., Heute, U., Muthuraman, M., 2013. Comparison of causality analysis on simultaneously measured fMRI and NIRS signals during motor tasks. IEEE Enginneering in Medicine and Biology Society 2013, 2628–2631.

Bakker, M., de Lange, F.P., Helmich, R.C., Scheeringa, R., Bloem, B.R., Toni, I., 2008. Cerebral correlates of motor imagery of normal and precision gait. NeuroImage 41, 998–1010.

Bhambhani, Y., Malik, R., Mookerjee, S., 2007. Cerebral oxygenation declines at exercise intensities above the respiratory compensation threshold. Respiratory in Physiology and Neurobiology 156, 196–202.

Billaut, F., Davis, J.M., Smith, K.J., Marino, F.E., Noakes, T.D., 2010. Cerebral oxygenation decreases but does not impair performance during self-paced, strenuous exercise. Acta Physiology 198, 477–486.

Boecker, H., Hillman, C.H., Scheef, L., Strüder, H.K., 2012. Functional Neuroimaging in Exercise and Sport Sciences. Springer, New York.

Brümmer, V., Schneider, S., Abel, T., Vogt, T., Strüder, H.K., 2011a. Brain cortical activity is influenced by exercise mode and intensity. Medicine and Science in Sports and Exercise 43, 1863–1872.

Brümmer, V., Schneider, S., Strüder, H.K., Askew, C.D., 2011b. Primary motor cortex activity is elevated with incremental exercise intensity. Neuroscience 181, 150–162.

Christensen, L.O., Johannsen, P., Sinkjaer, T., Petersen, N., Pyndt, H.S., Nielsen, J.B., 2000. Cerebral activation during bicycle movements in man. Experimental Brain Research 135, 66–72.

Dai, T.H., Liu, J.Z., Sahgal, V., Brown, R.W., Yue, G.H., 2001. Relationship between muscle output and functional MRI-measured brain activation. Experimental Brain Research 140, 290–300.

Dalsgaard, M.K., Secher, N.H., 2007. The brain at work: a cerebral metabolic manifestation of central fatigue? Journal of Neuroscience Research 85, 3334–3339.

Derosière, G., Alexandre, F., Bourdillon, N., Mandrick, K., Ward, T.E., Perrey, S., 2014. Similar scaling of contralateral and ipsilateral cortical responses during graded unimanual force generation. NeuroImage 85, 471–477.

Dettmers, C., Connelly, A., Stephan, K.M., Turner, R., Friston, K.J., Frackowiak, R.S., Gadian, D.G., 1996. Quantitative comparison of functional magnetic resonance imaging with positron emission tomography using a force-related paradigm. NeuroImage 4, 201–209.

Dietrich, A., Sparling, P.B., 2004. Endurance exercise selectively impairs prefrontal-dependent cognition. Brain and Cognition 55, 516–524.

Fang, Y., Daly, J.J., Sun, J., Hvorat, K., Fredrickson, E., Pundik, S., Sahgal, V., Yue, G.H., 2009. Functional corticomuscular connection during reaching is weakened following stroke. Clinical Neurophysiology 120, 994–1002.

Fontes, E.B., Okano, A.H., De Guio, F., Schabort, E.J., Min, L.L., Basset, F.A., Stein, D.J., Noakes, T.D., 2013. Brain activity and perceived exertion during cycling exercise: an fMRI study. British Journal in Sports Medicine 49, 556–560.

Fukuyama, H., Ouchi, Y., Matsuzaki, S., Nagahama, Y., Yamauchi, H., Ogawa, M., Kimura, J., Shibasaki, H., 1997. Brain functional activity during gait in normal subjects: a SPECT study. Neuroscience Letters 228, 183–186.

Gandevia, S.C., 2001. Spinal and supraspinal factors in human muscle fatigue. Physiological Review 81, 1725–1789.

Gerloff, C., Bushara, K., Sailer, A., Wassermann, E.M., Chen, R., Matsuoka, T., Waldvogel, D., Wittenberg, G.F., Ishii, K., Cohen, L.G., Hallett, M., 2006. Multimodal imaging of brain reorganization in motor areas of the contralesional hemisphere of well recovered patients after capsular stroke. Brain 129, 791–808.

Hilty, L., Langer, N., Pascual-Marqui, R., Boutellier, U., Lutz, K., 2011. Fatigue-induced increase in intracortical communication between mid/anterior insular and motor cortex during cycling exercise. European Journal of Neuroscience 34, 2035–2042.

Hiura, M., Nariai, T., Ishii, K., Sakata, M., Oda, K., Toyohara, J., Ishiwata, K., 2014. Changes in cerebral blood flow during steady-state cycling exercise: a study using oxygen-15-labeled water with PET. Journal of Cerebral Blood Flow and Metabolism 34, 389–396.

Jiang, Z., Wang, X.F., Kisiel-Sajewicz, K., Yan, J.H., Yue, G.H., 2012. Strengthened functional connectivity in the brain during muscle fatigue. NeuroImage 60, 728–737.

Jones, A.M., Poole, D.C., 2005. Oxygen Uptake Kinetics in Sport, Exercise and Medicine. Taylor & Francis Inc., New York.

Jung, R., Moser, M., Baucsek, S., Dern, S., Schneider, S., 2015. Activation patterns of different brain areas during incremental exercise measured by near-infrared spectroscopy. Experimental Brain Research 233, 1175–1180.

Kayser, B., 2003. Exercise starts and ends in the brain. European Journal of Applied Physiology 90, 411–419.

Kicić, D., Lioumis, P., Ilmoniemi, R.J., Nikulin, V.V., 2008. Bilateral changes in excitability of sensorimotor cortices during unilateral movement: combined electroencephalographic and transcranial magnetic stimulation study. Neuroscience 152, 1119–1129.

Kokotilo, K.J., Eng, J.J., Boyd, L.A., 2009. Reorganization of brain function during force production after stroke: a systematic review of the literature. Journal of Neurologic Physical Therapy 33, 45–54.

Kristeva, R., Patino, L., Omlor, W., 2007. Beta-range cortical motor spectral power and corticomuscular coherence as a mechanism for effective corticospinal interaction during steady-state motor output. NeuroImage 36, 785–792.

Lin, P.Y., Chen, J.J., Lin, S.I., 2013. The cortical control of cycling exercise in stroke patients: an fNIRS study. Human Brain Mapping 34, 2381–2390.

Liu, J.Z., Shan, Z.Y., Zhang, L.D., Sahgal, V., Brown, R.W., Yue, G.H., 2003. Human brain activation during sustained and intermittent submaximal fatigue muscle contractions: an FMRI study. Journal of Neurophysiology 90, 300–312.

Luft, A.R., Forrester, L., Macko, R.F., McCombe-Waller, S., Whitall, J., Villagra, F., Hanley, D.F., 2005. Brain activation of lower extremity movement in chronically impaired stroke survivors. NeuroImage 26, 184–194.

Mima, T., Toma, K., Koshy, B., Hallett, M., 2001. Coherence between cortical and muscular activities after subcortical stroke. Stroke 32, 2597–2601.

Miyai, I., Yagura, H., Hatakenaka, M., Oda, I., Konishi, I., Kubota, K., 2003. Longitudinal optical imaging study for locomotor recovery after stroke. Stroke 34, 2866–2870.

Miyai, I., Suzuki, M., Hatakenaka, M., Kubota, K., 2006. Effect of body weight support on cortical activation during gait in patients with stroke. Experimental Brain Research 169, 85–91.

Muthalib, M., Anwar, A.R., Perrey, S., Dat, M., Galka, A., Wolff, S., Heute, U., Deuschl, G., Raethjen, J., Muthuraman, M., 2013. Multimodal integration of fNIRS, fMRI and EEG neuroimaging. Clinical Neurophysiology 124, 2060–2062.

Noakes, T.D., 2012. Fatigue is a brain-derived emotion that regulates the exercise behavior to ensure the protection of whole body homeostasis. Frontiers in Physiology 3, 82.

Nowak, D.A., Grefkes, C., Ameli, M., Fink, G.R., 2009. Interhemispheric competition after stroke: brain stimulation to enhance recovery of function of the affected hand. Neurorehabiliation and Neural Repair 23, 641–656.

Nybo, L., Nielsen, B., 2001. Perceived exertion is associated with an altered brain activity during exercise with progressive hyperthermia. Journal of Applied Physiology 91, 2017–2023.

Omlor, W., Patino, L., Hepp-Reymond, M.C., Kristeva, R., 2007. Gamma-range corticomuscular coherence during dynamic force output. NeuroImage 34, 1191–1198.

Perrey, S., 2008. Non-invasive NIR spectroscopy of human brain function during exercise. Methods 45, 289–299.

Perrey, S., 2015. Editorial: investigating the human brain and muscle coupling during whole-body challenging exercise. Frontiers in Physiology 6, 285.

Pfurtscheller, G., 1981. Central beta rhythm during sensorimotor activities in man. Electroencephalography and Clinical Neurophysiology 51, 253–264.

Pontifex, M.B., Hillman, C.H., 2007. Neuroelectric and behavioral indices of interference control during acute cycling. Clinical Neurophysiology 118, 570–580.

Promjunyakul, N.O., Schmit, B.D., Schindler-Ivens, S.M., 2015. A novel fMRI paradigm suggests that pedaling-related brain activation is altered after stroke. Frontiers in Human Neuroscience 9, 324.

Robertson, C.V., Marino, F.E., 2015. Prefrontal and motor cortex EEG responses and their relationship to ventilatory thresholds during exhaustive incremental exercise. European Journal of Applied Physiology 115, 1939–1948.

Robertson, C.V., Marino, F.E., 2016. A role for the prefrontal cortex in exercise tolerance and termination. Journal of Applied Physiology 120, 464–466.

Robertson, A.D., Crane, D.E., Rajab, A.S., Swardfager, W., Marzolini, S., Shirzadi, Z., Middleton, L.E., MacIntosh, B.J., 2015. Exercise intensity modulates the change in cerebral blood flow following aerobic exercise in chronic stroke. Experimental Brain Research 233, 2467–2475.

Rooks, C.R., Thom, N.J., McCully, K.K., Dishman, R.K., 2010. Effects of incremental exercise on cerebral oxygenation measured by near-infrared spectroscopy: a systematic review. Progress in Neurobiology 92, 134–150.

Roy, C.S., Sherrington, C.S., 1890. On the regulation of the blood-supply of the brain. Journal of Physiology 11, 85–108.

Rupp, T., Perrey, S., 2008. Prefrontal cortex oxygenation and neuromuscular responses to exhaustive exercise. European Journal of Applied Physiology 102, 153–163.

Rupp, T., Jubeau, M., Millet, G.Y., Wuyam, B., Levy, P., Verges, S., Perrey, S., 2013. Muscle, prefrontal, and motor cortex oxygenation profiles during prolonged fatiguing exercise. Advances in Experimental Medicine and Biology 789, 149–155.

Santos-Concejero, J., Billaut, F., Grobler, L., Oliván, J., Noakes, T.D., Tucker, R., 2015. Maintained cerebral oxygenation during maximal self-paced exercise in elite Kenyan runners. Journal of Applied Physiology 118, 156–162.

Shibuya, K., Sadamoto, T., Sato, K., Moriyama, M., Iwadate, M., 2008. Quantification of delayed oxygenation in ipsilateral primary motor cortex compared with contralateral side during a unimanual dominant-hand motor task using near-infrared spectroscopy. Brain Research 1210, 142–147.

St Clair Gibson, A., Lambert, E.V., Rauch, L.H., Tucker, R., Baden, D.A., Foster, C., Noakes, T.D., 2006. The role of information processing between the brain and peripheral physiological systems in pacing and perception of effort. Sports Medicine 36, 705–722.

Stern, P., 2009. Neuroscience methods. So you want to learn how to network? Introduction. Science 326, 385.

van Duinen, H., Renken, R., Maurits, N., Zijdewind, I., 2007. Effects of motor fatigue on human brain activity, an fMRI study. NeuroImage 35, 1438–1449.

Verstynen, T., Diedrichsen, J., Albert, N., Aparicio, P., Ivry, R.B., 2005. Ipsilateral motor cortex activity during unimanual hand movements relates to task complexity. Journal of Neurophysiology 93, 1209–1222.

Voss, M.W., Weng, T.B., Burzynska, A.Z., Wong, C.N., Cooke, G.E., Clark, R., Fanning, J., Awick, E., Gothe, N.P., Olson, E.A., McAuley, E., Kramer, A.F., 2015. Fitness, but not physical activity, is related to functional integrity of brain networks associated with aging. NeuroImage 1, 113–125 pii:S1053-8119(15) 00955-6.

Ward, N., 2011. Assessment of cortical reorganisation for hand function after stroke. Journal of Physiology 589, 5625–5632.

Yang, Q., Fang, Y., Sun, C.K., Siemionow, V., Ranganathan, V.K., Khoshknabi, D., Davis, M.P., Walsh, D., Sahgal, V., Yue, G.H., 2009. Weakening of functional corticomuscular coupling during muscle fatigue. Brain Research 1250, 101–112.

Zama, T., Shimada, S., 2015. Simultaneous measurement of electroencephalography and near-infrared spectroscopy during voluntary motor preparation. Science Reports 5, 16438.

16

Exercise Enhances Cognitive Capacity in the Aging Brain

S. Snigdha, G.A. Prieto

University of California-Irvine, Irvine, CA, United States

Abstract

The aging brain undergoes several changes, which result in cognitive decline and memory impairments. However, this does not mean that the aged brain has lost its capablility of learning and remembering. There are means to achieve successful brain aging specifically via physical exercise. Physical exercise triggers several molecular and cellular cascades which support and maintain brain plasticity over time and lead to the improved cognitive capacity of the brain. By understanding the mechanisms by which exercise can improve cognitive function allows for causal and conclusive indicators about the effects of exercise on learning and memory in the aged brain. In this chapter, we discuss what changes in the aging brain result in cognitive decline and then explore how exercise primes the brain to access mechanisms that can improve cognitive faculties in the aging brain.

INTRODUCTION

The aging brain undergoes several changes, which result in cognitive decline and memory impairments. These changes include, but are not limited to, reduced volume, cellular loss, reduced synaptic firing, accumulation of reactive oxygen species (ROS), and in many cases leading to dementia. In fact, age-related dementia is one of the world's fastest growing medical catastrophe in the making with no easy solution. Indeed, while the numbers and statistics surrounding dementia are staggering, with an estimation of 24 million people living with some form of dementia worldwide, it is predicted that this number could jump to as many as 84 million by the year 2040 if no major breakthrough occurs.

However, this does not mean that no aged brain is capable of learning and remembering. While in some individuals age-related changes are excessive, other individuals show successful brain aging with little to no cognitive decline. Indeed, several factors may have a role in successful brain aging and one key modifiable risk factor for developing dementia that has now been identified is the physical activity or exercise (Barnes and Yaffe, 2011).

In this chapter, we will start by discussing on what changes in the aging brain result in cognitive decline and in many cases, dementia. We will then explore the brain body connections and determine how exercise primes the brain to access mechanisms that can improve cognitive faculties.

THE AGING BRAIN

Over the past few decades, researchers have studied and discovered much about how the brain changes both in healthy aging and a result of neurodegenerative disease such as Parkinson's disease, AD, or other dementias.
Some key changes that occur in the brain as a result of aging are:

- Reduction in brain volume, especially in regions involved in learning and memory such as the prefrontal cortex and the hippocampus.
- Changes in the brain's blood vessels occur. Blood flow can be reduced because arteries narrow and less growth of new capillaries occurs.

Physical Activity and the Aging Brain
http://dx.doi.org/10.1016/B978-0-12-805094-1.00016-2

- Cell loss, particularly neuronal loss occurs.
- There is a loss of synaptic connectivity due to reduction in neurotransmitters levels, or degradation of the myelin sheath or loss of receptors on synapses.
- Increase in accumulation of reactive oxygen species (ROS).
- Occurrence of a chronic inflammation state.

MAKING THE CONNECTION—MOVING THE BODY BUILDS THE BRAIN

Our understanding of how physical activity can positively impact most if not all of these brain changes has increased significantly in the past two decades. Exercise is now known to promote brain health and delay the onset of cognitive decline in aging and AD. Exercise has been reported to increase brain volume, improve synaptic plasticity and long-term potentiation (LTP) (van Praag et al., 1999a; Adams et al., 2000; Liu et al., 2011; Dao et al., 2013), trigger neurogenesis (Pereira et al., 2007) upregulate brain-derived neurotrophic factor (BDNF) expression, and reduce accumulation of ROS (Radak et al., 2001; Berchtold et al., 2002; Weintraub et al., 2013) in the brain. Each of these can improve cognitive function to some degree, but together they can significantly improve learning and memory. Let us see how.

Exercise Increases Brain Volume

Two key brain regions that are involved in learning and memory function are the prefrontal cortex and the hippocampus. In both the hippocampus and the prefrontal cortex white matter shrinkage increases as much as 1–2% with age (Raz et al., 2005). And even when this loss does not directly correlate with cognitive performance, the reduction in volume leads to an increased risk for developing cognitive impairment (Jack et al., 2010). However, this loss of volume is not unavoidable, and can be reversed with moderate-intensity exercise. In an elegant study conducted by Erickson and colleagues in 2011, it was demonstrated that as little as 1 year of aerobic exercise could increase hippocampal volume by 2%. Since hippocampal volume decreases 1–2% annually, the 2% increase in hippocampal volume afforded by exercise amounts to adding between 1 and 2 years worth to the hippocampus in an aging population (Erickson et al., 2011).

The hippocampus is critically involved in various memory functions, including episodic memory and spatial memory (Snigdha et al., 2013). Thus, it stands to reason that increased hippocampal volume should lead to improved performance of these aspects of cognition. This has been demonstrated in studies where people with higher levels of aerobic fitness display greater hippocampal volume and better spatial memory performance than individuals with lower fitness levels. Furthermore, exploratory analyses has also revealed that hippocampal volume mediates the relationship between fitness and spatial memory. In fact, it has been shown that neurons in the anterior hippocampus are selectively associated with spatial memory acquisition (Moser et al., 1995), and also that the effect of exercise on hippocampal volume is selective for the anterior hippocampus (Erickson et al., 2011).

Another region that has been known to benefit from even mild-intensity exercise is the medial prefrontal cortex (mPFC) (Colcombe and Kramer, 2003; Colcombe et al., 2003). Tamura et al. (2015) showed that volume reduction in the PFC (due to aging) can be countered by a 2 year program of physical activity, and that the benefits last for even after 6 months of cessation of the exercise regime all the while impeding cognitive decline (Tamura et al., 2015). Specifically, improvements in the attentional shift task and memory were positively correlated with the prefrontal volumetric changes.

While it is clear that exercise does not influence all brain regions uniformly, there is evidence to suggest that greatest volumetric changes appear to be in regions that decline fastest with age, such as the anterior hippocampus and medial prefrontal cortex. Thus it is likely that regions demonstrating less age-related decay might also be less amenable to growth, making exercise as one of the few intervention strategies that can selectively target brain regions most susceptible to age-related cognitive decline. Overall this body of work supports the idea that engaging in physical activity and moving our skeletal muscles can actually result in rebuilding of the brain 1 cubic mm by cubic mm at a time.

PHYSICAL EXERCISE FOR PREVENTING AGE-RELATED COGNITIVE DECLINE

We have already seen that exercise can help counter age-related loss of brain volume. This increase is a result of building new brain cells and forging new connections between the cells of the brain-a powerful determinant of cognitive capacity. Cognitive capacity is an umbrella term for several different aspects of cognitive function including

TABLE 16.1 Effect of Physical Exercise on Different Cognitive Domains

Domain	Definition	Effect of Exercise	References
Executive function	Top–down cognitive modulation of goal-directed activity	+ humans Supported by preclinical work	Smith et al. (2010), Colcombe and Kramer (2003), Wilbur et al. (2012), and Snigdha et al. (2014)
Episodic memory	Memory of personal experiences along with the context in which they occurred, often called the "what-when-where" memory	+ humans Supported by preclinical work	Nouchi et al. (2014), Hayes et al. (2015), Nichol et al. (2007), and Snigdha et al. (2014)
Processing speed	The amount of time it takes to process a set amount of information or the amount of information that can be processed within a certain unit of time.	+ human	Kelly et al. (2014), Nouchi et al. (2014), Smith et al. (2010), and Rosano et al. (2010)
Attention	Allocation of one's limited capacities to deal with an abundance of environmental stimulation	+ human	Kelly et al. (2014) and Smith et al. (2010)
Working memory	A short-term memory (in the order of seconds) together with an active computational workspace	Inconsistent	Smith et al. (2010)

episodic memory, attention, executive function, processing speed, working memory, language, and reading (Snigdha et al., 2013). Data drawn from both human studies and animal research demonstrate that while almost all of these cognitive abilities are impaired with age; exercise can improve the ability of the brain to resist to age-related brain insult, resulting in enhanced learning and contributing to maintenance of cognitive capacity in almost all of these domains (See Table 16.1).

Next we will see how exercise influence individual aspects of cognitive function.

Exercise Improves Episodic Memory

Episodic memory refers to the ability to remember information about personal experiences along with the context in which they occurred (Tulving and Thomson, 1972; Tulving, 1983; Dickerson and Eichenbaum, 2010). The common cognitive demand in episodic memory is to remember where (or when) a specific event occurred in any given context. This capacity involves distinguishing similar events and/or spatial locations and is thought to depend on pattern separation processes (Gilbert et al., 1998; Yassa et al., 2011a,b). The "where" component can refer to a specific place in an environment, or to a specific location on a screen or complex visual scene for tests which aim to study the episodic memory processes.

Exercise has been shown to have a huge impact on these processes in both human (Hayes et al., 2015; Smith et al., 2015) and animal studies (Nichol et al., 2007; Snigdha et al., 2014). In fact the animal literature on at least "episodic like" and hippocampal-dependent memory has consistently shown a positive association between voluntary running and performance on the memory tasks (van Praag et al., 2005; Nichol et al., 2007). Similarly most human studies using verbal recall and delayed word list recognition, visual episodic memory tests as well as face–name associations have been shown to improve with exercise in older adults (Nouchi et al., 2014; Hayes et al., 2015), however, there are some interesting exceptions (Wilbur et al., 2012). The study by Wilbur et al. demonstrated an improvement in several other aspects of cognition including processing speed and executive function, but did not report positive associations of exercise with episodic memory. Since this study was focused only on the Latino population, it may be possible (as suggested by the authors themselves) that the "rich tradition of oral history that is characteristic of the Latino community may provide some protective effects on episodic memory." This idea, supports our earlier suggestion that exercise does not influence all brain regions uniformly, and that when there is less age-related decay in any given cognitive domain, that domain may also be less amenable to growth and improvement. This finding also makes a case for cognitive stimulation (mental exercise) as a useful intervention to prevent age-related cognitive decline (discussed in other chapters in this book).

Exercise Improves Executive Function

Similar to episodic memory, executive function also refers to a combination of cognitive faculties that come together to control top–down modulation of goal-directed activity. It involves several different components including set shifting, pre-potent response inhibition, updating/working memory, and processing speed (Snigdha et al., 2014; NIH toolbox).

Several studies have shown the beneficial effects of exercise on executive function (Sabia et al., 2009; Chang et al., 2010). A meta-analysis by Colcombe and Kramer (2003) revealed that while several domains of cognition could be improved by exercise, the largest gains were observed on executive control mechanisms. This is a key point because executive control is one of the most important sub domains of cognition and is needed for almost all for everyday functions of an individual. In fact, executive functions can help people to engage in an activity like exercise which requires some effortful work to achieve a longer-term benefits (Daly et al., 2014; Hall and Fong, 2015). For example, in starting new exercise regime, the shorter-term inconvenience and/or distress needs to be overlooked to achieve long-term (but not immediately apparent) paybacks such as weight loss, improved physical, and mental health. Aspects of executive function such as volition, planning, and purposive action are thus necessary for initiating and maintaining a program of exercise. The need for an efficient executive function is apparent for both the adoption and maintenance of physical activity (Marteau and Hall, 2013; Hall and Fong, 2015) and creates a bi-directional positive relationship between exercise and executive function.

Not just humans, but even animals respond well to exercise and show improved executive function and inhibitory response abilities. For instance, aged dogs that have been trained to run on a treadmill, show improvement in executive function and improve performance on a reversal learning task following as little as 10 min of running/day (Snigdha et al., 2014). In addition, we have observed that once trained to run on the treadmills, the dogs usually look forward to the daily running sessions, enforcing the positive bi-directional relationship as mentioned earlier. Similarly rats and mice also are all very likely to run if given access to running wheels—this is contrast to what is seen in people, where motivation becomes a key determinant for sticking to an exercise program. However, the good news is that the bi-directional relationship between exercise and executive function should encourage persistence with any exercise program.

Exercise Improves Attention and Processing Speed

Exercise is also associated with enhancements in two different aspects of executive function-attention and processing speed in older adults. Both attention and processing speed are cognitive sub-domains critically linked to executive function. Older people can experience a decline in executive functions, processing speed (Cahn-Weiner et al., 2000) and attention, which are all often measured by simple reaction time (RT) tasks. Decline in processing speed can result in compromised ability to react, control behaviors, and even perform basic daily activities. Thus studies to evaluate interventions which can result in improved processing speed are critical for the aging population. While preclinical studies in this have been very limited, two large meta-analytic studies reported that aerobic exercise is effective in increasing cognitive performance, in general, and executive function in particular in older adults (Colcombe and Kramer, 2003; Smith et al., 2010). Both these studies evaluated the effects of aerobic exercise on measure on executive functions, a more recent meta-analysis on pooled data revealed that the most significant differences between "exercise" and "no exercise" control groups can be observed on processing speed (Kelly et al., 2014). It should be noted that the "exercise" group for this analysis comprised of Tai Chi which essentially combines aerobic exercise and resistance training. This meta-analysis supports the idea that combining aerobic exercise, with resistance training and flexibility training may improve performance on executive tasks including attention and working memory and processing speed more than one form of exercise by itself.

Over the last several years many studies have tested the efficacy of both single and longer term (e.g., 3- or 6-month) exercise interventions in the aging population. A study comparing middle aged and older individuals who completed a 4-month aerobic training program to age-matched controls showed significant improvements on a simple RT task several decades ago (Dustman et al., 1984). Similar results were obtained by Hawkins et al. who reported that, in older adults, a water fitness regime could lead to improved dual-task and context switching abilities (Hawkins et al., 1992). These studies have been included in the 18 studies review of Colcombe and Kramer (mentioned earlier), assessing performance on various cognitive tasks following aerobic exercise. A more recent finding, however, suggests that just like reaction measures, attention function is also more likely to be positively impacted if there is a combination of aerobic and resistance training (Kelly et al., 2014). Across individual trials, in a summary of 25 studies, Kelly et al. reported some significant improvements for exercise versus controls on most measures of executive function (including processing speed and attention). All told that there is much evidence supporting the benefits of exercise on processing speed and consequently on executive function and attention. This clearly points to exercise as an effective, low-cost intervention for improving mental prowess.

Acute Exercise and Memory Consolidation

Several studies have shown how chronic exercise improves cognitive function (van Praag et al., 2005; Chang and Etnier, 2009; Tsai et al., 2015); however, a single bout of exercise can also serve to improve brain function and more specifically-memory consolidation. Memory consolidation is a post-learning phenomenon where novel information goes from being labile to being stable. One effective way to examine memory consolidation is the use of post-trial interventions (Cahill and Alkire, 2003; Segal et al., 2012). By introducing exercise after the learning phase, it is possible to test effects of exercise on memory storage and consolidation selectively in such intervention studies. Studies using this type of post-trial learning paradigms now demonstrated that a single session of physical exercise following a learning paradigm can improve memory consolidation across different species including humans, dogs, and rats (Snigdha et al., 2014; Weinberg et al., 2014; Fernandes et al., 2016). This improvement is accompanied by increase in levels of both pre- and post-synaptic proteins implicated in memory consolidation and LTP. Overall, it stands to reason that even as little as a single session of exercise can activate the synaptic machinery required for LTP and memory consolidation and lead to improved cognitive function at least temporarily. Although it should be noted that single bouts or even short-term programs of exercise may not result in improvements in overall fitness and thus may be insufficient to realize the benefits that can be achieved by high levels of fitness. Thus it is likely that transient improvements in cognitive function following the single session (acute) exercise may be driven by mechanisms other than physical fitness.

Contradictory Findings

Despite evidence from epidemiological, cross-sectional, and neuroimaging works which consistently find physical exercise to be beneficial for cognitive function in the elderly (Colcombe et al., 2003; Barnes et al., 2008; Middleton et al., 2010; Erickson et al., 2011), data from randomized controlled trials (RCTs) still remain largely inconsistent (Clifford et al., 2010; Snowden et al., 2011). There may be several reasons for this inconsistency including differences in baseline levels of physical activity and cognitive status of participants (inclusion criterion), length, intensity and frequency of exercise intervention, and variation in methodologies and cognitive outcome measures across trials.

Variations in inclusion criteria include factors such as some studies recruiting physically active participants (Oken et al., 2006), while others recruiting physically weaker or even sedentary participants (Barnes et al., 2008; Langlois et al., 2013); not surprisingly then trials that evaluate effects of exercise on sedentary or frail older adults report more positive results. A similar observation can be made for trials recruiting participants with no cognitive impairment versus those that are cognitively impaired (reviewed in Kelly et al., 2014). In addition, RCTs are normally much shorter in duration and may not capture the benefits that longer interventions such as 1 year may report. This is also relevant because many studies report that while cognitive performance in control groups declined over time while exercise groups improve or sustain cognitive performance over time (Barnes et al., 2008; Liu-Ambrose et al., 2010; Muscari et al., 2010). Thus, short-term programs of exercise may not be sufficient to realize the benefits that can be achieved overtime. In fact, it may be the case that transient improvements in cognitive function in RCTs may be driven by mechanisms other than physical fitness all together (Kramer et al., 2001; Angevaren et al., 2008; Etnier and Chang, 2009). Future research will be key to determining what factors, other than fitness, might mediate the relationship between physical activity and cognitive function in the short term.

Finally, RCT interventions many a times do not meet the current public health exercise recommendations for the aged, which is 150 min of moderate intensity aerobic activity per week (Haskell et al., 2007) and two sessions per week of moderate intensity strength training working (American College of Sports, 2009). This is in contrast to epidemiological/cross-sectional studies where participants in "high activity" groups reported engaging in 4–7 h of exercise per week (Schuit et al., 2001; Sumic et al., 2007) at moderate to high intensity levels (Brown et al., 2012). This and the other earlier mentioned explanations for potential confounds may provide some (but not necessarily all) insight into the validity of comparisons of RCTs with epidemiological data.

MOLECULAR AND CELLULAR BUILDING BLOCKS FOR BRAIN REMODELING BY EXERCISE

Given the compelling evidence showing benefits of physical activity on cognitive capacity, it is critical to elucidate the neurobiological mechanisms through which exercise modifies the brain and facilitates neuronal functions. While much of the behavioral effects of exercise can be seen in human studies and clinical trials, animal models allow for examination of the cellular and molecular basis that are quite simply impossible to study in humans. In this section we will summarize research on animal models that support the notion that physical activity promotes brain remodeling at many levels including changes in gene and protein expression, as well as modifications at cellular and subcellular levels that ultimately impact physiological processes (e.g., LTP and rewiring). Notably, the positive effects of exercise on basic physiological processes might be reflected in neuronal circuitries, thus leading to protective effects against cognitive decline in aging. Because the most pronounced changes with physical activity are in the hippocampus, this section will focus on data showing exercise-induced changes in hippocampal molecular and structural remodeling, as well as in synaptic plasticity and rewiring.

New Neurons, New Circuitries: New Memories

For a long time, neurons were thought to be born at birth and lost with aging but an amazing discovery in 1965 pointed out that neurons can be generated in the adult brain (Altman and Das, 1965). The bad news is that neurogenesis is diminished with aging (Kuhn et al., 1996), and this is associated with cognitive deficits (Drapeau et al., 2003). The good news comes from the work done by Van Praag and colleagues, who over several years have shown that rodents given access to a running wheel for several weeks show increased neurogenesis together with improvements in learning (van Praag et al., 1999b). Running influences all aspects of new neuron maturation, including cell proliferation, survival, and neuronal differentiation in the dentate gyrus (DG) (Voss et al., 2013). Indeed, it has been proposed that exercise sets up several crucial conditions to maintain a niche for neurogenesis, such as facilitating the access to growth and trophic factors (Jin et al., 2002) while increasing blood vessels in the hippocampus (Palmer et al., 2000). The growth factors VEGF and IGF-1 are upregulated as a result of exercise and then travel through the blood stream and reach to the brain which promotes growth and survival of neurons, and build the vascular system in the brain. Indeed, some cognitive benefits of exercise can be prevented by blocking IGF-1 or VEGF signaling in the brain (Carro et al., 2000; Fabel et al., 2003).

Importantly, the enhancement in hippocampal neurogenesis and learning is observed in both young and aged mice (van Praag et al., 2005), and extended to mouse models of AD (Rodriguez et al., 2011). For instance, after 1 month of voluntary wheel running aged mice showed faster acquisition and better retention in a spatial memory test, while the decline in neurogenesis was reversed to 50% of young control levels (van Praag et al., 2005). The idea that exercise can induce formation of neurons is both spectacular and exciting, and has lead to further research to investigate the underlying mechanisms and to test if the exercise-induced neurons have the ability to be integrated into functional circuitries.

In the adulthood, granule cells generated in the subgranular zone are incorporated into pre-existing circuits (Deng et al., 2010). Indeed, new DG neurons form new synapses not only with their CA3 partners (canonical DG-CA3 circuit) but also with more distant regions of the brain, thus promoting brain rewiring that improve several brain functions including learning and memory processes (Bergami et al., 2015). Running increased input from lateral and caudo-medial entorhinal cortex (Vivar et al., 2016), regions important for spatial memory and theta rhythm generation (an oscillation critical for temporal coding/decoding of active neuronal ensembles (Buzsaki, 2002)). Interestingly, as part of rewiring it has been recently shown that newly generated axon terminals can juxtapose with or displace previously established synapses, thus degrading pre-existing memory circuits and resulting in forgetting (Akers et al., 2014). Thus, by adding new cells and promoting rewiring in hippocampus, exercise-induced neurogenesis may facilitate the functional dynamic of the hippocampus, which is constantly generating new memories while at the same time constantly erasing memories that are not exported and consolidated in cortical modules (Kitamura and Inokuchi, 2014).

Exercise Boosts Synaptic Plasticity

Plasticity of synaptic connections provides the basis for brain's ability to adapt or modify itself in response to novel experiences and/or environmental changes both in the short- and long-terms, and thus underlies memory and learning. One of the most widely used models for studying molecular mechanisms of hippocampal synaptic plasticity is LTP, a rapid and remarkably persistent increase in synaptic transmission elicited by brief patterns of afferent activity (Bliss and Collingridge, 1993). A growing body of data suggests that LTP is causally linked to synaptic processes underlying memory (Roman et al., 1987; Rioult-Pedotti et al., 2000; Whitlock et al., 2006; Nabavi et al., 2014). Indeed, the analysis of LTP is commonly used for the initial evaluation of behavioral and pharmacological interventions for age-related memory problems, as it is generally believed that memory deficits arise from synaptic dysfunction and declines in synaptic plasticity (Selkoe, 2002; Nicholson et al., 2004; Morrison and Baxter, 2012). In rodents, impairments in hippocampal LTP and synaptic vulnerability are present by middle age (Rex et al., 2006; Prieto et al., 2015), thus providing a candidate explanation for memory losses during normal aging. Consistent with the benefits of exercise on memory, it has been shown that physical activity reverses the age-related decline in LTP in DG (O'Callaghan et al., 2009) and CA1 (Kumar et al., 2012). Moreover, the effect of treadmill exercise on hippocampal LTP has also been observed in an aged-transgenic mouse model of AD (Zhao et al., 2015). How exercise improves hippocampal LTP is not fully understood; however, experimental work on this area has provided crucial elements to fill the gap between the widely observed effects of exercise in behavioral tests and the main cellular and molecular pathways involved in synaptic plasticity.

The critical initial elements for establishing LTP involve membrane depolarization and activation of NMDA receptors (NMDAR), which allows Ca^{2+} influx, drives intracellular signaling and insertion of AMPA receptors (AMPAR) into the postsynaptic surface; these biochemical changes lead to morphological adaptations in spines (Park et al., 2004; Fortin et al., 2010; Jurado et al., 2013). It has been shown that exercise increases mRNA hippocampal levels of NMDAR2B (Farmer et al., 2004), a subunit that facilitates LTP, and protein levels of GluR1 (Real et al., 2010), a key AMPAR subunit for the potentiation of synaptic transmission (Shi et al., 1999). Microarray analysis confirmed the upregulation of NMDAR2B subunit by exercise, and further showed an increased expression of genes involved with synaptic trafficking (synapsin I, synaptotagmin and syntaxin) and signal transduction pathways including $Ca^{2+}/$ calmodulin-dependent protein kinase II (CaMKII), mitogen-activated/extracellular signal-regulated protein kinase (MAPK-ERK), protein kinase C (PKCδ), and transcription factor cAMP response element binding protein (CREB), as well as BDNF (Molteni et al., 2002). Notably, following Ca^{2+} influx, CaMKII activation and its downstream actions (e.g., an increase in AMPAR conductance via GluA1 phosphorylation (Derkach et al., 1999)) are crucial for LTP (Malinow et al., 1989; Silva et al., 1992). Similarly, an important pathway for enduring LTP depends on PKA/CREB activation (Nguyen and Woo, 2003). Thus, exercise may engage hippocampus on LTP by increasing gene expression on crucial molecules for plasticity. It has also been suggested that the increased neurogenesis in DG following physical activity (van Praag et al., 1999b) facilitates DG LTP. Consistent with this idea, newborn granule cells from DG have a lower induction threshold and enhanced LTP induction compared to mature granule cells and running increases induction of the expression of immediate early genes (e.g., Arc) in new and preexisting DG neurons (Clark et al., 2011).

In contrast to the enhancement of the glutamatergic system by exercise, genes related to the GABAergic (inhibitory) system (GABA$_A$ receptor and glutamate decarboxylase GAD65) are downregulated by physical activity. Consistent with this finding it has been shown that running differentially affects synaptic inputs and reduces the ratio of innervation from inhibitory interneurons and glutamatergic mossy cells to new neurons (Vivar et al., 2016), thus switching the excitatory/inhibitory balance on new neurons. In addition to neurotransmitter systems, exercise also influences neuromodulation. By activating second messengers neuromodulators are critical elements for LTP, as they control many intracellular pathways associated with synaptic plasticity (e.g., PKA and PKC). Of note, brain levels of serotonin, endogenous opioids, and cannabinoids are elevated in mice that received exercise training (Vivar et al., 2013).

Although methods to study LTP in humans have not developed yet, using innovative approaches it has been also studied the effects of physical activity on plasticity at the network level. For instance, recent imaging literature demonstrates that exercise increases the coherence of brain networks in older adults (Voss et al., 2010a,b). Notably, fMRI assessment of brain network coherence and stability after participation in a 1 year aerobic exercise intervention trial revealed that exercise increased functional connectivity within the Default Mode Network and a Frontal Executive Network, two higher level cognitive networks central to brain dysfunction in aging (Celone et al., 2006; Miller et al., 2008; Voss et al., 2010b; Jin et al., 2012). In addition, increased functional connectivity of the Default Mode Network as a function of aerobic fitness is associated with better cognitive performance on tests of memory and executive function in the aged population (Voss et al., 2010a), suggesting that effects of physical activity on network coherence are highly relevant to cognitive benefits of exercise and elevated activity levels.

BDNF, a Molecular Hub for Connecting Most Brain Benefits by Exercise

Studies conducted by Cotman and his group at University of California–Irvine, have shown that exercise increases brain levels of molecules that can promote growth, development, function, and survival of neurons. Chief among these factors is BDNF. Indeed, one of the most consistent effects of exercise is the upregulation of hippocampal BDNF levels (Cotman and Berchtold, 2002). Work done by the Cotman lab for over two decades has demonstrated that exercise induces an upregulation of BDNF that can persist for up to a week even with just 2 days of wheel running (Neeper et al., 1995, 1996). BDNF is a crucial factor in most hippocampal functions (Park and Poo, 2013).

Consistent with the central role of BDNF in hippocampus, virtually all the benefits of exercise (e.g., increased neurogenesis, aniogenesis, and synaptic plasticity) could be recapitulated by enhancing BDNF signaling. It is also noteworthy that most of the effects of exercise in the brain impact closely related hippocampal function that depends on BDNF. Indeed, the strongest molecular relationship of exercise and functional connectivity was identified for BDNF (Foster, 2015).

BDNF signaling follows three canonical pathways (PI3K/Akt, MAPK/ERK, and PLC/CaMK), which can crosstalk with different signal transduction systems activated by neuromodulators (e.g., serotonin and cannabinoids) to target molecular effectors and finally modulate neuronal functions. For instance, in hippocampal neurons the PI3-K/Akt pathway is fundamental for the BDNF-induced protein synthesis and survival (Smith et al., 2014). BDNF plays a crucial role in most biochemical and structural changes for enduring LTP (Park and Poo, 2013). Indeed, BDNF has been shown to be crucial for basal synaptic transmission and for synaptic plasticity (Rex et al., 2007; Lynch et al., 2008). Importantly, BDNF induction can rescue LTP deficits in middle-aged rats (Rex et al., 2006). Neuronal activity on the other hand can enhance local synthesis and secretion of BDNF, which in turn adjusts synaptic efficacy and spine growth. This simple idea supports the possibility that exercise, by participating in BDNF regulation can mediate synapse development, plasticity and neurogenesis, and finally impact cognitive capacity (Intlekofer and Cotman, 2013).

CONCLUSION

In conclusion, physical exercise triggers several molecular and cellular cascades which support and maintain brain plasticity and lead to the improved cognitive capacity of the aging brain. In addition, the beneficial effects of exercise include a reciprocal relationship between physical activity and executive function such that physical activity induced changes in executive function can enhance and promote physical activity over time and these changes in activity level can improve future learning and prevent memory decline.

References

Adams, B., Chan, A., Callahan, H., Milgram, N.W., 2000. The canine as a model of human cognitive aging: recent developments. Progress in Neuro-Psychopharmacology & Biological Psychiatry 24, 675–692.

Akers, K.G., Martinez-Canabal, A., Restivo, L., Yiu, A.P., De Cristofaro, A., Hsiang, H.L., Wheeler, A.L., Guskjolen, A., Niibori, Y., Shoji, H., Ohira, K., Richards, B.A., Miyakawa, T., Josselyn, S.A., Frankland, P.W., 2014. Hippocampal neurogenesis regulates forgetting during adulthood and infancy. Science 344, 598–602.

Altman, J., Das, G.D., 1965. Autoradiographic and histological evidence of postnatal hippocampal neurogenesis in rats. Journal of Comparative Neurology 124, 319–335.

American College of Sports Medicine, 2009. American College of Sports Medicine position stand. Progression models in resistance training for healthy adults. Medicine and Science in Sports and Exercise 41, 687–708.

Angevaren, M., Aufdemkampe, G., Verhaar, H.J.J., Aleman, A., Vanhees, L., 2008. Physical activity and enhanced fitness to improve cognitive function in older people without known cognitive impairment. Cochrane Database of Systematic Reviews, CD005381.

Barnes, D.E., Blackwell, T., Stone, K.L., Goldman, S.E., Hillier, T., Yaffe, K., Study of Osteoporotic Fractures, 2008. Cognition in older women: the importance of daytime movement. Journal of the American Geriatrics Society 56, 1658–1664.

Barnes, D.E., Yaffe, K., 2011. The projected effect of risk factor reduction on Alzheimer's disease prevalence. The Lancet Neurology 10, 819–828.

Berchtold, N.C., Kesslak, J.P., Cotman, C.W., 2002. Hippocampal brain-derived neurotrophic factor gene regulation by exercise and the medial septum. Journal of Neuroscience Research 68, 511–521.

Bergami, M., Masserdotti, G., Temprana, S.G., Motori, E., Eriksson, T.M., Gobel, J., Yang, S.M., Conzelmann, K.K., Schinder, A.F., Gotz, M., Berninger, B., 2015. A critical period for experience-dependent remodeling of adult-born neuron connectivity. Neuron 85, 710–717.

Bliss, T.V., Collingridge, G.L., 1993. A synaptic model of memory: long-term potentiation in the hippocampus. Nature 361, 31–39.

Brown, B.M., Peiffer, J.J., Sohrabi, H.R., Mondal, A., Gupta, V.B., Rainey-Smith, S.R., Taddei, K., Burnham, S., Ellis, K.A., Szoeke, C., Masters, C.L., Ames, D., Rowe, C.C., Martins, R.N., AIBL Research Group, 2012. Intense physical activity is associated with cognitive performance in the elderly. Translational Psychiatry 2.

Buzsaki, G., 2002. Theta oscillations in the hippocampus. Neuron 33, 325–340.

Cahill, L., Alkire, M.T., 2003. Epinephrine enhancement of human memory consolidation: interaction with arousal at encoding. Neurobiology of Learning and Memory 79, 194–198.

Cahn-Weiner, D.A., Malloy, P.F., Boyle, P.A., Marran, M., Salloway, S., 2000. Prediction of functional status from neuropsychological tests in community-dwelling elderly individuals. Clinical Neuropsychology 14, 187–195.

Carro, E., Nunez, A., Busiguina, S., Torres-Aleman, I., 2000. Circulating insulin-like growth factor I mediates effects of exercise on the brain. Journal of Neuroscience 20, 2926–2933.

Celone, K.A., Calhoun, V.D., Dickerson, B.C., Atri, A., Chua, E.F., Miller, S.L., DePeau, K., Rentz, D.M., Selkoe, D.J., Blacker, D., Albert, M.S., Sperling, R.A., 2006. Alterations in memory networks in mild cognitive impairment and Alzheimer's disease: an independent component analysis. Journal of Neuroscience 26, 10222–10231.

Chang, Y.K., Etnier, J.L., 2009. Exploring the dose-response relationship between resistance exercise intensity and cognitive function. Journal of Sport & Exercise Psychology 31, 640–656.

Chang, Y.L., Jacobson, M.W., Fennema-Notestine, C., Hagler Jr., D.J., Jennings, R.G., Dale, A.M., McEvoy, L.K., 2010. Level of executive function influences verbal memory in amnestic mild cognitive impairment and predicts prefrontal and posterior cingulate thickness. Cerebral Cortex 20, 1305–1313.

Clark, P.J., Bhattacharya, T.K., Miller, D.S., Rhodes, J.S., 2011. Induction of c-Fos, Zif268, and Arc from acute bouts of voluntary wheel running in new and pre-existing adult mouse hippocampal granule neurons. Neuroscience 184, 16–27.

Clifford, A., Bandelow, S., Hogervorst, E., 2010. The effects of physical exercise on cognitive function in the elderly: a review. In: Handbook of Cognitive Aging: Causes, Processes and Effects, pp. 109–150.

Colcombe, S., Kramer, A.F., 2003. Fitness effects on the cognitive function of older adults: a meta-analytic study. Psychological Science 14, 125–130.

Colcombe, S.J., Erickson, K.I., Raz, N., Webb, A.G., Cohen, N.J., McAuley, E., Kramer, A.F., 2003. Aerobic fitness reduces brain tissue loss in aging humans. Journals of Gerontology Series A: Biological Sciences and Medical Sciences 58, 176–180.

Cotman, C.W., Berchtold, N.C., 2002. Exercise: a behavioral intervention to enhance brain health and plasticity. Trends in Neurosciences 25, 295–301.

Daly, R.M., Duckham, R.L., Gianoudis, J., 2014. Evidence for an interaction between exercise and nutrition for improving bone and muscle health. Current Osteoporosis Reports 12, 219–226.

Dao, A.T., Zagaar, M.A., Levine, A.T., Salim, S., Eriksen, J.L., Alkadhi, K.A., 2013. Treadmill exercise prevents learning and memory impairment in Alzheimer's disease-like pathology. Current Alzheimer Research 10, 507–515.

Deng, W., Aimone, J.B., Gage, F.H., 2010. New neurons and new memories: how does adult hippocampal neurogenesis affect learning and memory? Nature Reviews Neuroscience 11, 339–350.

Derkach, V., Barria, A., Soderling, T.R., 1999. Ca^{2+}/calmodulin-kinase II enhances channel conductance of alpha-amino-3-hydroxy-5-methyl-4-isoxazolepropionate type glutamate receptors. Proceedings of the National Academy of Sciences of the United States of America 96, 3269–3274.

Dickerson, B.C., Eichenbaum, H., 2010. The episodic memory system: neurocircuitry and disorders. Neuropsychopharmacology: Official Publication of the American College of Neuropsychopharmacology 35, 86–104.

Drapeau, E., Mayo, W., Aurousseau, C., Le Moal, M., Piazza, P.V., Abrous, D.N., 2003. Spatial memory performances of aged rats in the water maze predict levels of hippocampal neurogenesis. Proceedings of the National Academy of Sciences of the United States of America 100, 14385–14390.

Dustman, R.E., Ruhling, R.O., Russell, E.M., Shearer, D.E., Bonekat, H.W., Shigeoka, J.W., Wood, J.S., Bradford, D.C., 1984. Aerobic exercise training and improved neuropsychological function of older individuals. Neurobiology of Aging 5, 35–42.

Erickson, K.I., Voss, M.W., Prakash, R.S., Basak, C., Szabo, A., Chaddock, L., Kim, J.S., Heo, S., Alves, H., White, S.M., Wojcicki, T.R., Mailey, E., Vieira, V.J., Martin, S.A., Pence, B.D., Woods, J.A., McAuley, E., Kramer, A.F., 2011. Exercise training increases size of hippocampus and improves memory. Proceedings of the National Academy of Sciences of the United States of America 108, 3017–3022.

Etnier, J.L., Chang, Y.K., 2009. The effect of physical activity on executive function: a brief commentary on definitions, measurement issues, and the current state of the literature. Journal of Sport & Exercise Psychology 31, 469–483.

Fabel, K., Tam, B., Kaufer, D., Baiker, A., Simmons, N., Kuo, C.J., Palmer, T.D., 2003. VEGF is necessary for exercise-induced adult hippocampal neurogenesis. European Journal of Neuroscience 18, 2803–2812.

Farmer, J., Zhao, X., van Praag, H., Wodtke, K., Gage, F.H., Christie, B.R., 2004. Effects of voluntary exercise on synaptic plasticity and gene expression in the dentate gyrus of adult male Sprague-Dawley rats in vivo. Neuroscience 124, 71–79.

Fernandes, J., Kramer Soares, J.C., Zaccaro do Amaral Baliego, L.G., Arida, R.M., 2016. A single bout of resistance exercise improves memory consolidation and increases the expression of synaptic proteins in the hippocampus. Hippocampus, 1096–1103.

Fortin, D.A., Davare, M.A., Srivastava, T., Brady, J.D., Nygaard, S., Derkach, V.A., Soderling, T.R., 2010. Long-term potentiation-dependent spine enlargement requires synaptic Ca^{2+}-permeable AMPA receptors recruited by CaM-kinase I. Journal of Neuroscience 30, 11565–11575.

Foster, P.P., 2015. Role of physical and mental training in brain network configuration. Frontiers in Aging Neuroscience 7, 117.

Gilbert, P.E., Kesner, R.P., DeCoteau, W.E., 1998. Memory for spatial location: role of the hippocampus in mediating spatial pattern separation. The Journal of Neuroscience: the Official Journal of the Society for Neuroscience 18, 804–810.

Hall, P.A., Fong, G.T., 2015. Temporal self-regulation theory: a neurobiologically informed model for physical activity behavior. Frontiers in Human Neuroscience 9, 117.

Haskell, W.L., Lee, I.M., Pate, R.R., Powell, K.E., Blair, S.N., Franklin, B.A., Macera, C.A., Heath, G.W., Thompson, P.D., Bauman, A., 2007. Physical activity and public health: updated recommendation for adults from the American College of Sports Medicine and the American Heart Association. Medicine and Science in Sports and Exercise 39, 1423–1434.

Hawkins, H.L., Kramer, A.F., Capaldi, D., 1992. Aging, exercise, and attention. Psychology and Aging 7, 643–653.

Hayes, S.M., Alosco, M.L., Hayes, J.P., Cadden, M., Peterson, K.M., Allsup, K., Forman, D.E., Sperling, R.A., Verfaellie, M., 2015. Physical activity is positively associated with episodic memory in aging. Journal of the International Neuropsychological Society 21, 780–790.

Intlekofer, K.A., Cotman, C.W., 2013. Exercise counteracts declining hippocampal function in aging and Alzheimer's disease. Neurobiology of Disease 57, 47–55.

Jack Jr., C.R., Wiste, H.J., Vemuri, P., Weigand, S.D., Senjem, M.L., Zeng, G., Bernstein, M.A., Gunter, J.L., Pankratz, V.S., Aisen, P.S., Weiner, M.W., Petersen, R.C., Shaw, L.M., Trojanowski, J.Q., Knopman, D.S., 2010. Brain beta-amyloid measures and magnetic resonance imaging atrophy both predict time-to-progression from mild cognitive impairment to Alzheimer's disease. Brain 133, 3336–3348.

Jin, K., Zhu, Y., Sun, Y., Mao, X.O., Xie, L., Greenberg, D.A., 2002. Vascular endothelial growth factor (VEGF) stimulates neurogenesis in vitro and in vivo. Proceedings of the National Academy of Sciences of the United States of America 99, 11946–11950.

Jin, M., Pelak, V.S., Cordes, D., 2012. Aberrant default mode network in subjects with amnestic mild cognitive impairment using resting-state functional MRI. Magnetic Resonance Imaging 30, 48–61.

Jurado, S., Goswami, D., Zhang, Y., Molina, A.J., Sudhof, T.C., Malenka, R.C., 2013. LTP requires a unique postsynaptic SNARE fusion machinery. Neuron 77, 542–558.

Kelly, M.E., Loughrey, D., Lawlor, B.A., Robertson, I.H., Walsh, C., Brennan, S., 2014. The impact of exercise on the cognitive functioning of healthy older adults: a systematic review and meta-analysis. Ageing Research Reviews 16, 12–31.

IV. EXERCISE AS THERAPY FOR NEUROLOGICAL DISEASES

Kitamura, T., Inokuchi, K., 2014. Role of adult neurogenesis in hippocampal-cortical memory consolidation. Molecular Brain 7, 13.

Kramer, A.F., Hahn, S., McAuley, E., Cohen, N.J., Banich, M.T., Harrison, C., Chason, J., Boileau, R.A., Bardell, L., Colcombe, A., Vakil, E., 2001. Exercise, aging, and cognition: healthy body, healthy mind? In: Human Factors Interventions for the Health Care of Older Adults, pp. 91–120.

Kuhn, H.G., Dickinson-Anson, H., Gage, F.H., 1996. Neurogenesis in the dentate gyrus of the adult rat: age-related decrease of neuronal progenitor proliferation. Journal of Neuroscience 16, 2027–2033.

Kumar, A., Rani, A., Tchigranova, O., Lee, W.H., Foster, T.C., 2012. Influence of late-life exposure to environmental enrichment or exercise on hippocampal function and CA1 senescent physiology. Neurobiology of Aging 33 (828), 828 e1–e17.

Langlois, F., Vu, T.T.M., Chasse, K., Dupuis, G., Kergoat, M.J., Bherer, L., 2013. Benefits of physical exercise training on cognition and quality of life in frail older adults. Journals of Gerontology Series B: Psychological Sciences and Social Sciences 68, 400–404.

Liu-Ambrose, T., Nagamatsu, L.S., Graf, P., Beattie, B.L., Ashe, M.C., Handy, T.C., 2010. Resistance training and executive functions: a 12-month randomized controlled trial. Archives of Internal Medicine 170, 170–178.

Liu, H.L., Zhao, G., Cai, K., Zhao, H.H., Shi, L.D., 2011. Treadmill exercise prevents decline in spatial learning and memory in APP/PS1 transgenic mice through improvement of hippocampal long-term potentiation. Behavioural Brain Research 218, 308–314.

Lynch, G., Rex, C.S., Chen, L.Y., Gall, C.M., 2008. The substrates of memory: defects, treatments, and enhancement. European Journal of Pharmacology 585, 2–13.

Malinow, R., Schulman, H., Tsien, R.W., 1989. Inhibition of postsynaptic PKC or CaMKII blocks induction but not expression of LTP. Science 245, 862–866.

Marteau, T.M., Hall, P.A., 2013. Breadlines, brains, and behaviour. BMJ 347, f6750.

Middleton, L.E., Barnes, D.E., Lui, L.Y., Yaffe, K., 2010. Physical activity over the life course and its association with cognitive performance and impairment in old age. Journal of the American Geriatrics Society 58, 1322–1326.

Miller, S.L., Celone, K., DePeau, K., Diamond, E., Dickerson, B.C., Rentz, D., Pihlajamaki, M., Sperling, R.A., 2008. Age-related memory impairment associated with loss of parietal deactivation but preserved hippocampal activation. Proceedings of the National Academy of Sciences of the United States of America 105, 2181–2186.

Molteni, R., Ying, Z., Gomez-Pinilla, F., 2002. Differential effects of acute and chronic exercise on plasticity-related genes in the rat hippocampus revealed by microarray. European Journal of Neuroscience 16, 1107–1116.

Morrison, J.H., Baxter, M.G., 2012. The ageing cortical synapse: hallmarks and implications for cognitive decline. Nature Reviews Neuroscience 13, 240–250.

Moser, M.B., Moser, E.I., Forrest, E., Andersen, P., Morris, R.G.M., 1995. Spatial-learning with a minislab in the dorsal hippocampus. Proceedings of the National Academy of Sciences of the United States of America 92, 9697–9701.

Muscari, A., Giannoni, C., Pierpaoli, L., Berzigotti, A., Maietta, P., Foschi, E., Ravaioli, C., Poggiopollini, G., Bianchi, G., Magalotti, D., Tentoni, C., Zoli, M., 2010. Chronic endurance exercise training prevents aging-related cognitive decline in healthy older adults: a randomized controlled trial. International Journal of Geriatric Psychiatry 25, 1055–1064.

Nabavi, S., Fox, R., Proulx, C.D., Lin, J.Y., Tsien, R.Y., Malinow, R., 2014. Engineering a memory with LTD and LTP. Nature 511, 348–352.

Neeper, S.A., Gomez-Pinilla, F., Choi, J., Cotman, C., 1995. Exercise and brain neurotrophins. Nature 373, 109.

Neeper, S.A., Gomez-Pinilla, F., Choi, J., Cotman, C.W., 1996. Physical activity increases mRNA for brain-derived neurotrophic factor and nerve growth factor in rat brain. Brain Research 726, 49–56.

Nguyen, P.V., Woo, N.H., 2003. Regulation of hippocampal synaptic plasticity by cyclic AMP-dependent protein kinases. Progress in Neurobiology 71, 401–437.

Nichol, K.E., Parachikova, A.I., Cotman, C.W., 2007. Three weeks of running wheel exposure improves cognitive performance in the aged Tg2576 mouse. Behavioural Brain Research 184, 124–132.

Nicholson, D.A., Yoshida, R., Berry, R.W., Gallagher, M., Geinisman, Y., 2004. Reduction in size of perforated postsynaptic densities in hippocampal axospinous synapses and age-related spatial learning impairments. Journal of Neuroscience 24, 7648–7653.

Nouchi, R., Taki, Y., Takeuchi, H., Sekiguchi, A., Hashizume, H., Nozawa, T., Nouchi, H., Kawashima, R., 2014. Four weeks of combination exercise training improved executive functions, episodic memory, and processing speed in healthy elderly people: evidence from a randomized controlled trial. Age (Dordrecht) 36, 787–799.

O'Callaghan, R.M., Griffin, E.W., Kelly, A.M., 2009. Long-term treadmill exposure protects against age-related neurodegenerative change in the rat hippocampus. Hippocampus 19, 1019–1029.

Oken, B.S., Zajdel, D., Kishiyama, S., Flegal, K., Dehen, C., Haas, M., Kraemer, D.F., Lawrence, J., Leyva, J., 2006. Randomized, controlled, six-month trial of yoga in healthy seniors: effects on cognition and quality of life. Alternative Therapies in Health and Medicine 12, 40–47.

Palmer, T.D., Willhoite, A.R., Gage, F.H., 2000. Vascular niche for adult hippocampal neurogenesis. Journal of Comparative Neurology 425, 479–494.

Park, H., Poo, M.M., 2013. Neurotrophin regulation of neural circuit development and function. Nature Reviews Neuroscience 14, 7–23.

Park, M., Penick, E.C., Edwards, J.G., Kauer, J.A., Ehlers, M.D., 2004. Recycling endosomes supply AMPA receptors for LTP. Science 305, 1972–1975.

Pereira, A.C., Huddleston, D.E., Brickman, A.M., Sosunov, A.A., Hen, R., McKhann, G.M., Sloan, R., Gage, F.H., Brown, T.R., Small, S.A., 2007. An in vivo correlate of exercise-induced neurogenesis in the adult dentate gyrus. Proceedings of the National Academy of Sciences of the United States of America 104, 5638–5643.

Prieto, G.A., Snighda, S., Baglietto-Vargas, D., Smith, E.D., Berchtold, N., Tong, L., Ajami, D., LaFerla, F.M., Rebek, J., Cotman, C.W., 2015. Synapse-specific IL-1 receptor subunit reconfiguration augments vulnerability to IL-1β in the aged hippocampus. Proceedings of the National Academy of Sciences of the United States of America 112, E5078–E5087.

Radak, Z., Kaneko, T., Tahara, S., Nakamoto, H., Pucsok, J., Sasvari, M., Nyakas, C., Goto, S., 2001. Regular exercise improves cognitive function and decreases oxidative damage in rat brain. Neurochemistry International 38, 17–23.

Raz, N., Lindenberger, U., Rodrigue, K.M., Kennedy, K.M., Head, D., Williamson, A., Dahle, C., Gerstorf, D., Acker, J.D., 2005. Regional brain changes in aging healthy adults: general trends, individual differences and modifiers. Cerebral Cortex 15, 1676–1689.

Real, C.C., Ferreira, A.F., Hernandes, M.S., Britto, L.R., Pires, R.S., 2010. Exercise-induced plasticity of AMPA-type glutamate receptor subunits in the rat brain. Brain Research 1363, 63–71.

Rex, C.S., Lauterborn, J.C., Lin, C.Y., Kramar, E.A., Rogers, G.A., Gall, C.M., Lynch, G., 2006. Restoration of long-term potentiation in middle-aged hippocampus after induction of brain-derived neurotrophic factor. Journal of Neurophysiology 96, 677–685.

Rex, C.S., Lin, C.Y., Kramar, E.A., Chen, L.Y., Gall, C.M., Lynch, G., 2007. Brain-derived neurotrophic factor promotes long-term potentiation-related cytoskeletal changes in adult hippocampus. Journal of Neuroscience 27, 3017–3029.

Rioult-Pedotti, M.S., Friedman, D., Donoghue, J.P., 2000. Learning-induced LTP in neocortex. Science 290, 533–536.

Rodriguez, J.J., Noristani, H.N., Olabarria, M., Fletcher, J., Somerville, T.D., Yeh, C.Y., Verkhratsky, A., 2011. Voluntary running and environmental enrichment restores impaired hippocampal neurogenesis in a triple transgenic mouse model of Alzheimer's disease. Current Alzheimer Research 8, 707–717.

Roman, F., Staubli, U., Lynch, G., 1987. Evidence for synaptic potentiation in a cortical network during learning. Brain Research 418, 221–226.

Rosano, C., Venkatraman, V.K., Guralnik, J., Newman, A.B., Glynn, N.W., Launer, L., Taylor, C.A., Williamson, J., Studenski, S., Pahor, M., Aizenstein, H., 2010. Psychomotor speed and functional brain MRI 2 years after completing a physical activity treatment. Journals of Gerontology Series A: Biological Sciences and Medical Sciences 65(6), 639–647. http://dx.doi.org/10.1093/gerona/glq038.

Sabia, S., Nabi, H., Kivimaki, M., Shipley, M.J., Marmot, M.G., Singh-Manoux, A., 2009. Health behaviors from early to late midlife as predictors of cognitive function: the Whitehall II study. American Journal of Epidemiology 170, 428–437.

Schuit, A.J., Feskens, E.J., Launer, L.J., Kromhout, D., 2001. Physical activity and cognitive decline, the role of the apolipoprotein e4 allele. Medicine and Science in Sports and Exercise 33, 772–777.

Segal, S.K., Cotman, C.W., Cahill, L.F., 2012. Exercise-induced noradrenergic activation enhances memory consolidation in both normal aging and patients with amnestic mild cognitive impairment. Journal of Alzheimer's Disease 32, 1011–1018.

Selkoe, D.J., 2002. Alzheimer's disease is a synaptic failure. Science 298, 789–791.

Shi, S.H., Hayashi, Y., Petralia, R.S., Zaman, S.H., Wenthold, R.J., Svoboda, K., Malinow, R., 1999. Rapid spine delivery and redistribution of AMPA receptors after synaptic NMDA receptor activation. Science 284, 1811–1816.

Silva, A.J., Stevens, C.F., Tonegawa, S., Wang, Y., 1992. Deficient hippocampal long-term potentiation in alpha-calcium-calmodulin kinase II mutant mice. Science 257, 201–206.

Smith, E.D., Prieto, G.A., Tong, L., Sears-Kraxberger, I., Rice, J.D., Steward, O., Cotman, C.W., 2014. Rapamycin and Interleukin-1beta impair brain-derived neurotrophic factor-dependent neuron survival by modulating autophagy. Journal of Biological Chemistry 289, 20615–20629.

Smith, J.C., Lancaster, M.A., Nielson, K.A., Woodard, J.L., Seidenberg, M., Durgerian, S., Sakaie, K., Rao, S.M., 2015. Interactive effects of physical activity and APOE-epsilon4 on white matter tract diffusivity in healthy elders. NeuroImage.

Smith, P.J., Blumenthal, J.A., Hoffman, B.M., Cooper, H., Strauman, T.A., Welsh-Bohmer, K., Browndyke, J.N., Sherwood, A., 2010. Aerobic exercise and neurocognitive performance: a meta-analytic review of randomized controlled trials. Psychosomatic Medicine 72, 239–252.

Snigdha, S., de Rivera, C., Milgram, N.W., Cotman, C.W., 2014. Exercise enhances memory consolidation in the aging brain. Frontiers in Aging Neuroscience 6, 3.

Snigdha, S., Milgram, N.W., Willis, S.L., Albert, M., Weintraub, S., Fortin, N.J., Cotman, C.W., 2013. A preclinical cognitive test battery to parallel the National Institute of Health Toolbox in humans: bridging the translational gap. Neurobiology of Aging 34, 1891–1901.

Snowden, M., Steinman, L., Mochan, K., Grodstein, F., Prohaska, T.R., Thurman, D.J., Brown, D.R., Laditka, J.N., Soares, J., Zweiback, D.J., Little, D., Anderson, L.A., 2011. Effect of exercise on cognitive performance in community-dwelling older adults: review of intervention trials and recommendations for public health practice and research. Journal of the American Geriatrics Society 59, 704–716.

Sumic, A., Michael, Y.L., Carlson, N.E., Howieson, D.B., Kaye, J.A., 2007. Physical activity and the risk of dementia in oldest old. Journal of Aging and Health 19, 242–259.

Tamura, M., Nemoto, K., Kawaguchi, A., Kato, M., Arai, T., Kakuma, T., Mizukami, K., Matsuda, H., Soya, H., Asada, T., 2015. Long-term mild-intensity exercise regimen preserves prefrontal cortical volume against aging. International Journal of Geriatric Psychiatry 30, 686–694.

Tsai, C.L., Wang, C.H., Pan, C.Y., Chen, F.C., 2015. The effects of long-term resistance exercise on the relationship between neurocognitive performance and GH, IGF-1, and homocysteine levels in the elderly. Frontiers in Behavioral Neuroscience 9, 23.

Tulving, E., 1983. Ecphoric processes in episodic memory. Philosophical Transactions of the Royal Society B 302, 361–371.

Tulving, E., Thomson, D.M., 1972. Word-blindness in episodic memory. Psychonomic Science 29, 262.

van Praag, H., Christie, B.R., Sejnowski, T.J., Gage, F.H., 1999a. Running enhances neurogenesis, learning, and long-term potentiation in mice. Proceedings of the National Academy of Sciences of the United States of America 96, 13427–13431.

van Praag, H., Kempermann, G., Gage, F.H., 1999b. Running increases cell proliferation and neurogenesis in the adult mouse dentate gyrus. Nature Neuroscience 2, 266–270.

van Praag, H., Shubert, T., Zhao, C., Gage, F.H., 2005. Exercise enhances learning and hippocampal neurogenesis in aged mice. The Journal of Neuroscience: the Official Journal of the Society for Neuroscience 25, 8680–8685.

Vivar, C., Peterson, B.D., van Praag, H., 2016. Running rewires the neuronal network of adult-born dentate granule cells. NeuroImage 131, 29–41.

Vivar, C., Potter, M.C., van Praag, H., 2013. All about running: synaptic plasticity, growth factors and adult hippocampal neurogenesis. Current Topics in Behavioral Neurosciences 15, 189–210.

Voss, M.W., Erickson, K.I., Prakash, R.S., Chaddock, L., Malkowski, E., Alves, H., Kim, J.S., Morris, K.S., White, S.M., Wojcicki, T.R., Hu, L., Szabo, A., Klamm, E., McAuley, E., Kramer, A.F., 2010a. Functional connectivity: a source of variance in the association between cardiorespiratory fitness and cognition? Neuropsychologia 48, 1394–1406.

Voss, M.W., Prakash, R.S., Erickson, K.I., Basak, C., Chaddock, L., Kim, J.S., Alves, H., Heo, S., Szabo, A.N., White, S.M., Wojcicki, T.R., Mailey, E.L., Gothe, N., Olson, E.A., McAuley, E., Kramer, A.F., 2010b. Plasticity of brain networks in a randomized intervention trial of exercise training in older adults. Frontiers in Aging Neuroscience 2.

Voss, M.W., Vivar, C., Kramer, A.F., van Praag, H., 2013. Bridging animal and human models of exercise-induced brain plasticity. Trends in Cognitive Sciences 17, 525–544.

Weinberg, L., Hasni, A., Shinohara, M., Duarte, A., 2014. A single bout of resistance exercise can enhance episodic memory performance. Acta Psychologica 153, 13–19.

Weintraub, S., Dikmen, S.S., Heaton, R.K., Tulsky, D.S., Zelazo, P.D., Bauer, P.J., Carlozzi, N.E., Slotkin, J., Blitz, D., Wallner-Allen, K., Fox, N.A., Beaumont, J.L., Mungas, D., Nowinski, C.J., Richler, J., Deocampo, J.A., Anderson, J.E., Manly, J.J., Borosh, B., Havlik, R., Conway, K., Edwards, E., Freund, L., King, J.W., Moy, C., Witt, E., Gershon, R.C., 2013. Cognition assessment using the NIH Toolbox. Neurology 80, S54–S64.

IV. EXERCISE AS THERAPY FOR NEUROLOGICAL DISEASES

Whitlock, J.R., Heynen, A.J., Shuler, M.G., Bear, M.F., 2006. Learning induces long-term potentiation in the hippocampus. Science 313, 1093–1097.

Wilbur, J., Marquez, D.X., Fogg, L., Wilson, R.S., Staffileno, B.A., Hoyem, R.L., Morris, M.C., Bustamante, E.E., Manning, A.F., 2012. The relationship between physical activity and cognition in older Latinos. Journals of Gerontology Series B: Psychological Sciences and Social Sciences 67, 525–534.

Yassa, M.A., Lacy, J.W., Stark, S.M., Albert, M.S., Gallagher, M., Stark, C.E., 2011a. Pattern separation deficits associated with increased hippocampal CA3 and dentate gyrus activity in nondemented older adults. Hippocampus 21, 968–979.

Yassa, M.A., Mattfeld, A.T., Stark, S.M., Stark, C.E., 2011b. Age-related memory deficits linked to circuit-specific disruptions in the hippocampus. Proceedings of the National Academy of Sciences of the United States of America 108, 8873–8878.

Zhao, G., Liu, H.L., Zhang, H., Tong, X.J., 2015. Treadmill exercise enhances synaptic plasticity, but does not alter beta-amyloid deposition in hippocampi of aged APP/PS1 transgenic mice. Neuroscience 298, 357–366.

LIFESTYLE EXERCISE AFFECTING NEUROLOGICAL STRUCTURE AND FUNCTION IN OLDER ADULTS

17

Synergistic Effects of Combined Physical Activity and Brain Training on Neurological Functions

T.M. Shah[1,2], R.N. Martins[1,2,3]

[1]McCusker Alzheimer's Research Foundation, Hollywood Medical Centre, Nedlands, WA, Australia; [2]Edith Cowan University, Joondalup, WA, Australia; [3]University of Western Australia, Crawley, WA, Australia

Abstract

Aging is a well-documented risk factor for cognitive decline and other neurodegenerative disorders such as Alzheimer's disease (AD) and Parkinsonism. Lifestyle factors, for example, staying physically and mentally active are associated with enhanced cognition and can lower the risk of certain neurological disorders including AD. In particular, both, physical and mental activities can modulate neuro-cognitive benefits via specific mechanisms that are directly linked to the classical pathological features of some neurological disorders. This chapter discusses the relationship between staying active and its association with brain health and cognition. The combined training mediated mechanisms are discussed in context to peripheral biomarkers, neurological functions, and brain structure. We conclude that combined physical and cognitive training can provide stronger cognitive benefits and could assist in slowing neurodegeneration. Clinical evidence is further required to show that this combined training can alter the disease trajectory in pathological cognitive decline such as that found in AD.

INTRODUCTION

Aging is a well-documented risk factor for cognitive decline and can lead to dementia and neurological disorders such as Alzheimer's disease (AD) and Parkinsonism. AD is the most common neurodegenerative disorder of the central nervous system (Yuan et al., 2015). Currently, therapeutics is administered at an advanced stage of AD where irreversible brain damage may have already occurred. Thus, research into successful brain aging by identifying the role of lifestyle strategies to enhance cognition and preserve brain health shows a significant interest (Mora, 2013). Poor lifestyle such as low education and physical inactivity are recognized as modifiable risk factors of AD (Barnes and Yaffe, 2011). Indeed, regular participation in leisure activities during middle-age is associated with 47% reduction in the risk of dementia (Dannhauser et al., 2014). Furthermore, there is evidence that exercise and cognitive training interventions can independently provide neuro-cognitive benefits (Ball et al., 2002; Erickson et al., 2011). Consequently, lifestyle interventions that include multimodal approach such as combining physical and cognitive training to optimize their potential as cognitive enhancers are highly recommended (Etnier et al., 2015).

In this chapter, we will evaluate the relationship between combined physical and mental activities and neurodegeneration, with an emphasis on human cognitive performance. The chapter discusses potential mechanisms of action through which combined training can promote healthy brain aging. Specifically, we examine the additive and/or synergistic mechanisms involving brain changes such as alterations in neurotransmitters, structural and functional changes in the central nervous system and other chemical, molecular and cellular mechanisms including the influence of genetic variants.

LEISURE ACTIVITIES IMPROVES COGNITION AND REDUCES THE RISK OF DEMENTIA AND AD

There is relevant evidence from observational studies suggesting a link between self-reported leisure activities and cognition. In a dose–response relationship, engaging in one type of activity can maintain cognitive health and engaging in two or more types of activities can improve cognition (Wang et al., 2013). Thus, engaging in a broad spectrum of leisure activities than any one type and the activities during middle-age are linked to better cognitive performance later in old age and can reduce the risk of dementia (Karp et al., 2006; Ihle et al., 2015). It is also suggested that individuals with low levels of education, spending over 1.25h behind physical activity per week and a 1-point increase in cognitive activity frequency (frequency rated on a 5-point composite scale of 7 activities) may benefit the most (Ihle et al., 2015; Rajan et al., 2015). Specifically, higher mental activity is associated with less decline in global cognition, language, processing speed, and executive functions; higher physical activity is associated with less decline in episodic memory and language, whereas higher social activity is associated with less decline in global cognition (Bielak et al., 2007; Wang et al., 2013). Social engagement, included as a component of leisure activities and rich social network, is also linked to improved cognition and reduced risk of dementia (Wang et al., 2002; Barnes et al., 2004; James et al., 2011). However, social engagement has not frequently been used in combined interventions. Table 17.1 provides an example of studies examining the relationship between activities and brain health in healthy older adults.

Engaging in higher levels of leisure activities is also linked to a lower risk of dementia, including AD and vascular dementia (Scarmeas et al., 2001; Friedland et al., 2001; Verghese et al., 2003; Paillard-Borg et al., 2009). Moreover, the risk of incident mild cognitive impairment (MCI, a diagnostic of AD) is lowered by combined activities including moderate exercise and computer use (Geda et al., 2012; Hughes et al., 2015). Furthermore, frequent engagement in intellectual, novel and diverse cognitive activities is linked to stronger cognitive benefits and reduced risk of dementia, MCI and AD; predominantly in the female gender (Wilson et al., 2002; Crowe et al., 2003; Fritsch et al., 2005; Verghese et al., 2006; Bielak et al., 2007). Besides gender differences, the interaction between the presence of genetic variants and activities also affects cognitive outcomes and this is discussed in the later sections of this chapter. Overall, if leisure activities can promote brain health, then it is reasonable to hypothesize that when used as a combined intervention, stronger cognitive benefits may be achieved. Such benefits could help prevent or delay the onset of pathological cognitive decline.

COMBINED PHYSICAL AND COGNITIVE TRAINING INTERVENTIONS SHOW STRONGER COGNITIVE BENEFITS

Observational studies showing the strength of relationship between cognition and leisure activities have led to clinical trials investigating the synergistic benefits and mechanisms behind combined physical and cognitive training. For example, 2months of combined aerobic (walking and running) and paper- and pencil-based cognitive training showed highest benefits for memory when compared to single intervention or a control group (Fabre et al., 2002). Similarly, 9months of combined training showed greater improvement in cognitive composite score, emotional status, and physical function with sustained benefits at 5years follow-up (Oswald et al., 1996, 2006).

More recently, cognitive training has become computerized, as such training is easy to administer, user friendly, adaptive and the training sessions can be timed and monitored uniformly for all participants. For example, healthy older adults completing mild aerobic exercise/walking and computerized cognitive training for 4months showed improved verbal episodic memory when compared to the control group (Shatil, 2013; Shah et al., 2014). In one of these studies, the cognitive training group also showed improved cognition which could indicate that when used in combination, there is a possibility of stronger cognitive training gains to that of physical training (Shatil, 2013). Moreover, in a dose–response relationship, (i.e., more training sessions resulted in more cognitive benefits) combined training for 6weeks appears to provide the greatest benefits in global cognition (Bamidis et al., 2015). However, when control group conditions simulates that of actual training condition, the results do not replicate to those discussed earlier. For instance, if control group is exposed to watching educational DVDs and performing stretching and toning exercises for 12weeks, then this could trigger actual intervention effects. As a consequence, the expected training gains observed for combined training is lost as both, the training and control group show improved cognition (Barnes et al., 2013).

Simultaneous administration of combined training or exergaming, i.e., virtual reality-enhanced exercises has potential benefits over sequenced training. The resulting complex dual-tasking can be more challenging and can

TABLE 17.1 Studies Showing the Relationship Between Activities, Cognition and Risk of Cognitive Decline in the Healthy Elderly

Study Type	Type of Activities	Combined Activity Levels/Intensity/Duration/Frequency	Associated Neuro-Cognitive Benefits (and References)
Observational	Fitness, cerebrovascular health and cognitively stimulating activities	Higher fitness levels, brain blood flow indices and cognitive activities is beneficial	Fitness, cerebrovascular health, and total number of mental activities is associated with improved cognition, attention, and executive functions; women-only study (Eskes et al., 2010)
	Leisure time physical, mental, and social activities:	Engaging in more types of activities; cognitively challenging/intellectual activities are most beneficial	Mental activities improved global cognition, language, processing speed, and executive functions; physical activity improved memory and language; and social activity improved global cognition; social activity was not associated with cognition in men (Bielak et al., 2007; Wang et al., 2013)
	Physical activities: Sports, gardening, walking, swimming, gymnastics, travelling, dancing etc.	1.25h of physical activity and 1-point increase in cognitive activity score (frequency rated on a 5-point composite scale of 7 activities); more activities during middle-age	Reduced risk of cognitive decline; individuals with low education shows more benefits (Rajan et al., 2015; Ihle et al., 2015)
	Mental activities: Reading, writing, playing cards, painting, drawing, bingo, crosswords, handicraft, using computer, etc.	Engaging in many types of activities; no association with intensity levels	Reduced dementia risk in individuals with highest activity scores and engaging in all or any two types of activities (Karp et al., 2006)
		Frequent participation and high levels of leisure activities; cognitive activities are more beneficial	Reduced dementia/AD risk (Scarmeas et al., 2001; Wang et al., 2002; Verghese et al., 2003)
	Social activities: Attending theatre, exhibition, concert, going to religious places, etc.	Engaging in moderate physical activities plus computer use	Reduced risk of mild cognitive impairment (Geda et al., 2012)
		Higher social activity/engagement, higher number of social network in later age	Reduced risk of cognitive decline/dementia (Wang et al., 2002; Barnes et al., 2004; James et al., 2011)
Interventional	Walking and jogging (aerobic) plus paper and pencil based cognitive training	Two, 1h exercise sessions per week for 2 months plus one 90-min brain training session per week for 2 months	Improved memory (Fabre et al., 2002)
	Balance, coordination and flexibility training with paper and pencil based cognitive training	60 sessions; 90 min of mental training activities followed by 45 min of physical training over 9 months	Improved cognition and emotional status; maintained at 5 years of follow-up (Oswald et al., 2006)
	Mild aerobic exercise and computerized cognitive training	56 training sessions for 16 weeks; exercise for 45-min 3 times per week and 48 min of cognitive training for 3 times per week	Cognitive training and combined groups improved on hand-eye coordination, global visual memory, processing speed, visual scanning, and naming (Shatil, 2013)
	Walking, resistance training and computerized cognitive training	160 training sessions for 16 weeks; 60 min of walking/resistance training for 5 days per week, 60 min of cognitive training for 5 days per week	Improved verbal episodic memory and increased brain glucose metabolism in the left primary sensorimotor cortex (Shah et al., 2014)
	Dance based aerobics, stretching exercise and computerized cognitive training	72 training sessions for 12 weeks; 1 h per day, 3 days per week for each training	No intervention-specific benefits (Barnes et al., 2013)
	Simultaneous treadmill exercise and computerized cognitive training	20 training session for 10 weeks; 30–40 min for each training; twice per week	Simultaneous combined group improved cognition and motor-cognitive dual task performance (Theill et al., 2013)
	Exergaming – stationary cycling with virtual reality tours	60 training sessions for 12 weeks; 45 min per session 5 times per week	Improved executive function; increased plasma BDNF levels, and risk reduction in clinical progression for mild cognitive impairment (Anderson-Hanley et al., 2012)
	Dancing, Tai chi	6 months	Improved cognition, balance, and quality of sleep (Nguyen and Kruse, 2012; Kattenstroth et al., 2013)

BDNF, brain derived neurotropic factor.

reduce the time for administering two separate interventions. Simultaneous training show improvement in executive functions (maintained at 1 year follow-up), paired association task, and visuospatial functions (Theill et al., 2013; Satoh et al., 2014; Eggenberger et al., 2015). Exergaming, such as cybercycling–stationary cycling with 3D-virtual tours or computerized cognitive training with Wii balance board exercises also report improved executive functions and increased brain signals in the prefrontal region (Anderson-Hanley et al., 2012; Frantzidis et al., 2014). Moreover, single-arm intervention integrating physical, cognitive, and social activity such as dancing or Tai Chi (Chinese martial art) for 6 months can improve cognition, balance, and quality of sleep in the elderly (Nguyen and Kruse, 2012; Kattenstroth et al., 2013). Although the combination and interactions between the type, intensity, duration, and frequency of physical and cognitive activities remain to be determined, the following mechanisms may provide an insight as to how combined training is beneficial in enhancing cognition.

MECHANISMS UNDERLYING THE SYNERGISTIC EFFECTS OF COMBINED PHYSICAL AND MENTAL ACTIVITIES FOR HEALTHY BRAIN AGING

The clinical significance of stronger associations observed between combined activities and cognition can only be established by identifying the underlying mechanisms induced by combined training. Besides the well-known cardiovascular health benefits of physical activity, there is evidence that physical and mental activities can cause direct alterations in the brain's structure and chemistry including changes in AD-related biomarkers. Table 17.2 show findings from human studies identifying mechanisms that can help protect the aging brain. The underpinning molecular and neurological mechanisms can come from diverse pathways and is further discussed in the following.

Identification of Activity-Induced Changes at Molecular and Cellular Level

The pathological hallmark feature of AD is the deposition of Aβ plaques in the cerebral cortex. If leisure activities can contribute to the reduced risk of dementia, then it is important to justify its role in mechanisms directly involved in the deposition or clearance of Aβ. Work from animal models show that mice genetically engineered to develop AD (and thus have high levels of brain Aβ) show reduced levels of brain Aβ following 16–20 weeks of wheel running/treadmill exercise or 8 weeks of cognitive stimulation (Adlard et al., 2005; Um et al., 2008; Gerenu et al., 2013). The combined training modulates of Aβ levels is not yet known; but mice exposed to environmental enrichment show increased secretion of Aβ degrading enzyme, neprilysin and plaque degradation and clearance (Lazarov et al., 2005; Herring et al., 2011). To further validate these findings in the aging human brain, the comparison between levels of activity and brain Aβ (measured using brain imaging) has been done and is further discussed later in this chapter.

There is now evidence that the brain has capability to undergo continuous change, form new cells and can compensate for injury or respond to a stimuli, also known as neuroplasticity (Bavelier and Neville, 2002; Gage and Temple, 2013). Activities can contribute to neural plasticity; for instance, voluntary wheel-running exercise increases cell proliferation in mice hippocampus, whereas cognitive stimulation facilitates the survival of adult neurons (Kempermann et al., 1997; Fabel et al., 2003; van Praag, 2008; Shors, 2013). Wheel-running, swimming, and sensory-motor learning have been reported to increase dendrite and synaptic connections in rodents leading to improved cognition (Pysh and Weiss, 1979; Greenough et al., 1986). Moreover, mental activities via higher levels of education and linguistic abilities also promotes cognitive reserve, which is an individual's resistance to impairment in cognitive processes under pathological conditions (Snowdon et al., 1996; Carret et al., 2005; Iacono et al., 2015).

Activity-induced secretion of neurotransmitters and neurotrophins can also promote brain health. For instance, acetylcholine levels (important for learning and memory and decreased in AD) are reported to be increased in exercising rats (Fordyce and Farrar, 1991). Following acute bout of exercise with simultaneous cognitive task, increased plasma levels of norepinephrine and dopamine metabolites have been reported (McMorris et al., 2008). In particular, activity-induced changes have been reported for neurochemicals such as serotonin, dopamine, growth and trophic factors including insulin-like growth factor 1 (IGF-1), vascular endothelial growth factor (VEGF), and brain-derived neurotrophic factor (BDNF) which are linked to either alleviation of depression, angiogenesis, neurogenesis or survival of neurons (Rogers et al., 1990; Vicario-Abejón et al., 1998; Russo-Neustadt et al., 2001; Cotman and Berchtold, 2002; McAuley et al., 2004). In humans, only peripheral levels of these neurological markers can be measured. Among these key proteins, BDNF shows convincing relationship in reference to the brain's functional connectivity network and BDNF activity can be modulated by IGF-1 and baseline levels of VEGF (Voss et al., 2013). Numerous studies show that BDNF is raised following exercise training (for a review see Szuhany et al., 2015), following cognitive

TABLE 17.2   Examples of Human Studies Showing Mechanisms by Which Physical and/or Cognitive Activities Can Protect the Aging Brain

Mechanism	Assessments	Biological Effects of Physical/Cognitive/Combined Activities (and References)
Regulation of brain Aβ levels	Observational: PET imaging	High levels of physical activity and greater time spent in lifetime of cognitive activities are independently associated with lower brain Aβ load (Liang et al., 2010; Brown et al., 2012; Landau et al., 2012)
Alterations in brain glucose metabolism	Interventional: PET imaging	Decreased brain glucose metabolism in the left dorsolateral prefrontal cortex following a 14-day lifestyle program (Small et al., 2006); increased brain glucose metabolism in the left primary sensorimotor cortex following 16 weeks of walking, resistance training, and computerized cognitive training (Shah et al., 2014)
Increased brain volume	Interventional: Structural MRI	Increased grey and white matter volume in the prefrontal and temporal cortex, increased hippocampal volume following 6 months–1 year of aerobic training (Colcombe et al., 2006; Erickson et al., 2011); increased hippocampal volume following 2 months of cognitive training (Engvig et al., 2014)
Enhancing functional brain networks	Interventional: Functional MRI	Increased functional connectivity in brain regions related to degenerative changes following 1 year of walking (Voss et al., 2010); increased resting state cerebral blood flow to the prefrontal cortex following 8 weeks of cognitive training (Mozolic et al., 2010); combined cognitive training, Tai chi exercise and counselling for 6 weeks improved resting state functional connectivity between the medial prefrontal cortex and medial temporal lobe (Li et al., 2014)
Increased BDNF secretion	Interventional: Plasma samples	Increased plasma BDNF levels following exergaming for 3 months (Anderson-Hanley et al., 2012)
Increased IGF-1 secretion	Interventional: Serum samples	Increased levels of serum IGF-1 following 6 months to 1 year of moderate to high-intensity physical training (Cassilhas et al., 2007; Tsai et al., 2015)
Increased neurotransmitter secretion	Interventional: Plasma samples	Higher concentration of norepinephrine and dopamine metabolites following acute bouts of simultaneous exercise with cognitive task (McMorris et al., 2008)
Increased brain metabolites	Interventional: MRS imaging	Increased choline and creatine signals following 5 weeks of memory training (Valenzuela et al., 2003)

Aβ, beta amyloid; *BDNF*, brain derived neurotropic factor; *IGF-1*, insulin growth like factor; *MRI*, magnetic resonant imaging; *MRS*, magnetic resonant spectroscopy; *PET*, positron emission tomography.

training in Parkinson's disease (Angelucci et al., 2015) and Schizophrenia (Fisher et al., 2016), and as a result of exergaming in healthy older adults (Anderson-Hanley et al., 2012).

Finally, there is an increasing evidence that activity-induced cognitive benefits can interact with specific genetic polymorphisms. For example, BDNF Val66Met polymorphism is linked to decreased activity-dependent BDNF secretion and synthesis of pro-BDNF to mature BDNF (Egan et al., 2003). Studies investigating whether engaging in different types of activities can compensate for the effects of these polymorphisms or whether non carriers only gain benefits showing inconsistent results (Erickson et al., 2013; Stuart et al., 2014; Canivet et al., 2015). Obviously, this complex issue of gene–environment interactions is in early stages of research and requires further validation.

Identification of Activity-Induced Changes in the Human Brain by Neuroimaging

As discussed in the previous section, findings from animal studies suggest a relationship between activity and reduced brain Aβ load. In humans, levels of Aβ load in the brain can be assessed by brain imaging. Observational studies show that higher physical activity levels and greater time spent in lifetime of cognitive activities are independently associated with lower brain Aβ load (Liang et al., 2010; Brown et al., 2012; Landau et al., 2012). In addition, individuals carrying the ε4 variant of apolipoprotein E (APOE ε4, a major genetic risk factor for late-onset AD) reporting higher levels of physical and cognitive activities show reduced brain Aβ load (Brown et al., 2012; Wirth et al., 2014). Thus, cognitively normal but sedentary APOE ε4 carriers may be at a higher risk for brain Aβ deposition (Head et al., 2012).

The brain consumes maximum glucose in the body and brain imaging to measure cerebral metabolic rate of glucose can provide a direct insight into neuronal activity. Cerebral glucose hypo metabolism has been reported in AD (Friedland et al., 1983; Foster et al., 1984; Minoshima et al., 1997; Mosconi et al., 2008). Following a 14-day lifestyle combined program that included diet and stress reduction activities, a significant reduction in glucose metabolism was reported in the left dorsolateral prefrontal cortex which are the regions related to working memory and verbal fluency (Small et al., 2006). Furthermore, increased cerebral glucose metabolism was reported in the left primary sensorimotor cortex after 16-weeks of combined intervention which was associated with improved verbal memory (Shah et al., 2014). This region is particularly spared in early AD pathology (Minoshima et al., 1997) and could indicate that such resistant brain areas in AD may be involved in compensatory mechanisms due to cognitive reserve and higher neuronal activity following combined interventions. It is argued that both, increased and decreased metabolism in certain brain regions could also be attributed to training-related (i.e., difficult versus easy training; short or prolonged training) compensatory mechanisms which could explain for the different findings in both studies (for a review see Belleville and Bherer, 2012). Future research involving AD or dementia patients will likely contribute to greater insights into the relationship between brain glucose metabolism and combined training.

A widely used parameter for determining age-related brain atrophy is magnetic resonance imaging (MRI) which can measure the brain volume. The extensively studied brain region associated with memory and spatial navigation is known as the hippocampus, and is severely affected in AD. Both physical (mainly walking) and mental activities are considered as moderators of hippocampal volume. For instance, 6 months–1 year of aerobic training showed an increase in grey and white matter volume in the prefrontal and temporal cortex and 2% increase in the hippocampus volume (Colcombe et al., 2006; Erickson et al., 2011). Likewise, frequent participation in playing games and puzzles and memory training for 2 months is associated with an increased hippocampus volume (Engvig et al., 2014; Schultz et al., 2015). Six months of combined training showed that fitness levels were associated with changes in neuronal activity in brain regions involved with spatial learning including the hippocampus, but only if subjects had additional spatial training (Holzschneider et al., 2012). Findings such as these support the notion that physical and mental activities could work in synergism to promote slowing of hippocampal atrophy.

In addition, the brain's functional connectivity can be measured using functional MRI (fMRI) which is measured by studying changes occurring in the brain's blood circulation and oxygenation at rest and in response to neural stimulus. For example, single-arm interventions such as 1 year of walking can result in an increased functional connectivity in brain networks related to degenerative changes (Voss et al., 2010). Furthermore, 8 weeks of cognitive training showed an increase in resting cerebral blood flow to the prefrontal cortex (Mozolic et al., 2010). A combination of cognitive training, Tai Chi exercise, and counselling for 6 weeks showed improved resting state functional connectivity between the medial prefrontal cortex and medial temporal lobe (Li et al., 2014). Both these regions are parts of the default mode network and are associated with age-related cognitive decline. Finally, the metabolic information in the images captured by MRI can be measured using magnetic resonance spectroscopy (MRS). For instance, MRS performed following 5 weeks of memory training in older adults showed increased choline and creatine signals (metabolites essential for intact neural function and cell membrane integrity) in the hippocampus (Valenzuela et al., 2003).

Thus, both mental and physical activities play an important role in modulating AD pathology through mechanisms discussed earlier. However, it must be noted that most of the brain imaging studies have assessed the effects of single activity or single-arm intervention. There are very few publications that has assessed the effects of combined training on brain's structure, function, and nervous system metabolite levels. Whether additive or synergistic benefits are observed in these mechanisms after combined training is an emerging research question and is clearly an area in need of further investigation.

FUTURE DIRECTIONS

In light of the current evidence presented in this chapter, it is suggested that combined training plays a stronger role in protecting the aging brain and in enhancing cognition than single activity. An important caveat to note is that most of the studies discussed in this chapter evaluated the effects of combined training in cognitively intact, healthy older adults. As a consequence, the effects of combined training on brain health under the influence of neurodegenerative diseases are not clearly understood. Nevertheless, the use of combined training as a protective factor also requires more evidence and many questions need to be addressed. For example, identification of the most beneficial type of activity combination and its intensity, duration, and frequency is required. An ideal combination may differ across individuals and the influence of genetic variants must be further assessed. Finally, inclusion of combined training as a preventative or delaying strategy for AD and other neurodegenerative diseases will require comprehensive understanding of combined training-induced changes in disease-specific biological markers.

References

Adlard, P.A., Perreau, V.M., Pop, V., Cotman, C.W., 2005. Voluntary exercise decreases amyloid load in a transgenic model of Alzheimer's disease. Journal of Neuroscience 25 (17), 4217–4221.

Anderson-Hanley, C., Arciero, P.J., Brickman, A.M., Nimon, J.P., Okuma, N., Westen, S.C., Merz, M.E., Pence, B.D., Woods, J.A., Kramer, A.F., 2012. Exergaming and older adult cognition: a cluster randomized clinical trial. American Journal of Preventive Medicine 42 (2), 109–119.

Angelucci, F., Peppe, A., Carlesimo, G.A., Serafini, F., Zabberoni, S., Barban, F., Shofany, J., Caltagirone, C., Costa, A., 2015. A pilot study on the effect of cognitive training on BDNF serum levels in individuals with Parkinson's disease. Frontiers in Human Neuroscience 9. http://dx.doi.org/10.3389/fnhum.2015.00130.

Ball, K., Berch, D.B., Helmers, K.F., Jobe, J.B., Leveck, M.D., Marsiske, M., Morris, J.N., Rebok, G.W., Smith, D.M., Tennstedt, S.L., 2002. Effects of cognitive training interventions with older adults: a randomized controlled trial. Journal of the American Medical Association 288 (18), 2271–2281.

Bamidis, P.D., Fissler, P., Papageorgiou, S.G., Zilidou, V., Konstantinidis, E.I., Billis, A.S., Romanopoulou, E., Karagianni, M., Bearatis, I., Tsapanou, A., Tsilikopoulou, G., Grigoriadou, E., Ladas, A., Kyrillidou, A., Tsolaki, A., Frantzidis, C., Sidiropoulos, E., Siountas, A., Matsi, S., Papatriantafyllou, J., Margioti, E., Nika, A., Schlee, W., Elbert, T., Tsolaki, M., Vivas, A.B., Kolassa, I.-T., 2015. Gains in cognition through combined cognitive and physical training: the role of training dosage and severity of neurocognitive disorder. Frontiers in Aging Neuroscience 7. http://dx.doi.org/10.3389/fnagi.2015.00152.

Barnes, D.E., Yaffe, K., 2011. The projected impact of risk factor reduction on Alzheimer's disease prevalence. Lancet Neurology 10 (9), 819–828. http://dx.doi.org/10.1016/S1474-4422(11)70072-2.

Barnes, L.L., Mendes de Leon, C.F., Wilson, R.S., Bienias, J.L., Evans, D.A., 2004. Social resources and cognitive decline in a population of older African Americans and whites. Neurology 63 (12), 2322–2326. Retrieved from: http://www.ncbi.nlm.nih.gov/pubmed/15623694.

Barnes, D.E., Santos-Modesitt, W., Poelke, G., Kramer, A.F., Castro, C., Middleton, L.E., Yaffe, K., 2013. The Mental Activity and eXercise (MAX) trial: a randomized controlled trial to enhance cognitive function in older adults. JAMA Internal Medicine 173 (9), 797–804.

Bavelier, D., Neville, H.J., 2002. Cross-modal plasticity: where and how? Nature Reviews. Neuroscience 3 (6), 443–452.

Belleville, S., Bherer, L., 2012. Biomarkers of cognitive training effects in aging. Current Translational Geriatrics and Gerontology Reports 1 (2), 104–110.

Bielak, A.A., Hughes, T.F., Small, B.J., Dixon, R.A., 2007. It's never too late to engage in lifestyle activities: significant concurrent but not change relationships between lifestyle activities and cognitive speed. Journal of Gerontology 62 (6), P331–P339.

Brown, B.M., Peiffer, J.J., Taddei, K., Lui, J.K., Laws, S.M., Gupta, V.B., Taddei, T., Ward, V.K., Rodrigues, M.A., Burnham, S., Rainey-Smith, S., Villemagne, V.L., Bush, A., Ellis, K.A., Masters, C.L., Ames, D., Macaulay, S.L., Szoeke, C., Rowe, C.C., Martins, R.N., 2012. Physical activity and amyloid-β plasma and brain levels: results from the Australian Imaging, Biomarkers and Lifestyle Study of Ageing. Molecular Psychiatry 18 (8), 875–881. http://dx.doi.org/10.1038/mp.2012.107.

Canivet, A., Albinet, C.T., André, N., Pylouster, J., Rodríguez-Ballesteros, M., Kitzis, A., Audiffren, M., 2015. Effects of BDNF polymorphism and physical activity on episodic memory in the elderly: a cross sectional study. European Review of Aging and Physical Activity 12 (1), 1–9. http://dx.doi.org/10.1186/s11556-015-0159-2.

Carret, N.L., Auriacombe, S., Letenneur, L., Bergua, V., Dartigues, J.F., Fabrigoule, C., 2005. Influence of education on the pattern of cognitive deterioration in AD patients: the cognitive reserve hypothesis. Brain and Cognition 57 (2), 120–126.

Cassilhas, R.C., Viana, V.A., Grassmann, V., Santos, R.T., Santos, R.F., Tufik, S., Mello, M.T., 2007. The impact of resistance exercise on the cognitive function of the elderly. Medicine & Science in Sports & Exercise 39 (8), 1401.

Colcombe, S.J., Erickson, K.I., Scalf, P.E., Kim, J.S., Prakash, R., McAuley, E., Elavsky, S., Marquez, D.X., Hu, L., Kramer, A.F., 2006. Aerobic exercise training increases brain volume in aging humans. Journal of Gerontology, Series A 61 (11), 1166–1170.

Cotman, C.W., Berchtold, N.C., 2002. Exercise: a behavioral intervention to enhance brain health and plasticity. Trends Neuroscience 25 (6), 295–301.

Crowe, M., Andel, R., Pedersen, N.L., Johansson, B., Gatz, M., 2003. Does participation in leisure activities lead to reduced risk of Alzheimer's disease? A prospective study of Swedish twins. Journal of Gerontology 58 (5), P249–P255.

Dannhauser, T.M., Cleverley, M., Whitfield, T.J., Fletcher, B., Stevens, T., Walker, Z., 2014. A complex multimodal activity intervention to reduce the risk of dementia in mild cognitive impairment–ThinkingFit: pilot and feasibility study for a randomized controlled trial. BMC Psychiatry 14 (1), 1–9. http://dx.doi.org/10.1186/1471-244x-14-129.

Egan, M.F., Kojima, M., Callicott, J.H., Goldberg, T.E., Kolachana, B.S., Bertolino, A., Zaitsev, E., Gold, B., Goldman, D., Dean, M., 2003. The BDNF val66met polymorphism affects activity-dependent secretion of BDNF and human memory and hippocampal function. Cell 112 (2), 257–269.

Eggenberger, P., Schumacher, V., Angst, M., Theill, N., de Bruin, E.D., 2015. Does multicomponent physical exercise with simultaneous cognitive training boost cognitive performance in older adults? A 6-month randomized controlled trial with a 1-year follow-up. Clinical Interventions in Aging 10, 1335.

Engvig, A., Fjell, A.M., Westlye, L.T., Skaane, N.V., Dale, A.M., Holland, D., Due-Tonnessen, P., Sundseth, O., Walhovd, K.B., 2014. Effects of cognitive training on gray matter volumes in memory clinic patients with subjective memory impairment. Journal of Alzheimer's Disease 41 (3), 779–791. http://dx.doi.org/10.3233/jad-131889.

Erickson, K.I., Voss, M.W., Prakash, R.S., Basak, C., Szabo, A., Chaddock, L., Kim, J.S., Heo, S., Alves, H., White, S.M., 2011. Exercise training increases size of hippocampus and improves memory. Proceedings of the National Academy of Sciences of the United States of America 108 (7), 3017–3022.

Erickson, K.I., Banducci, S.E., Weinstein, A.M., MacDonald, A.W., Ferrell, R.E., Halder, I., Flory, J.D., Manuck, S.B., 2013. The brain-derived neurotrophic factor Val66Met polymorphism moderates an effect of physical activity on working memory performance. Psychological Science 24 (9), 1770–1779. http://dx.doi.org/10.1177/0956797613480367.

Eskes, G.A., Longman, S., Brown, A.D., McMorris, C.A., Langdon, K.D., Hogan, D.B., Poulin, M., 2010. Contribution of physical fitness, cerebrovascular reserve and cognitive stimulation to cognitive function in post-menopausal women. Frontiers in Aging Neuroscience 2 (1), 137.

Etnier, J.L., Shih, C.-H., Piepmeier, A., Etnier, J., Shih, C., Piepmeier, A., 2015. Behavioral interventions to benefit cognition (intervenciones cognitivas para beneficiar la cognición). RETOS [Challenges. New Trends in Physical Education, Sport and Recreation] 27, 197–202.

Fabel, K., Tam, B., Kaufer, D., Baiker, A., Simmons, N., Kuo, C.J., Palmer, T.D., 2003. VEGF is necessary for exercise induced adult hippocampal neurogenesis. European Journal of Neuroscience 18 (10), 2803–2812.

Fabre, C., Chamari, K., Mucci, P., Masse-Biron, J., Prefaut, C., 2002. Improvement of cognitive function by mental and/or individualized aerobic training in healthy elderly subjects. International Journal of Sports Medicine 23 (6), 415–421.

Fisher, M., Mellon, S.H., Wolkowitz, O., Vinogradov, S., 2016. Neuroscience-informed auditory training in schizophrenia: a final report of the effects on cognition and serum brain-derived neurotrophic factor. Schizophrenia Research. Cognition 3, 1–7. http://dx.doi.org/10.1016/j.scog.2015.10.006.

Fordyce, D., Farrar, R., 1991. Enhancement of spatial learning in F344 rats by physical activity and related learning-associated alterations in hippocampal and cortical cholinergic functioning. Behavioural Brain Research 46 (2), 123–133.

Foster, N.L., Chase, T.N., Mansi, L., Brooks, R., Fedio, P., Patronas, N.J., Di Chiro, G., 1984. Cortical abnormalities in Alzheimer's disease. Annals of Neurology 16 (6), 649–654.

Frantzidis, C.A., Ladas, A.-K.I., Vivas, A.B., Tsolaki, M., Bamidis, P.D., 2014. Cognitive and physical training for the elderly: evaluating outcome efficacy by means of neurophysiological synchronization. International Journal of Psychophysiology 93 (1), 1–11.

Friedland, R.P., Budinger, T.F., Ganz, E., Yano, Y., Mathis, C.A., Koss, B., Ober, B.A., Huesman, R.H., Derenzo, S.E., 1983. Regional cerebral metabolic alterations in dementia of the Alzheimer type: positron emission tomography with [18F] fluorodeoxyglucose. Journal of Computer Assisted Tomography 7 (4), 590–598.

Friedland, R.P., Fritsch, T., Smyth, K.A., Koss, E., Lerner, A.J., Chen, C.H., Petot, G.J., Debanne, S.M., 2001. Patients with Alzheimer's disease have reduced activities in midlife compared with healthy control-group members. Proceedings of the National Academy of Sciences of the United States of America 98 (6), 3440–3445. http://dx.doi.org/10.1073/pnas.061002998.

Fritsch, T., Smyth, K.A., Debanne, S.M., Petot, G.J., Friedland, R.P., 2005. Participation in novelty-seeking leisure activities and Alzheimer's disease. Journal of Geriatric Psychiatry and Neurology 18 (3), 134–141. http://dx.doi.org/10.1177/0891988705277537.

Gage, F.H., Temple, S., 2013. Neural stem cells: generating and regenerating the brain. Neuron 80 (3), 588–601.

Geda, Y.E., Silber, T.C., Roberts, R.O., Knopman, D.S., Christianson, T.J., Pankratz, V.S., Boeve, B.F., Tangalos, E.G., Petersen, R.C., 2012. Computer activities, physical exercise, aging, and mild cognitive impairment: a population-based study. Mayo Clinic Proceedings 87 (5), 437–442. http://dx.doi.org/10.1016/j.mayocp.2011.12.020.

Gerenu, G., Dobarro, M., Ramirez, M.J., Gil-Bea, F.J., 2013. Early cognitive stimulation compensates for memory and pathological changes in Tg2576 mice. Biochimica et Biophysica Acta (BBA). Molecular Basis of Disease 1832 (6), 837–847.

Greenough, W.T., McDonald, J.W., Parnisari, R.M., Camel, J.E., 1986. Environmental conditions modulate degeneration and new dendrite growth in cerebellum of senescent rats. Brain Research 380 (1), 136–143.

Head, D., Bugg, J.M., Goate, A.M., Fagan, A.M., Mintun, M.A., Benzinger, T., Holtzman, D.M., Morris, J.C., 2012. Exercise Engagement as a Moderator of APOE Effects on Amyloid Deposition. Archives of Neurology 69 (5), 636–643. http://dx.doi.org/10.1001/archneurol.2011.845.

Herring, A., Lewejohann, L., Panzer, A.-L., Donath, A., Kröll, O., Sachser, N., Paulus, W., Keyvani, K., 2011. Preventive and therapeutic types of environmental enrichment counteract beta amyloid pathology by different molecular mechanisms. Neurobiology of Disease 42 (3), 530–538.

Holzschneider, K., Wolbers, T., Röder, B., Hötting, K., 2012. Cardiovascular fitness modulates brain activation associated with spatial learning. NeuroImage 59 (3), 3003–3014.

Hughes, T.F., Becker, J.T., Lee, C.-W., Chang, C.-C.H., Ganguli, M., 2015. Independent and combined effects of cognitive and physical activity on incident MCI. Alzheimer's Dementia 11 (11), 1377–1384.

Iacono, D., Zandi, P., Gross, M., Markesbery, W.R., Pletnikova, O., Rudow, G., Troncoso, J.C., 2015. APOε2 and education in cognitively normal older subjects with high levels of AD pathology at autopsy: findings from the Nun Study. Oncotarget 6 (16), 14082.

Ihle, A., Oris, M., Fagot, D., Baeriswyl, M., Guichard, E., Kliegel, M., 2015. The association of leisure activities in middle adulthood with cognitive performance in old age: the moderating role of educational level. Gerontology 61 (6), 543–550.

James, B.D., Wilson, R.S., Barnes, L.L., Bennett, D.A., 2011. Late-life social activity and cognitive decline in old age. Journal of the International Neuropsychological Society 17 (6), 998–1005. http://dx.doi.org/10.1017/S1355617711000531.

Karp, A., Paillard-Borg, S., Wang, H.-X., Silverstein, M., Winblad, B., Fratiglioni, L., 2006. Mental, physical and social components in leisure activities equally contribute to decrease dementia risk. Dementia and Geriatric Cognitive Disorders 21 (2), 65–73.

Kattenstroth, J.-C., Kalisch, T., Holt, S., Tegenthoff, M., Dinse, H.R., 2013. Six months of dance intervention enhances postural, sensorimotor, and cognitive performance in elderly without affecting cardio-respiratory functions. Frontiers in Aging Neuroscience 5, 5. http://dx.doi.org/10.3389/fnagi.2013.00005.

Kempermann, G., Kuhn, H.G., Gage, F.H., 1997. More hippocampal neurons in adult mice living in an enriched environment. Nature 386 (6624), 493–495.

Landau, S.M., Marks, S.M., Mormino, E.C., Rabinovici, G.D., Oh, H., O'Neil, J.P., Wilson, R.S., Jagust, W.J., 2012. Association of lifetime cognitive engagement and low β-amyloid deposition. Archives of Neurology 69 (5), 623–629.

Lazarov, O., Robinson, J., Tang, Y.-P., Hairston, I.S., Korade-Mirnics, Z., Lee, V.M.-Y., Hersh, L.B., Sapolsky, R.M., Mirnics, K., Sisodia, S.S., 2005. Environmental enrichment reduces Aβ levels and amyloid deposition in transgenic mice. Cell 120 (5), 701–713.

Li, R., Zhu, X., Yin, S., Niu, Y., Zheng, Z., Huang, X., Wang, B., Li, J., 2014. Multimodal intervention in older adults improves resting-state functional connectivity between the medial prefrontal cortex and medial temporal lobe. Frontiers in Aging Neuroscience 6, 39. http://dx.doi.org/10.3389/fnagi.2014.00039.

Liang, K.Y., Mintun, M.A., Fagan, A.M., Goate, A.M., Bugg, J.M., Holtzman, D.M., Morris, J.C., Head, D., 2010. Exercise and Alzheimer's disease biomarkers in cognitively normal older adults. Annals of Neurology 68 (3), 311–318.

McAuley, E., Kramer, A.F., Colcombe, S.J., 2004. Cardiovascular fitness and neurocognitive function in older adults: a brief review. Brain, Behavior, and Immunity 18 (3), 214–220.

McMorris, T., Collard, K., Corbett, J., Dicks, M., Swain, J., 2008. A test of the catecholamines hypothesis for an acute exercise–cognition interaction. Pharmacology, Biochemistry, and Behavior 89 (1), 106–115.

Minoshima, S., Giordani, B., Berent, S., Frey, K.A., Foster, N.L., Kuhl, D.E., 1997. Metabolic reduction in the posterior cingulate cortex in very early Alzheimer's disease. Annals of Neurology 42 (1), 85–94.

Mora, F., 2013. Successful brain aging: plasticity, environmental enrichment, and lifestyle. Dialogues in Clinical Neuroscience 15 (1), 45–52.

Mosconi, L., Pupi, A., De Leon, M.J., 2008. Brain glucose hypometabolism and oxidative stress in preclinical Alzheimer's disease. Annals of New York Academy of Sciences 1147 (1), 180–195.

Mozolic, J.L., Hayasaka, S., Laurienti, P.J., 2010. A cognitive training intervention increases resting cerebral blood flow in healthy older adults. Frontiers in Human Neuroscience 4, 16. http://dx.doi.org/10.3389/neuro.09.016.2010.

Nguyen, M.H., Kruse, A., 2012. A randomized controlled trial of Tai chi for balance, sleep quality and cognitive performance in elderly Vietnamese. Clinical Interventions in Aging 7, 185–190. http://dx.doi.org/10.2147/cia.s32600.

Oswald, W.D., Rupprecht, R., Gunzelmann, T., Tritt, K., 1996. The SIMA-project: effects of 1 year cognitive and psychomotor training on cognitive abilities of the elderly. Behavioural Brain Research 78 (1), 67–72.

Oswald, W.D., Gunzelmann, T., Rupprecht, R., Hagen, B., 2006. Differential effects of single versus combined cognitive and physical training with older adults: the SimA study in a 5-year perspective. European Journal of Ageing 3 (4), 179–192.

Paillard-Borg, S., Fratiglioni, L., Winblad, B., Wang, H.X., 2009. Leisure activities in late life in relation to dementia risk: principal component analysis. Dementia and Geriatric Cognitive Disorders 28 (2), 136–144. http://dx.doi.org/10.1159/000235576.

Pysh, J., Weiss, G., 1979. Exercise during development induces an increase in Purkinje cell dendritic tree size. Science 206 (4415), 230–232.

Rajan, K.B., Barnes, L.L., Skarupski, K.A., Mendes de Leon, C.F., Wilson, R.S., Evans, D.A., 2015. Physical and cognitive activities as deterrents of cognitive decline in a biracial population sample. The American Journal of Geriatric Psychiatry 23 (12), 1225–1233. http://dx.doi.org/10.1016/j.jagp.2015.07.008.

Rogers, R.L., Meyer, J.S., Mortel, K.F., 1990. After reaching retirement age physical activity sustains cerebral perfusion and cognition. Journal of the American Geriatrics Society 38 (2), 123–128.

Russo-Neustadt, A., Ha, T., Ramirez, R., Kesslak, J.P., 2001. Physical activity-antidepressant treatment combination: impact on brain-derived neurotrophic factor and behavior in an animal model. Behavioural Brain Research 120 (1), 87–95.

Satoh, M., Ogawa, J.-i., Tokita, T., Nakaguchi, N., Nakao, K., Kida, H., Tomimoto, H., 2014. The effects of physical exercise with music on cognitive function of elderly people: Mihama-Kiho project. PLoS One 9 (4), e95230.

Scarmeas, N., Levy, G., Tang, M.-X., Manly, J., Stern, Y., 2001. Influence of leisure activity on the incidence of Alzheimer's disease. Neurology 57 (12), 2236–2242.

Schultz, S.A., Larson, J., Oh, J., Koscik, R., Dowling, M.N., Gallagher, C.L., Carlsson, C.M., Rowley, H.A., Bendlin, B.B., Asthana, S., 2015. Participation in cognitively-stimulating activities is associated with brain structure and cognitive function in preclinical Alzheimer's disease. Brain, Imaging, and Behavior 9 (4), 729–736.

Shah, T., Verdile, G., Sohrabi, H., Campbell, A., Putland, E., Cheetham, C., Dhaliwal, S., Weinborn, M., Maruff, P., Darby, D., 2014. A combination of physical activity and computerized brain training improves verbal memory and increases cerebral glucose metabolism in the elderly. Translational Psychiatry 4 (12), e487.

Shatil, E., 2013. Does combined cognitive training and physical activity training enhance cognitive abilities more than either alone? A four-condition randomized controlled trial among healthy older adults. Frontiers in Aging Neuroscience 5 (8).

Shors, T., 2013. Training your brain: do mental and physical (MAP) training enhance cognition through the process of neurogenesis in the hippocampus? Neuropharmacology 64, 506–514.

Small, G.W., Silverman, D.H.S., Siddarth, P., Ercoli, L.M., Miller, K.J., Lavretsky, H., Wright, B.C., Bookheimer, S.Y., Barrio, J.R., Phelps, M.E., 2006. Effects of a 14-day healthy longevity lifestyle program on cognition and brain function. The American Journal of Geriatric Psychiatry 14 (6), 538–545.

Snowdon, D.A., Kemper, S.J., Mortimer, J.A., Greiner, L.H., Wekstein, D.R., Markesbery, W.R., 1996. Linguistic ability in early life and cognitive function and Alzheimer's disease in late life: findings from the nun study. Journal of the American Medical Association 275 (7), 528–532. http://dx.doi.org/10.1001/jama.1996.03530310034029.

Stuart, K., Summers, M.J., Valenzuela, M.J., Vickers, J.C., 2014. BDNF and COMT polymorphisms have a limited association with episodic memory performance or engagement in complex cognitive activity in healthy older adults. Neurobiology of Learning and Memory 110, 1–7. http://dx.doi.org/10.1016/j.nlm.2014.01.013.

Szuhany, K.L., Bugatti, M., Otto, M.W., 2015. A meta-analytic review of the effects of exercise on brain-derived neurotrophic factor. Journal of Psychiatric Research 60, 56–64. http://dx.doi.org/10.1016/j.jpsychires.2014.10.003.

Theill, N., Schumacher, V., Adelsberger, R., Martin, M., Jäncke, L., 2013. Effects of simultaneously performed cognitive and physical training in older adults. BMC Neuroscience 14 (1), 1.

Tsai, C.-L., Wang, C.-H., Pan, C.-Y., Chen, F.-C., 2015. The effects of long-term resistance exercise on the relationship between neurocognitive performance and GH, IGF-1, and homocysteine levels in the elderly. Frontiers in Behavioral Neuroscience 9. http://dx.doi.org/10.3389/fnbeh.2015.00023.

Um, H.S., Kang, E.B., Leem, Y.H., Cho, I.H., Yang, C.H., Chae, K.R., Hwang, D.Y., Cho, J.Y., 2008. Exercise training acts as a therapeutic strategy for reduction of the pathogenic phenotypes for Alzheimer's disease in an NSE/APPsw-transgenic model. International Journal of Molecular Medicine 22 (4), 529–539.

Valenzuela, M.J., Jones, M., Rae, W.W.C., Graham, S., Shnier, R., Sachdev, P., 2003. Memory training alters hippocampal neurochemistry in healthy elderly. Neuroreport 14 (10), 1333–1337.

van Praag, H., 2008. Neurogenesis and exercise: past and future directions. Neuromolecular Medicine 10 (2), 128–140.

Verghese, J., Lipton, R.B., Katz, M.J., Hall, C.B., Derby, C.A., Kuslansky, G., Ambrose, A.F., Sliwinski, M., Buschke, H., 2003. Leisure activities and the risk of dementia in the elderly. The New England Journal of Medicine 348 (25), 2508–2516.

Verghese, J., LeValley, A., Derby, C., Kuslansky, G., Katz, M., Hall, C., Buschke, H., Lipton, R.B., 2006. Leisure activities and the risk of amnestic mild cognitive impairment in the elderly. Neurology 66 (6), 821–827. http://dx.doi.org/10.1212/01.wnl.0000202520.68987.48.

Vicario-Abejón, C., Collin, C., McKay, R.D.G., Segal, M., 1998. Neurotrophins induce formation of functional excitatory and inhibitory synapses between cultured hippocampal neurons. Journal of Neuroscience 18 (18), 7256–7271.

Voss, M.W., Prakash, R.S., Erickson, K.I., Basak, C., Chaddock, L., Kim, J.S., Alves, H., Heo, S., Szabo, A.N., White, S.M., Wójcicki, T.R., Mailey, E.L., Gothe, N., Olson, E.A., McAuley, E., Kramer, A.F., 2010. Plasticity of brain networks in a randomized intervention trial of exercise training in older adults. Frontiers in Aging Neuroscience 2, 32. http://dx.doi.org/10.3389/fnagi.2010.00032.

Voss, M.W., Erickson, K.I., Prakash, R.S., Chaddock, L., Kim, J.S., Alves, H., Szabo, A., Phillips, S.M., Wójcicki, T.R., Mailey, E.L., 2013. Neurobiological markers of exercise-related brain plasticity in older adults. Brain, Behavior, and Immunity 28, 90–99.

Wang, H.-X., Karp, A., Winblad, B., Fratiglioni, L., 2002. Late-life engagement in social and leisure activities is associated with a decreased risk of dementia: a longitudinal study from the Kungsholmen project. American Journal of Epidemiology 155 (12), 1081–1087.

Wang, H.-X., Jin, Y., Hendrie, H.C., Liang, C., Yang, L., Cheng, Y., Unverzagt, F.W., Ma, F., Hall, K.S., Murrell, J.R., 2013. Late life leisure activities and risk of cognitive decline. Journal of Gerontology, Series A 68 (2), 205–213.

Wilson, R.S., Bennett, D.A., Bienias, J.L., Aggarwal, N.T., Mendes De Leon, C.F., Morris, M.C., Schneider, J.A., Evans, D.A., 2002. Cognitive activity and incident AD in a population-based sample of older persons. Neurology 59 (12), 1910–1914.

Wirth, M., Villeneuve, S., La Joie, R., Marks, S.M., Jagust, W.J., 2014. Gene–environment interactions: lifetime cognitive activity, APOE genotype, and beta-amyloid burden. Journal of Neuroscience 34 (25), 8612–8617.

Yuan, M., Xu, L., Yin, X., 2015. Uric acid and the risk of Alzheimer's disease is there an association? American Journal of Alzheimer's Disease and Other Dementias 31 (3), 294–295. http://dx.doi.org/10.1177/1533317515602550.

Physical Activity: Effects of Exercise on Neurological Function

R. Beurskens[1,2], M. Dalecki[3]

[1]Geriatric Center at the University of Heidelberg, Bethanien Hospital, Heidelberg, Germany; [2]University of Potsdam, Germany; [3]York University, Toronto, ON, Canada

Abstract

Motor performance in humans is controlled by higher-order cognitive functions located in the frontal lobes and the motor cortex. Injuries (e.g., concussion, traumatic brain injuries), diseases (e.g., Alzheimer's disease, dementia) as well as aging deteriorate these brain structures, thereby impairing adequate brain functioning. Consequences of improper brain functioning are impaired motor and/or cognitive performance. Physical exercise has been shown to positively modulate brain functions by increasing neural activity and/or by activating additional brain areas (e.g., neural plasticity, neural compensation), thereby counteracting degenerative processes and improving motor and/or cognitive functions in young and older adults alike. This chapter will evaluate adaptations in brain function following various adverse effects (i.e., aging, cognitive impairment, brain injuries), describe underlying mechanisms and theories, and demonstrate that physical exercise is a suitable tool to influence neural plasticity and motor/cognitive behavior in young and older adults.

INTRODUCTION

Experimental studies suggest that human motor performance is under control of higher-order cognitive processes, primarily located in the frontal lobes, the motor cortex, and the hippocampus. On the one hand, injuries (e.g., concussion, traumatic brain injuries), diseases (e.g., Alzheimer's disease, dementia), and aging deteriorate those brain structures, impairing proper brain functioning. The consequences are impaired motor and/or cognitive performance. On the other hand, physical exercise has been shown to positively modulate brain functions (e.g., neural plasticity, neural compensation), thereby counteracting degenerative processes and improving motor and/or cognitive performance in young and older adults alike. This chapter will investigate changes and adaptations in brain function following various adverse effects (aging, cognitive impairment, brain injuries), describe underlying mechanisms and theories, and demonstrate how physical exercise affects neural plasticity and motor/cognitive behavior in young and older adults.

AGE-RELATED FUNCTIONAL AND STRUCTURAL CHANGES IN THE HUMAN BRAIN

Early studies in the 1990s were already able to show age-related changes in the human brain. Older people are affected by a general loss of brain mass and a distinctive atrophy of frontal gray and white matter. Thus, aging is accompanied by structural cortical changes that may compromise cognitive and motor functions. A structure-specific shrinkage of white and gray matter is particularly evident in the prefrontal cortex, the hippocampus, and the cerebellum (Resnick et al., 2003). In the past, primarily cross-sectional experimental paradigms were used to assess brain volume and structure in older compared to young adults. However, unlike longitudinal investigations, these studies are not suited to directly investigate effects of aging on brain volume change because they primarily estimate the effects of aging from correlations with age. Throughout the lifespan, the human brain shows distinct age-related changes in whole brain volume beginning with exponential growth by 25% between early childhood and adolescents. Subsequently, brain volume steadily declines climaxing in a decrease of 26% at the age of 71–80 years. Similarly, from early childhood, gray matter volume increases, reaching a plateau in the 4th decade of life and subsequently decreases by 13% until the age of 70+ years (Courchesne et al., 2000). These findings were confirmed in several imaging studies. For example, using magnetic resonance tomography in a sample of older adults (age range: 59–84 years), brain volume in the prefrontal lobes decreased by 2.6 cm^3 ($\triangleq$2.9%) annually. When reviewing changes in gray and white matter separately, the annual decline amounted to 1.7% and 2.1%, respectively (Resnick et al., 2003). The same authors also found a trend toward reduced volume loss in a very healthy subsample (i.e., no medical conditions or cognitive impairment at 5 year follow-up), indicating that brain atrophy was postponed in individuals who remain in sound medical and cognitive condition. Besides the frontal lobes, other brain areas are affected by a loss in gray and white matter structures with advancing age as well. Older adults aged 55 years and older show a 1–2% decline in hippocampal volume each year (Erickson et al., 2011). This decrease in hippocampal structures is mainly attributed to (1) reductions in the neuropil part of the brain structure, (2) to cell body shrinkage, and (3) to changes in vascularization. The hippocampus is located in the medial temporal lobe and is keenly involved in cognitive processing and motor sequence consolidation. During training of a sequence learning task, activity in the hippocampus was directly related to gains in motor performance (Albouy et al., 2008). These findings indicate that hippocampal structures are activated during motor sequence learning to optimize behavior. Summing up, the available literature suggests that the anatomical decrease of brain mass, particularly in the frontal lobes and hippocampus, contributes to decreased cognitive processing capacities with advancing age and thus limits to what extent neural plasticity can compensate for age-related decrements of locomotion.

There is an extensive amount of literature illustrating that cognitive functions change with advancing age. Studies investigating task-related cortical adaptation and neural activation primarily focused on cognitive function as a behavioral outcome. That is, diminished speed of information processing or lower capacity of higher-order cognitive functions (i.e., working memory, executive functions). Park et al. (2002) investigated 345 persons, ranging from 20 to 92 years of age and measured perceptual speed (i.e., Digit Symbol test: remembering figure/digit combinations), visuospatial working memory (i.e., Spatial Span task: remembering the order of presented targets), and verbal working memory (i.e., Digit Span test: verbally repeating a series of digits). The authors demonstrated that all three cognitive domains decline with advancing age. Interestingly, speed of processing showed the best results in mediating age-related variance during the performance of working memory tasks, indicating the importance of processing speed for understanding the association between aging and cognition. In line with this assumption, Earles and Kersten (1999) showed that the age-related variance in long-term memory was reduced by 52% when controlling for performance in a perceptual speed task (using a similar task as Park et al. (2002)). Regarding short-term memory, this effect was even more pronounced and the reduction in age-related variance amounted to 91%. Thus, long- and short-term memory performance has been shown to be associated with limitations in perceptual speed in elderly subjects.

So far, experiments investigating the effects of age-related cortical shrinkage on motor performance have not received much attention in the scientific community. Thus, the question: *What are functional consequences of age-related cortical shrinkage?* remains largely unanswered. Nowadays, researchers started to focus on the neural basis underlying declines in motor performance in older adults (Goble et al., 2010; Van Impe et al., 2012). In a cross-sectional approach, Goble et al. (2010) were able to show that older adults maintained motor performance in complex movement tasks but increased neural activity in several brain areas. Affected brain areas included the supplementary motor area and cortical regions specifically related to cognitive functions (e.g., parietal cortex/dorsolateral prefrontal cortex). This age-related increase in activity in the supplementary motor area was associated with an improved ability to coordinate complex movements (i.e., parallel motions of the hands), suggesting a compensation mechanism to maintain motor performance. Recent research on aging revealed stronger frontal activation in older as compared to young adults, which is indicative of a compensatory process during aging (Reuter-Lorenz and Cappell, 2008). In elderly persons, it has been widely recognized that postural control declines with advancing age, leading to an increased risk of falling and reduced mobility. Postural control depends on several sensory systems (i.e., somatosensory, visual and vestibular systems), the motor system, and multiple neural systems to control and process these various sensory inputs. All of them are known to be affected by aging (Du Pasquier et al., 2003). Muscle strength and muscle volume decrease and alterations in the motor unit firing frequency occur, resulting in an impaired ability to maintain postural control. In addition to these peripheral changes, efficient processing of different sensory inputs might be affected by the age-related decline in gray and white matter integrity (Sullivan and Pfefferbaum, 2007). Previous research highlights the involvement of various brain regions (i.e., frontal gyri, precentral gyrus, parietal lobe) in postural control (Slobounov et al., 2005), confirming that postural control is a complex sensorimotor coordination task requiring the integration of sensory information and the execution of corrective motor commands. This integration is implemented by forwarding relevant information across cortical and subcortical pathways (Van Impe et al., 2012). An age-related degeneration of white matter impairs efficient transmission and processing of sensorimotor information, thus affecting postural control in the elderly. More specifically, older adults show lower-white matter integrity in frontal, parietal, and occipital brain regions. In addition, correlations between white matter integrity and postural control have been shown in balance control tasks involving proprioceptive and/or visual feedback in older, but not in young adults (Van Impe et al., 2012). These findings imply that an age-related decline in motor performance is not only triggered by peripheral and musculoskeletal changes or altered postural strategies, but is also caused by changes in neural processing pathways and the associated decline in cognitive functioning.

In the past, dual-task paradigms were used to investigate the interaction of motor performance and cognitive function in young and older adults. That is, when simultaneously performing a motor task (e.g., standing or walking) and a cognitive interference task (e.g., serial subtraction of numbers, memorizing words), decrements in motor performance (i.e., reduced walking speed) or in cognitive performance (i.e., increased error rate) could be observed (Beurskens and Bock, 2012). These decreases in motor performance can partly be compensated for by cognitive work around strategies, thus replacing automated sensorimotor processing with effortful higher-order cognitive functions (Beurskens and Bock, 2012). This mechanism represents a fairly good example of neural plasticity, as deficits emerging in one part of the nervous system can be overcome by activating another part of that system. Even young adults show dual-task-related adaptations of neural activation patterns.

Figs. 18.1A and B illustrate behavioral and neurophysiological data (i.e., electroencephalographic data; EEG) obtained from young adults aged 20–30 years when walking while concurrently performing an additional cognitive (i.e., auditory Go/NoGo task) or a motor interference task (i.e., holding two interlocked rings) compared to single-task walking (Beurskens et. al., 2016). Results indicated that neural activation in frontal brain regions is modulated while walking in dual-task situations. In frontal brain areas, neural activity is lower in alpha and beta frequencies during walking while concurrently performing a cognitive interference task compared to walking only. This decrease can similarly be seen when walking while performing a motor interference task. Lower alpha frequencies are indicative of an increased cognitive load during dual-task walking (Basar, 2012). Thus, impaired motor performance during dual-task walking is mirrored in neural activation patterns of the brain of young adults. Human walking and the associated neural activation patterns are also affected by advancing age. Walking speed and stride length decrease, while lateral sway and stride time variability increase. Some of these changes are used to stabilize posture (i.e., compensation), while others are dysfunctional. The observed deteriorations in motor performance have been attributed, among others, to cognitive decline. This assumption is supported by the fact that age-related changes in walking behavior are more pronounced in people with cognitive impairment and accentuated under dual-task conditions (Beurskens and Bock, 2012). On the cortical level, activity in frontal brain areas increased during dual-task walking in older adults and correlated with executive function performance (Doi et al., 2013). In older age, shifts in neural activity patterns may help to overcome age-related impairments in locomotion. However, there is a price to pay. As mentioned before,

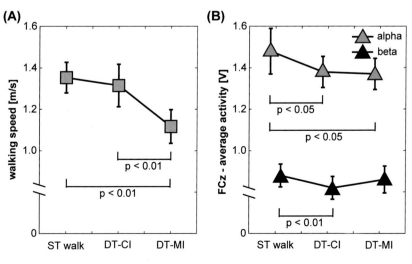

FIGURE 18.1 Young adults walking speed (A) and the associated neural activity in frontal brain regions (B), displayed separately for single-task walking (ST walk), walking while performing a cognitive interference task (DT-CI), and walking while performing a motor interference task (DT-MI). FCz represents an EEG electrode located above the medial frontal and the medial central cortex.

cognitive functioning is impaired in older adults, thus fewer resources are available to compensate for deterioration in walking performance. As a consequence, older adults show larger problems than young adults when walking and concurrently being engaged in another activity (Beurskens and Bock, 2012). These findings indicate that the central ability to simultaneously process walking requirements and cognitive demands decreases with age. The deterioration might arise from insufficient central processing capabilities in older people or from disorders in the coordination of multiple sensory and motor processing demands (Wickens, 2008), caused by changes in brain structures.

THEORIES OF NEURAL PLASTICITY IN OLDER ADULTS

Neural plasticity describes functional (e.g., altered activity patterns) and structural (e.g., cortical reorganization) adaptations of the human brain in response to training as well as in response to injury or aging. During the past four decades, several theories emerged that tried to explain age-related shifts in activation patterns. During the early 1960s, Joseph Altman was one of the first researchers to propose the hypothesis of neurogenesis, i.e., the regeneration of neurons, in the aging brain. Using animals, he proposed that in adult rats with and without experimental lesions, an increasing number of neurons in the hippocampus can be derived from cells multiplying at high rates in the ependymal and subependymal walls located next to the hippocampus (Altman and Das, 1965). These results showed that the neoformation of neurons is possible in specific neural structures. However, the question of where these cells originated from (e.g., the availability of stem cells in the respective brain regions), remained unsolved for the following decades. Not until the beginning of the 1990s, Reynolds and Weiss (1992) described stem cells found in the hippocampus of the adult brain. These findings confirm the early hypotheses postulated by Joseph Altman. Consequently, the theory of adult neurogenesis seemed plausible and was widely accepted in the scientific community.

A wide-ranged discussion about the consequences of adult neurogenesis started to form. The main questions were: *What is adult neurogenesis good for? What are the consequences of adult neurogenesis?* Several theories have been proposed naming possible functions of adult neurogenesis, including the neurogenic reserve theory (Kempermann, 2008). It postulated that adult neurogenesis might produce a base for sustained cellular plasticity with increasing age, resulting from activity and experience throughout the lifespan. Thus, continued neurogenesis could provide improved capacity and efficiency of cognitive processes at higher ages. Experiments in animals showed that both physical and cognitive activity experienced in early to mid-life reduced age-related decrements in the cleavage of cells. For example, exposure to a complex environment, including social interaction, the stimulation of exploratory behavior (i.e., using tunnels and toys), and higher physical activity improved learning performance. It has been shown that neurogenesis was five-times higher in the group exposed to enriched environments compared to a control group exposed to standard environments (i.e., no social interaction, no additional physical activity) (Kempermann et al., 2002). These findings support the observation that adult neurogenesis promotes successful aging by showing that an active life style increased neural functioning. According to Kempermann (2008), the main principle is that physical and/or cognitive activity maintained the potential for cell-based plasticity by preserving adult neurogenesis. Feedback from systems involved in locomotion serves as a communicator between peripheral systems and processes involved in brain plasticity. This feedback communicates to the brain that the recruitment of more neurons will add substantial benefit when coping with specific motor demands. As a consequence, adult neurogenesis utilizes locomotion as an indicator of cognitive challenge or demand. Thus, locomotion is a non-specific trigger related to specific cognitive events and creates the prerequisite for the cognitive stimuli to recruit new neurons. Evidence for neurogenesis is mainly restricted to the hippocampus and olfactory bulb, but current research has revealed that other parts of the brain, including the cerebellum, may be involved as well (Ponti et al., 2008).

Adult neurogenesis is now a widely accepted phenomenon in biological sciences and has received a lot of attention in recent years. However, consequences of adult neurogenesis in humans need to be further explored. If the aforementioned findings of animal experiments are also observed in humans, one could argue that physical and cognitive activity started early in the life will help to develop highly-optimized brain networks that are capable of solving cognitively-demanding and complex situations. Further, lifelong activity contributes to a neurogenic reserve. That is, generating new neurons that can be recruited for specific motor and/or cognitive demands. Thus, adult neurogenesis counteracts potential cognitive overload caused by overstrained cognitive systems due to high task demands. Certainly, increasing physical and cognitive activity throughout the lifespan only represents one side of the coin when neural plasticity is discussed. There are more mechanisms and processes on the neural and biological level (i.e., expansion of white-matter tracts in childhood and adolescence) contributing to neural plasticity. However, the individual alone can accomplish the modulation of physical activity. Taking the necessary steps to optimize activity-dependent plasticity by building a neurogenic reserve might represent one key to successful aging.

In general, the adult brain does not represent a hardwired structure consisting solely of fixed neural circuits. Rather, it has the capability of rewiring different instances of cortical and subcortical neural circuits in response to specific training interventions as well as in response to injury. It has clearly been demonstrated that the capacity of the central nervous system is able to structurally and functionally adapt in response to previous experiences. The basic principle behind neural plasticity is the theory that individual connections between neurons are constantly established or removed, depending on how they are stimulated. The underlying mechanisms have been summarized in the *cell assembly theory* or *Hebb's postulate* proposed by the Canadian psychologist Donald Hebb (Hebb, 1949). Whenever there are two or more nearby neurons that produce an impulse simultaneously, their cortical maps can be considered as one. The theory is often summarized by the phrase "Neurons wire together if they fire together" as postulated by Lowel and Singer (1992).

Nowadays, neural plasticity has been defined as any change in neural structures or functions that can be observed from measures of individual neurons or deduced from measures taken across populations of multiple neurons (Warraich and Kleim, 2010). It thus reflects changes in neural circuitry. Basically, each motor behavior that we perform in everyday life (i.e., speaking, grasping, walking) or during sports activities (i.e., running, dancing) involves the combination of acquired motor skills and neural control. The capacity to produce movements also persists during the absence of continued training and stimulation, which shows that specific motor skills exist as stable and lasting neurobiological pathways within the central nervous systems (Warraich and Kleim, 2010). Empirical evidence shows the existence of motor learning-dependent neural plasticity within various motor regions of the brain. For example, performing a one-handed, five-finger exercise on the piano over the course of 1 week (5 sessions per week for 2 h each session) in middle-aged adults resulted in enlarged representation of the trained hand in motor areas and increased cortical excitability within these regions (Pascual-Leone et al., 1995). Thus, behavior seems to reflect the activity of neural circuits within specific brain areas. The activity pattern of individual neurons within these neural circuits is determined by the synaptic inputs they receive (Warraich and Kleim, 2010). Changes in motor outcome thus represent changes in cortical activity patterns. It has previously been shown that the human brain is significantly interconnected (Wickens, 2008) and this interconnectivity plays an important role in the reorganization of cortical structures after training or following an injury or disease. The acquisition of complex motor skills, the integration of additional cognitive demands during motor tasks, and the functional recovery from neural damage and aging provide good examples of neural plasticity.

Several theories have been proposed to explain age-related changes in cognitive function, in motor function, and in cortical activation patterns. Current theories on neural plasticity in older adults include the theory of cognitive reserve (Stern, 2009), the compensation-related utilization of neural circuits model (CRUNCH) (Reuter-Lorenz and Cappell, 2008), and the HAROLD model (Hemispheric Asymmetry Reduction in Older Adults) (Cabeza, 2002).

Briefly, the concept of cognitive reserve is subdivided into *neural reserve* and *neural compensation* (Stern, 2009). The former (*neural reserve*) comprises the ability to optimize performance in cognitive paradigms and reflects individual differences as well as modulations that occur due to task difficulty in the healthy brain. That is, a more efficient recruitment of brain networks, higher capacities, and/or more flexibility when activating neural circuits. The latter (*neural compensation*) describes the ability to compensate for brain injuries and the associated impairments of standard processing networks. That is, brain structures or networks that are not normally used by an individual with an intact brain are activated, which helps to maintain or improve task performance. Thus, alterations in neural recruitment develop to overcome functional or structural limitations. The CRUNCH model, proposed by Reuter-Lorenz and Cappell (2008), states that inefficient processing causes the brain of older adults to recruit more brain regions (i.e., additional neural resources) to achieve task performances equivalent to that of younger adults. However, the newly recruited networks are not as optimal as the primary one to maintain task performance. As task demands increase, a resource ceiling is reached, leading to insufficient processing and age-related decrements. Finally, the HAROLD model posits that neural activity during cognitive performance tends to be less lateralized in older compared to young adults. This model primarily describes the lateralization of activity during cognitive performances, i.e., an activation shift from one hemisphere to another. Evidence shows that increased bilateral activity in older adults is associated with enhanced performance in a cognitive task. For example, older adults showing a bilateral pattern of prefrontal activity were faster in a verbal working memory task than those who did not (Reuter-Lorenz et al., 2000).

Besides the aforementioned theories on neural plasticity, another underlying mechanism that is capable of enabling the human brain to adapt to various stimuli (i.e., aging, disease, training, etc.) is *functional redundancy*. According to Warraich and Kleim (2010), functional redundancy can be observed within specific brain areas (i.e., internal redundancy) and across various brain areas (i.e., external redundancy). For example, motor representations of body parts are laid out multiple times within the human primary somatosensory cortex. Thus, stimulating different areas within the primary motor cortex can trigger the same movements. In addition, increased complexity of finger movements resulted in a distribution of movement-related activation from the primary motor cortex towards more arm-related representations (Lotze et al., 2000), indicating that complex movements lead to shifts in motor cortex activation from one somatosensory area to another (i.e., external redundancy). In summary, external redundancy can be observed as the same motor or cognitive functions being represented across different brain areas (Warraich and Kleim, 2010), which is also referred to as parallel processing. External redundancy may occur across brain regions that work in one general modality (e.g., trunk movements) or across brain regions that work in different modalities (audition versus vision). External redundancy can also be found across two or more sensory modalities (i.e., cross-modal processing) (Wallace et al., 2004). This internal and external redundancy enhances neural integration of various information, improves sensory and/or motor functions and may also serve as a function to enhance the brain's ability to restore/improve motor function after cognitive decline (i.e., dementia) or acute brain injuries (i.e., concussion, stroke).

EXERCISE AND NEUROLOGICAL CHANGES

As described in the previous chapter, neural plasticity serves as a process to restore motor and cognitive functions. A general decline in these functions can often be seen following specific degenerating maladies or injuries. The following section will describe the effects of exercise and physical activity on neurological function as a result of aging. Training and exercise applied in older age or throughout the life span may increase available brain resources and compensatory potential to counteract the previously described decrements in cognitive and motor performance.

There is consensus in the scientific community that physical exercise is beneficial for various motor (Correa et al., 2013) and cognitive functions (Colcombe and Kramer, 2003). These positive effects have equally been shown in young (Taube, 2012) and older adults (Beurskens et al., 2015), for aerobic exercise (Lakatta, 2002), strength training, and balance training (Beurskens et al., 2015). For example, 13 weeks of heavy-resistance strength training at 80% of the one-repetition maximum (i.e., the maximum amount of force that can be generated in one maximal contraction) in older adults aged 65+ years increased maximal isometric force production of the leg extensors (Beurskens et al., 2015). Others have found similar effects for measures of muscle volume and muscle quality (Correa et al., 2013), and functional performance and mobility (i.e., gait speed, transfer) (Holviala et al., 2012). However, physical exercise not only affects motor functions. As early as in 1978, Spirduso and Clifford (1978) found that endurance-trained, physically active older adults showed a similar level of cognitive functioning (i.e., performance in a simple and a complex reaction time task) compared to young adults and outperformed non-active young adults that were almost 40 years younger. Since then, similar results (i.e., better cognitive performance of active older compared to non-active older adults) have been found in a large number of cross-sectional studies (Etnier et al., 1997 for a review). The presented findings represent landmarks in research on the interaction of motor and cognitive functions.

Effects of Aerobic Exercise on Brain Function

Studies looking at the relationship between fitness level and brain functions showed that higher aerobic fitness scores (as measured by maximum oxygen uptake) are associated with better executive function, faster processing speed, and greater volume of different brain structures (Erickson et al., 2014). Voelcker-Rehage et al. (2011) showed that 12 months of cardiovascular (i.e., heart rate-based walking) or sensorimotor training (balance, eye–hand coordination, leg–arm coordination, spatial orientation) in older adults improves executive function (as assessed by a modified version of the Flanker Task) and perceptual speed (measured by a Visual Search Task) compared to an active control group (i.e., relaxing and stretching exercises). These findings are in line with Colcombe et al. (2004) demonstrating that aerobic exercises conducted for 6 months improved executive function performance, measured by a Flanker Task (subjects were asked to respond to a central arrow cue embedded in an array of five arrows that pointed either to the left or right) in older adults aged 58–77 years. Recently, Antunes et al. (2015) confirmed the beneficial effects of aerobic exercise in older adults by showing that 6 months of cycle ergometer training improved performance in several cognitive domains (i.e., attentional processes, short-term working memory, and general intelligence). In a review and meta-analysis, Colcombe and Kramer (2003) compared 18 different intervention studies published between 1966 and 2001. Fitness training was shown to produce robust benefits for subjects' cognitive capacity, primarily increasing performance in executive control processes. The magnitude of effects was modulated by the total intervention duration, i.e., interventions of more than 6 months lead to more pronounced improvements in cognitive performance compared to shorter training durations. Interestingly, training interventions combining strength training and aerobic exercises are more effective in improving cognitive capacity than cardiovascular training alone. These findings indicate that the combination of two or more types of training puts higher demands on subjects' cognitive processing capabilities than one type of training alone (i.e., strength or balance or endurance) (Colcombe and Kramer, 2003).

Nowadays, advances in neurophysiological and imaging technologies (i.e., widespread availability of fMRI, shielded EEG electrodes, and artifact removal algorithms) allow the examination of neural activation during behavioral tasks. Thus, it is possible to combine and correlate electrophysiological brain measures and behavioral data to evaluate potential underlying neural processes that modulate motor and/or cognitive performance in humans. In the aforementioned study by Voelcker-Rehage et al. (2011), the control group did not show improvements in executive function performance following stretching and relaxing exercises. However, their neural activation patterns revealed an increased task-related activation in frontal, parietal, and sensorimotor cortical areas, indicating the necessity to recruit additional resources as a compensation mechanism to preserve cognitive performance. On the other hand, sensorimotor exercises increased cognitive performance in the balance-training group, albeit neural activation patterns remained unchanged. The authors concluded that older adults performing sensorimotor and/or coordinative exercise may need less compensatory activation to perform executive function tasks. Similar findings were observed for the cardiovascular training group (i.e., less prefrontal activation or no increase in brain activation), indicating a reduced need for compensation. These changes lead to more automated and thus more effective motor responses and more effective processing and integration of visuo-spatial information. Furthermore, cardiovascular training was associated with increased activation of the sensorimotor network, whereas coordination training was associated with increased activation in the visual–spatial network. Colcombe et al. (2004) were able to demonstrate that participants conducting aerobic exercises alter their neural activation patterns while performing an executive function task (i.e., Flanker task), compared with participants performing stretching and toning exercises. After 6 months of training, participants in the aerobic group showed significantly higher levels of task-related activity in brain areas responsible for attentional control (i.e., middle and superior frontal gyrus, superior parietal lobe) and a reduced level of activity in the anterior cingulate cortex. This enhanced recruitment in frontal and parietal brain regions seemed to be accompanied by an increased control of task-related activation in posterior cortex regions and in the frontal attentional circuitry. These findings also indicate that higher cardiovascular capacity (as acquired by the cardiovascular intervention) reduced neural activity in the anterior cingulate cortex, a region of the brain that is strongly associated with attention control processes and the resolving of behavioral conflicts. Also, cardiovascular-trained persons had higher levels of cortical activation in regions involved in executive functioning and processing (Voelcker-Rehage et al., 2010). Higher cardiovascular fitness was positively correlated with activation of the right inferior frontal gyrus and the superior temporal gyrus, regions thought to be involved in the maintenance of interference control (Colcombe et al., 2004) and visuo-spatial awareness (Karnath et al., 2001), respectively.

Processes that affect neural plasticity can be found on several physiological and structural levels. Aerobic exercise modulates neural plasticity or adult neurogenesis by increasing the production of neurotrophic factors. For example, the production of proteins promoting growth and differentiation of neurons, such as brain-derived neurotrophic factor (BDNF), are promoted. In their 2015 review, Szuhany et al. (2015) demonstrated a moderate increase in BDNF levels following one single session of aerobic exercise. This increase was further intensified by regularly conducted sessions over a period of 3–24 weeks. Hence, research provides evidence for the beneficial role of BDNF in hippocampal neurogenesis, synaptic plasticity, and neural repair (Erickson et al., 2014). Furthermore, it has been shown that gray matter volume is increased following aerobic exercise, thereby counteracting the natural shrinking of the human brain that occurs in late adulthood (Guiney and Machado, 2013). A study by Colcombe et al. (2006), using a sample of 59 older adults revealed that participating in regular aerobic exercise over a period of 6 months increased prefrontal cortex volume. This finding is in line with previously reported results, indicating that brain regions involved in coordinating and processing information, such as the prefrontal cortex (Erickson et al., 2014) and the hippocampus (Erickson et al., 2011), are affected by aerobic exercises. Erickson et al. (2011) showed that hippocampal volume in older adults aged 55–80 years increases by about 2% following 12 months of cardiovascular training. This increase was associated with improvement of cardiovascular fitness (i.e., maximum oxygen uptake) and spatial memory performance. Furthermore, the hippocampal brain structure is of specific interest since exercise-induced increases in gray matter volume (i.e., neurogenesis) in the hippocampus are significantly associated with learning and memory processes. In a sample of 56 adults between 59 and 81-years-old, higher cardiovascular fitness levels (assessed by a graded treadmill protocol) were associated with larger hippocampal volumes and better performance in a spatial memory task (i.e., remembering the location of black dots on a screen) (Erickson et al., 2009).

V. LIFESTYLE EXERCISE AFFECTING NEUROLOGICAL STRUCTURE AND FUNCTION IN OLDER ADULTS

Effects of Balance and Strength Training Exercise on Brain Function

Cardiovascular and endurance training primarily involves adaptations in metabolic and energetic processes. However, physical activity also involves balance and strength training, which put more demands to the motor system (i.e., coordination, muscle activation, etc.). These types of training might also affect brain function in humans. Beurskens et al. (2015) showed that bilateral force production of the leg extensor increased following 13 weeks of bilateral heavy resistance training (3 sessions/week for 60 min per session) in older adults aged 60–80 years. The authors argue that the underlying mechanisms resulting in improved bilateral leg strength can be found in the adaptation of cortical activation patterns. Bilateral heavy-resistance training seems to increase cortical activation and more brain regions are recruited in both hemispheres when performing bilateral contractions (Noble et al., 2014), thereby reducing cortical inhibition. Following short-term resistance training (2 weeks, 3 sessions/week), cortical inhibition is reduced in older adults (Christie and Kamen, 2014) and increased cortical activity and the recruitment of additional brain regions have been shown during bilateral compared to unilateral contractions (Noble et al., 2014). These findings indicate that bilateral resistance training might ramp up the activation of more brain regions, leading to increased muscular output triggered through direct cortico-spinal pathways (Aune et al., 2013). Following balance training, reduced cortical excitability has been shown during the performance of a balance task and increased cortical excitability during the execution of an explosive strength task (Beck et al., 2007). When balance-trained subjects executed a postural control task (i.e., stance perturbations on an accelerating treadmill), cortical excitability was reduced. On the other hand, when balance-trained subjects were measured in a strength task that required dorso-flexion of the ankle, enhanced cortical excitability was evident. Thus, cortical adaptation to balance training seems to be highly task-specific. In addition, Taube (2012) argued that balance training and the accompanied improvement in postural control leads to adaptations in subcortical structures of the brain such as the basal ganglia and cerebellum. For example, activity in subcortical brain regions increased with increasing task automatization (Puttemans et al., 2005) and also after 6 weeks of balance training (Taubert et al., 2011). Following this argument, balance training induces a shift in neural activation from cortical to more subcortical areas. Further, Niemann et al. (2014) demonstrated that balance and strength training also require various cognitive functions, such as perceptual and higher-level information processing. Thus, exercises incorporating balance and strength might also effect cognitive functioning. There is evidence in the literature that balance, strength, and aerobic training similarly improve cognitive functions (Liu-Ambrose et al., 2012; Niemann et al., 2014; Voelcker-Rehage et al., 2011).

Regarding strength training, results by Liu-Ambrose et al. (2010) suggest that 12 months of regular high-intensity strength and resistance training showed positive effects on leg strength and executive function performance in older adults aged 65–75 years. Performance in a Stroop task (which involves naming the color in which words are printed, while ignoring the potentially conflicting word meaning, e.g., the word "red" printed in blue) improved by 12.6% in the resistance training group; a finding that was not present in the active control group conducting stretching and toning exercises. In another study, Liu-Ambrose et al. (2012) showed that selective attention and conflict resolution performance (as assessed by a modified Flanker task, i.e., responding to an arrow presented on a computer screen, based on its pointing direction) improved in a sample of 155 older women aged 65–75 years, following 12 months of high-intensity resistance training (2 sessions per week). Further, the improvement in cognitive capability was accompanied by enhanced cortical activity, particularly obvious in brain regions commonly associated with response inhibition, such as the prefrontal cortex and the anterior portion of the left middle temporal gyrus.

Besides strength and resistance training, balance and coordination exercises represent promising candidates to prevent cognitive decline and improve cognitive functioning in older adults. The aforementioned study by Niemann et al. (2014) demonstrated that overall hippocampal volume in older adults (age range: 62–79 years) increased by 2.8% and specifically, right hippocampal volume increased by 3.9% following 12 months of coordinative training. The coordinative training mainly included balance, eye-hand coordination, leg-arm coordination, as well as spatial orientation, and reaction to moving objects/persons. In particular, the right hippocampus has shown to be responsible for cognitive processes involving spatial and episodic memory (Burgess et al., 2002). In addition, Voelcker-Rehage et al. (2010) showed that not only cardiovascular fitness (measured using a submaximal graded exercise test on a motor-driven treadmill) but also motor fitness (i.e., movement speed, balance performance, motor coordination) in older adults showed strong associations with executive control (i.e., Flanker task and n-back task) and perceptual speed (i.e., visual search task). Also, increased activity in parietal areas of the brain was found in participants with high motor fitness. These areas have been shown to be involved in visuo-motor coordination and the processing of visuo-spatial information. Thus, higher motor fitness seems to go hand in hand with more automated motor responses and more effective processing and integration of visuo-spatial information.

Summarizing, aerobic exercise as well as balance and strength training are well-suited to improve higher-order cognitive functioning and to modulate associated cortical structures in prefrontal and hippocampal brain areas in older adults. Seniors showed improved executive function and memory performance following various training regimens and increased brain volume in the frontal lobes and the hippocampus; two brain areas significantly associated with executive functions and memory processes.

EXERCISE AS THERAPY FOR NEUROLOGICAL DISEASES

The following section will briefly demonstrate the effects of physical exercise in therapeutic and rehabilitative settings. Therefore, we are going to highlight changes in cortical structures and the associated patterns of neural activity (1) following dementia, representing a distinct age-related decline in cognitive function and (2) following concussion, which represents an injury that can primarily be found in young adults following sport accidents. In addition, concussion and traumatic brain injury have the potential to negatively affect brain functions both immediately after the injury and later in life. Thus, this section addresses the neurological impacts of exercise and physical activity from two different perspectives.

Dementia

According to the international classification of diseases (ICD-10), dementia can be considered an umbrella term describing a group of progressive symptoms, including deficits in memory, attention and language skills, (complex) motor skills, and other higher-order cognitive functions (i.e., orientation, executive function). These impairments develop due to permanent damage to neural structures, and are most commonly induced by diseases like Alzheimer's (the most common cause of dementia in people over the age of 65 years) or by congestion of blood supply (i.e., vascular dementia). Recently, strategies to prevent Alzheimer's disease have been discussed in conjunction with several protective factors present throughout the life-span that may prevent the development of cognitive impairments. Hence, the so-called *brain reserve theory* was formulated (Valenzuela and Sachdev, 2006). Brain reserve is defined as a neurological phenomenon where (1) the available brain volume affects the development of brain diseases and injuries (i.e., neurological brain reserve) and (2) mental activity across the life-span allows flexible cognitive resource allocation despite the occurrence of neural dysfunctions (i.e., behavioral brain reserve). The latter definition is closely related to the theory of cognitive reserve proposed by Stern (2009). Briefly, the theory of brain reserves argues that sufficient structural and/or cognitive resources are available to postpone the onset of Alzheimer's disease and dementia. These additional resources primarily depend on factors such as the level of education, the complexity of occupational work, and other cognitively stimulating lifestyle pursuits (Valenzuela and Sachdev, 2006) and are associated with a lowered risk of dementia. Also, increased mental activity in middle-aged and older adults was associated with lower dementia rates. These findings indicate that the risk of dementia can be modulated by an individuals' life style. Interestingly, regular physical activity throughout the life span might prevent cognitive decline and dementia, and is associated with a reduced risk of developing mild cognitive impairment and Alzheimer's disease in middle-aged adults (Geda et al., 2010).

Similar to the results in healthy older adults, strength and functional training has been shown to improve motor functions (for example, increased leg strength, improved gait function) in patients suffering from cognitive decline and dementia (Hauer et al., 2012) while cardiovascular training facilitates physical fitness (Heyn et al., 2008). Physical exercise is also considered to induce a positive neurophysiological effect that helps to maintain normal brain activity in the elderly, indicating the potential of exercise for attenuation of neurodegenerative processes caused by dementia. Thus, training interventions seem to be a feasible intervention in this vulnerable patient group. Physical exercise (i.e., cardiovascular training) is associated with a reduced incidence of Alzheimer's disease and improved cognitive functions in older adults at risk for Alzheimer's disease (Lautenschlager et al., 2008). On the behavioral level, aerobic training improved conflict resolution, processing speed, memory performance, and verbal fluency performance while resistance training additionally improved executive functions in older women with mild cognitive impairment. Aerobic training also positively modulated regional patterns of functional brain plasticity (i.e., hemodynamic activity) during the performance of an associative memory task (Nagamatsu et al., 2012). However, only a few studies have examined the impact of exercise intervention on brain structure (e.g., hippocampal volume) in older adults with mild cognitive impairment. Animal studies showed that physical exercise in a running wheel improved sensorimotor function, increased coordination, and reduced cognitive deterioration in mice suffering from Alzheimer's disease. On the cortical level, dementia-related changes in cortical structures were reversed and a reduction in oxidative stress (i.e., improved neuroprotection) was present. These effects were most pronounced after 6 months of physical exercise (Garcia-Mesa et al., 2011). In human studies, physical activity has been shown to have a beneficial impact on brain aging and preventing the development of cognitive impairment and dementia. Investigating 86 women aged 70–80 years, ten Brinke et al. (2015) demonstrated that 6 months of aerobic exercise (i.e., performing a walking program at 70–80% of the individual's heart rate reserve) but not resistance or balance training significantly increased hippocampal volume by 4% in older women with mild cognitive impairment. The hippocampus of the human brain is a region of specific interest, as it is sensitive to ageing effects and hippocampal atrophy represents an important indicator of Alzheimer's disease (Jack et al., 2010). Thus, maintaining hippocampal volume will presumably help to prevent the development of dementia. As mentioned before (cf. subchapter "*Effects of Aerobic Exercise on Brain Function*"), aerobic exercise conducted over a period of 6 months has been shown to significantly increase hippocampal (Erickson et al., 2011) and prefrontal cortex volume (Colcombe et al., 2006) among healthy community-dwelling older adults. This structural increase in brain volume was associated with improved cardiovascular fitness and cognitive performance (i.e., spatial memory). Erickson et al. (2011) demonstrated that regular walking exercises (12 months, 3 days/week) significantly increased brain volume in the left and right hippocampus by 2.1% and 1.9%, respectively. This increase was associated with a reversal of the age-related loss in hippocampal volume by up to 2 years. These findings in healthy older adults showed that regular cardiovascular or aerobic exercise might reverse the structural loss of brain volume and the decline of cognitive functioning in older persons suffering from Alzheimer's disease and/or mild cognitive impairment.

Concussion

Concussion, or mild traumatic brain injury, is a complex pathophysiological process affecting the human brain, which can occur when linear and/or rotational forces directly or indirectly impinge upon the head. Recently, several studies have shown that sport-related concussions can lead to various effects on health and cognitive functioning. Directly after the impact, concussive injuries induce a complex cascade of metabolic and pathophysiological events (such as changes in ionic balance, decreased cerebral blood flow, and mitochondrial dysfunction, which all lead to an energy-crisis in the brain) accompanied by axonal degeneration (cf. Werner and Engelhard, 2007 for a review). Typical acute concussion symptoms include short-term memory loss, headache, dizziness, light sensitivity, and migraine. In 80–90% of the patients, the majority of these symptoms occur shortly after the impact and last for ~7–10 days. However, the remaining 10–20% of patients show long-lasting symptoms. Further, patients suffering from mild traumatic brain injury seem to have a five-fold increased risk of developing mild cognitive impairments, a greater risk of chronic traumatic encephalopathy, and a tendency toward an earlier onset of Alzheimer's disease compared to healthy adults (Guskiewicz et al., 2005). Over time, concussive injuries can lead to altered diffusion characteristics in white matter tracts of the human brain across the life span (Tremblay et al., 2014). Thus, the aforementioned impairments following mild traumatic brain injury can last for months or even years (a phenomenon known as post-concussion syndrome) and are potentially linked to chronic neuro-inflammation and progressive neuro-degeneration (Loane and Faden, 2010). In addition, recent studies showed that individuals with a history of concussion developed prolonged cognitive-motor integration deficits if they had to perform a motor and a cognitively demanding task concurrently. Notably, all participants of this experiment with a history of concussion were considered asymptomatic after standard clinical assessments, had been returned to their regular sport activities, and on average their most recent concussion was diagnosed 13–19 months ago (Brown et al., 2015; Dalecki et al., 2016).

In recent years, these findings have drawn increasing attention to the importance of gaining a better understanding of concussion recovery. Similar to other impairments affecting cortical structures (i.e., aging, dementia), training and exercise might be a valuable treatment tool and show beneficial effects on brain functions during the recovery from traumatic brain injury. However, research on the relationship between exercise and concussion in humans is scarce. Animal studies provide a first insight into potential benefits of exercise following concussion. For example, physical exercise is known to enhance cell survival and functional recovery after brain injuries in rodents (Fogelman and Zafonte, 2012). Benefits of exercise were reported for the facilitation of molecular markers of neuroplasticity and neurogenesis following traumatic brain injury in rats. Voluntary exercise on a running wheel improved BDNF regulation and recovery of cognitive function (i.e., Morris water maze performance). Of note, BDNF activation was significantly associated with exercise-induced improvements in cognitive performance and hippocampal volume change after TBI injury (Griesbach et al., 2009). In accordance with these findings, an earlier study by Hicks et al. (1998) showed that exercise improved BDNF levels in hippocampal regions after traumatic brain injury. Interestingly, following TBI, a combination of physical exercise (i.e., running on a wheel) and amphetamine treatment for 7 days was not effective in improving BNDF activation and did not reduce oxidative stress (Griesbach et al., 2008). Only when exercise and amphetamine treatments were applied separately, BNDF activation increased during TBI recovery. Furthermore, 10 days of treadmill exercise showed positive effects on Purkinje cell loss and astrocytic reaction in the cerebellum of rats suffering from traumatic brain injury (Seo et al., 2010). In line with this finding, voluntary running wheel exercise for 2 weeks after an induced mild fluid percussion injury in rats showed positive impacts on molecular systems that are involved in protein fate and function, which may be related to synaptic plasticity (Szabo et al., 2010). One of the rare human studies looking at the influence of exercise on recovery after concussion studied the influence of different activity levels after concussion on neurocognitive functions (i.e., attention, memory, reaction time, and information processing speed) and symptom recovery (Majerske et al., 2008). Findings indicated that moderate levels of exercise or activity (i.e., slow jogging) were best suited to improve recovery and neurocognitive functions in adolescents suffering from concussion. That is, visual memory performance and reaction times improved significantly.

Thus, human and animal studies both indicate that physical activity and exercise post-concussion can be an effective tool to enhance the recovery of impaired cortical functions following a concussion or traumatic brain injury. However, current findings also suggest that the effects of physical activity and exercise after concussions depend on the type and intensity of the exercises, the time of application and the nature of the brain injury (Griesbach, 2011). Traumatic brain injuries show a diverse range of characteristics, which further complicate the establishment of common treatment strategies and recovery guidelines (McCrory et al., 2013). In the past, guidelines recommended that symptoms need to detumesce before starting sports-related activities. In contrast to that, current guidelines only suggest an initial rest period for the acute symptomatic period following injury (i.e., 24–48 h). This revision of established guidelines indicates that active recovery following a traumatic brain injury is beneficial and seems, under specific circumstances, to enhance the recovery from concussion (Griesbach, 2011). It has also been demonstrated that physical exercise has a positive effect on various concussion-related symptoms. That is, among others, depression, migraine, and chronic fatigue (Lawlor and Hopker, 2001; Moss-Morris et al., 2005), each of them representing potential persistent symptoms of concussion. Further, evidence showed that cardiovascular exercises reduced symptoms of the post-concussion syndrome (such as headaches and dizziness), especially in populations who were slow to recover from mild traumatic brain injury (Leddy et al., 2010).

Summing up, current evidence demonstrates that exercise (especially cardiovascular exercise) can be a valuable treatment after traumatic brain injury, and may help to reduce concussion-related symptoms in the acute phase following the injury as well as in patients suffering from post-concussive syndrome. Thus, exercise may also be helpful in preventing potential long-term impacts of head injuries on neuro-cortical functions in people who have had a concussion. However, further research, especially in humans, is needed to evaluate the intensity, duration, and type of exercise that is most suitable as treatment for concussion and traumatic brain injury recovery.

CONCLUSION

Aging is accompanied by a distinct performance loss in motor and cognitive functions. Reasons for these age-related decreases in functional capacity are manifold and range from decreased muscle mass and function, reduced cortico-spinal activation and changes in neural activation patterns and the deterioration of cortical structures. A wide range of physical exercises, ranging from cardiovascular to coordination and strength training, have the capability to prevent functional impairments in motor and cognitive performance and counteract the cortical decay in older individuals with and without cognitive impairments. Engaging in regular cardiovascular, coordination and strengthening exercises is beneficial for several cortical structures (i.e., hippocampal and prefrontal regions, motor cortex) and restores injury-related and age-related degenerative processes in young and older adults. Particularly, neural activation patterns are modulated by physical exercise, which results in a more efficient use of the available cognitive resources.

References

Albouy, G., Sterpenich, V., Balteau, E., Vandewalle, G., Desseilles, M., Dang-Vu, T., Darsaud, A., Ruby, P., Luppi, P.H., Degueldre, C., Peigneux, P., Luxen, A., Maquet, P., 2008. Both the hippocampus and striatum are involved in consolidation of motor sequence memory. Neuron 58 (2), 261–272. http://dx.doi.org/10.1016/j.neuron.2008.02.008.

Altman, J., Das, G.D., 1965. Autoradiographic and histological evidence of postnatal hippocampal neurogenesis in rats. Journal of Comparative Neurology 124 (3), 319–335.

Antunes, H.K., De Mello, M.T., de Aquino Lemos, V., Santos-Galduroz, R.F., Camargo Galdieri, L., Amodeo Bueno, O.F., Tufik, S., D'Almeida, V., 2015. Aerobic physical exercise improved the cognitive function of elderly males but did not modify their blood homocysteine levels. Dementia and Geriatric Cognitive Disorders EXTRA 5 (1), 13–24. http://dx.doi.org/10.1159/000369160.

Aune, T.K., Aune, M.A., Ettema, G., Vereijken, B., 2013. Comparison of bilateral force deficit in proximal and distal joints in upper extremities. Human Movement Science 32 (3), 436–444. http://dx.doi.org/10.1016/j.humov.2013.01.005.

Basar, E., 2012. A review of alpha activity in integrative brain function: fundamental physiology, sensory coding, cognition and pathology. International Journal of Psychophysiology: Official Journal of the International Organization of Psychophysiology 86 (1), 1–24. http://dx.doi.org/10.1016/j.ijpsycho.2012.07.002.

Beck, S., Taube, W., Gruber, M., Amtage, F., Gollhofer, A., Schubert, M., 2007. Task-specific changes in motor evoked potentials of lower limb muscles after different training interventions. Brain Research 1179, 51–60. http://dx.doi.org/10.1016/j.brainres.2007.08.048.

Beurskens, R., Bock, O., 2012. Age-related deficits of dual-task walking: a review. Neural Plasticity 2012, 1–9.:131608. http://dx.doi.org/10.1155/2012/131608.

Beurskens, R., Gollhofer, A., Muehlbauer, T., Cardinale, M., Granacher, U., 2015. Effects of heavy-resistance strength and balance training on unilateral and bilateral leg strength performance in old adults. PLoS One 10 (2), e0118535. http://dx.doi.org/10.1371/journal.pone.0118535.

Beurskens, R., Steinberg, F., Antoniewicz, F., Wolff, W., Granacher, U., 2016. Neural correlates of dual-task walking: effects of cognitive versus motor interference in young adults. Neural Plasticity, p. 9, [Article ID 8032180]. http://dx.doi.org/10.1155/2016/8032180.

Brown, J.A., Dalecki, M., Hughes, C., Macpherson, A.K., Sergio, L.E., 2015. Cognitive-motor integration deficits in young adult athletes following concussion. BMC Sports Science, Medicine and Rehabilitation 7, 25. http://dx.doi.org/10.1186/s13102-015-0019-4.

Burgess, N., Maguire, E.A., O'Keefe, J., 2002. The human hippocampus and spatial and episodic memory. Neuron 35 (4), 625–641.

Cabeza, R., 2002. Hemispheric asymmetry reduction in older adults: the HAROLD model. Psychology and Aging 17 (1), 85–100.

Christie, A., Kamen, G., 2014. Cortical inhibition is reduced following short-term training in young and older adults. Age 36 (2), 749–758. http://dx.doi.org/10.1007/s11357-013-9577-0.

Colcombe, S.J., Kramer, A.F., 2003. Fitness effects on the cognitive function of older adults: a meta-analytic study. Psychological Sciences 14 (2), 125–130.

Colcombe, S.J., Kramer, A.F., Erickson, K.I., Scalf, P., McAuley, E., Cohen, N.J., Webb, A., Jerome, G.J., Marquez, D.Z., Elavsky, S., 2004. Cardiovascular fitness, cortical plasticity, and aging. Proceedings of the National Academy of Sciences of the United States of America 101 (9), 3316–3321. http://dx.doi.org/10.1073/pnas.0400266101.

Colcombe, S.J., Erickson, K.I., Scalf, P.E., Kim, J.S., Prakash, R., McAuley, E., Elavsky, S., Marquez, D.X., Hu, L., Kramer, A.F., 2006. Aerobic exercise training increases brain volume in aging humans. The Journals of Gerontology. Series A 61 (11), 1166–1170.

Correa, C.S., Baroni, B.M., Radaelli, R., Lanferdini, F.J., Cunha Gdos, S., Reischak-Oliveira, A., Vaz, M.A., Pinto, R.S., 2013. Effects of strength training and detraining on knee extensor strength, muscle volume and muscle quality in elderly women. Age 35 (5), 1899–1904. http://dx.doi.org/10.1007/s11357-012-9478-7.

Courchesne, E., Chisum, H.J., Townsend, J., Cowles, A., Covington, J., Egaas, B., Harwood, M., Hinds, S., Press, G.A., 2000. Normal brain development and aging: quantitative analysis at in vivo MR imaging in healthy volunteers. Radiology 216 (3), 672–682. http://dx.doi.org/10.1148/radiology.216.3.r00au37672.

Doi, T., Makizako, H., Shimada, H., Park, H., Tsutsumimoto, K., Uemura, K., Suzuki, T., 2013. Brain activation during dual-task walking and executive function among older adults with mild cognitive impairment: a fNIRS study. Aging Clinical and Experimental Research 25 (5), 539–544. http://dx.doi.org/10.1007/s40520-013-0119-5.

Dalecki, M., Albines, D., Macpherson, A., Sergio, L.E., 2016. Prolonged cognitive-motor impairments in children and adolescents with a history of concussion. Concussion 12. http://dx.doi.org/10.2217/cnc-2016-0001.

Du Pasquier, R.A., Blanc, Y., Sinnreich, M., Landis, T., Burkhard, P., Vingerhoets, F.J., 2003. The effect of aging on postural stability: a cross sectional and longitudinal study. Neurophysiologie Clinique/Clinical Neurophysiology 33 (5), 213–218.

Earles, J.L., Kersten, A.W., 1999. Processing speed and adult age differences in activity memory. Experimental Aging Research 25 (3), 243–253. http://dx.doi.org/10.1080/036107399244011.

Erickson, K.I., Prakash, R.S., Voss, M.W., Chaddock, L., Hu, L., Morris, K.S., White, S.M., Wójcicki, T.R., McAuley, E., Kramer, A.F., 2009. Aerobic fitness is associated with hippocampal volume in elderly humans. Hippocampus 19 (10), 1030–1039. http://dx.doi.org/10.1002/hipo.20547.

Erickson, K.I., Voss, M.W., Prakash, R.S., Basak, C., Szabo, A., Chaddock, L., Kim, J.S., Heo, S., Alves, H., White, S.M., Wojcicki, T.R., Mailey, E., Vieira, V.J., Martin, S.A., Pence, B.D., Woods, J.A., McAuley, E., Kramer, A.F., 2011. Exercise training increases size of hippocampus and improves memory. Proceedings of the National Academy of Sciences of the United States of America 108 (7), 3017–3022. http://dx.doi.org/10.1073/pnas.1015950108.

Erickson, K.I., Leckie, R.L., Weinstein, A.M., 2014. Physical activity, fitness, and gray matter volume. Neurobiology of Aging 35 (Suppl. 2), S20–S28. http://dx.doi.org/10.1016/j.neurobiolaging.2014.03.034.

Etnier, J.L., Salazar, W., Landers, D.M., Petruzzello, S.J., Han, M., Nowell, P., 1997. The influence of physical fitness and exercise upon cognitive functioning: a meta-analysis. Journal of Sport & Exercise Psychology 19 (3), 249–277.

Fogelman, D., Zafonte, R., 2012. Exercise to enhance neurocognitive function after traumatic brain injury. PM & R 4 (11), 908–913. http://dx.doi.org/10.1016/j.pmrj.2012.09.028.

Garcia-Mesa, Y., Lopez-Ramos, J.C., Gimenez-Llort, L., Revilla, S., Guerra, R., Gruart, A., Laferla, F.M., Cristòfol, R., Delgado-García, J.M., Sanfeliu, C., 2011. Physical exercise protects against Alzheimer's disease in 3xTg-AD mice. Journal of Alzheimer's Disease 24 (3), 421–454. http://dx.doi.org/10.3233/JAD-2011-101635.

Geda, Y.E., Roberts, R.O., Knopman, D.S., Christianson, T.J., Pankratz, V.S., Ivnik, R.J., Boeve, B.F., Tangalos, E.G., Petersen, R.C., Rocca, W.A., 2010. Physical exercise, aging, and mild cognitive impairment: a population-based study. Archives of Neurology 67 (1), 80–86. http://dx.doi.org/10.1001/archneurol.2009.297.

Goble, D.J., Coxon, J.P., Van Impe, A., De Vos, J., Wenderoth, N., Swinnen, S.P., 2010. The neural control of bimanual movements in the elderly: brain regions exhibiting age-related increases in activity, frequency-induced neural modulation, and task-specific compensatory recruitment. Human Brain Mapping 31 (8), 1281–1295. http://dx.doi.org/10.1002/hbm.20943.

Griesbach, G.S., Hovda, D.A., Gomez-Pinilla, F., Sutton, R.L., 2008. Voluntary exercise or amphetamine treatment, but not the combination, increases hippocampal brain-derived neurotrophic factor and synapsin I following cortical contusion injury in rats. Neuroscience 154 (2), 530–540. http://dx.doi.org/10.1016/j.neuroscience.2008.04.003.

Griesbach, G.S., Hovda, D.A., Gomez-Pinilla, F., 2009. Exercise-induced improvement in cognitive performance after traumatic brain injury in rats is dependent on BDNF activation. Brain Research 1288, 105–115. http://dx.doi.org/10.1016/j.brainres.2009.06.045.

Griesbach, G.S., 2011. Exercise after traumatic brain injury: is it a double-edged sword? PM & R 3 (6 Suppl. 1), S64–S72. http://dx.doi.org/10.1016/j.pmrj.2011.02.008.

Guiney, H., Machado, L., 2013. Benefits of regular aerobic exercise for executive functioning in healthy populations. Psychonomic Bulletin & Review 20 (1), 73–86. http://dx.doi.org/10.3758/s13423-012-0345-4.

Guskiewicz, K.M., Marshall, S.W., Bailes, J., McCrea, M., Cantu, R.C., Randolph, C., Jordan, B.D., 2005. Association between recurrent concussion and late-life cognitive impairment in retired professional football players. Neurosurgery 57 (4), 719–726 discussion 719–726.

Hauer, K., Schwenk, M., Zieschang, T., Essig, M., Becker, C., Oster, P., 2012. Physical training improves motor performance in people with dementia: a randomized controlled trial. Journal of the American Geriatrics Society 60 (1), 8–15. http://dx.doi.org/10.1111/j.1532-5415.2011.03778.x.

Hebb, D.O., 1949. The Organization of Behavior: A Neuropsychological Theory. Wiley & Sons, New York.

Heyn, P.C., Johnson, K.E., Kramer, A.F., 2008. Endurance and strength training outcomes on cognitively impaired and cognitively intact older adults: a meta-analysis. The Journal of Nutrition Health and Aging 12 (6), 401–409.

Hicks, R.R., Boggs, A., Leider, D., Kraemer, P., Brown, R., Scheff, S.W., Seroogy, K.B., 1998. Effects of exercise following lateral fluid percussion brain injury in rats. Restorative Neurology and Neuroscience 12 (1), 41–47.

Holviala, J., Kraemer, W.J., Sillanpaa, E., Karppinen, H., Avela, J., Kauhanen, A., Hakkinen, A., Hakkinen, K., 2012. Effects of strength, endurance and combined training on muscle strength, walking speed and dynamic balance in aging men. European Journal of Applied Physiology 112 (4), 1335–1347. http://dx.doi.org/10.1007/s00421-011-2089-7.

Jack Jr., C.R., Wiste, H.J., Vemuri, P., Weigand, S.D., Senjem, M.L., Zeng, G., Bernstein, M.A., Gunter, J.L., Pankratz, V.S., Aisen, P.S., Weiner, M.W., Petersen, R.C., Shaw, L.M., Trojanowski, J.Q., Knopman, D.S., Alzheimer's Disease Neuroimaging Initiative, 2010. Brain beta-amyloid measures and magnetic resonance imaging atrophy both predict time-to-progression from mild cognitive impairment to Alzheimer's disease. Brain 133 (11), 3336–3348. http://dx.doi.org/10.1093/brain/awq277.

Karnath, H.O., Ferber, S., Himmelbach, M., 2001. Spatial awareness is a function of the temporal not the posterior parietal lobe. Nature 411 (6840), 950–953. http://dx.doi.org/10.1038/35082075.

Kempermann, G., Gast, D., Gage, F.H., 2002. Neuroplasticity in old age: sustained fivefold induction of hippocampal neurogenesis by long-term environmental enrichment. Annals of Neurology 52 (2), 135–143. http://dx.doi.org/10.1002/ana.10262.

Kempermann, G., 2008. The neurogenic reserve hypothesis: what is adult hippocampal neurogenesis good for? Trends in Neurosciences 31 (4), 163–169. http://dx.doi.org/10.1016/j.tins.2008.01.002.

Lakatta, E.G., 2002. Age-associated cardiovascular changes in health: impact on cardiovascular disease in older persons. Heart Failure Reviews 7 (1), 29–49.

Lautenschlager, N.T., Cox, K.L., Flicker, L., Foster, J.K., van Bockxmeer, F.M., Xiao, J., Greenop, K.R., Almeida, O.P., 2008. Effect of physical activity on cognitive function in older adults at risk for Alzheimer disease: a randomized trial. JAMA 300 (9), 1027–1037. http://dx.doi.org/10.1001/jama.300.9.1027.

Lawlor, D.A., Hopker, S.W., 2001. The effectiveness of exercise as an intervention in the management of depression: systematic review and meta-regression analysis of randomised controlled trials. BMJ 322 (7289), 763–767.

Leddy, J.J., Kozlowski, K., Donnelly, J.P., Pendergast, D.R., Epstein, L.H., Willer, B., 2010. A preliminary study of subsymptom threshold exercise training for refractory post-concussion syndrome. Clinical Journal of Sport Medicine 20 (1), 21–27. http://dx.doi.org/10.1097/JSM.0b013e3181c6c22c.

Liu-Ambrose, T., Nagamatsu, L.S., Graf, P., Beattie, B.L., Ashe, M.C., Handy, T.C., 2010. Resistance training and executive functions: a 12-month randomized controlled trial. Archives of Internal Medicine 170 (2), 170–178.

Liu-Ambrose, T., Nagamatsu, L.S., Voss, M.W., Khan, K.M., Handy, T.C., 2012. Resistance training and functional plasticity of the aging brain: a 12-month randomized controlled trial. Neurobiology of Aging 33 (8), 1690–1698. http://dx.doi.org/10.1016/j.neurobiolaging.2011.05.010.

Loane, D.J., Faden, A.I., 2010. Neuroprotection for traumatic brain injury: translational challenges and emerging therapeutic strategies. Trends in Pharmacological. Sciences 31 (12), 596–604. http://dx.doi.org/10.1016/j.tips.2010.09.005.

Lotze, M., Erb, M., Flor, H., Huelsmann, E., Godde, B., Grodd, W., 2000. fMRI evaluation of somatotopic representation in human primary motor cortex. NeuroImage 11 (5 Pt 1), 473–481. http://dx.doi.org/10.1006/nimg.2000.0556.

Lowel, S., Singer, W., 1992. Selection of intrinsic horizontal connections in the visual cortex by correlated neuronal activity. Science 255 (5041), 209–212.

Majerske, C.W., Mihalik, J.P., Ren, D., Collins, M.W., Reddy, C.C., Lovell, M.R., Wagner, A.K., 2008. Concussion in sports: postconcussive activity levels, symptoms, and neurocognitive performance. Journal of Athletic Training 43 (3), 265–274. http://dx.doi.org/10.4085/1062-6050-43.3.265.

McCrory, P., Meeuwisse, W.H., Aubry, M., Cantu, B., Dvorak, J., Echemendia, R.J., Engebretsen, L., Johnston, K., Kutcher, J.S., Raftery, M., Sills, A., Benson, B.W., Davis, G.A., Ellenbogen, R.G., Guskiewicz, K., Herring, S.A., Iverson, G.L., Jordan, B.D., Kissick, J., McCrea, M., McIntosh, A.S., Maddocks, D., Makdissi, M., Purcell, L.M., Schneider, K., Tator, C.H., Turner, M., 2013. Consensus statement on concussion in sport: the 4th international conference on concussion in sport held in Zurich, November 2012. British Journal of Sports Medicine 47 (5), 250–258. http://dx.doi.org/10.1136/bjsports-2013-092313.

Moss-Morris, R., Sharon, C., Tobin, R., Baldi, J.C., 2005. A randomized controlled graded exercise trial for chronic fatigue syndrome: outcomes and mechanisms of change. Journal of Health Psychology 10 (2), 245–259. http://dx.doi.org/10.1177/1359105305049774.

Nagamatsu, L.S., Handy, T.C., Hsu, C.L., Voss, M., Liu-Ambrose, T., 2012. Resistance training promotes cognitive and functional brain plasticity in seniors with probable mild cognitive impairment. Archives of Internal Medicine 172 (8), 666–668. http://dx.doi.org/10.1001/archinternmed.2012.379.

Niemann, C., Godde, B., Voelcker-Rehage, C., 2014. Not only cardiovascular, but also coordinative exercise increases hippocampal volume in older adults. Frontiers in Aging Neuroscience 6, 170. http://dx.doi.org/10.3389/fnagi.2014.00170.

Noble, J.W., Eng, J.J., Boyd, L.A., 2014. Bilateral motor tasks involve more brain regions and higher neural activation than unilateral tasks: an fMRI study. Experimental Brain Research 232 (9), 2785–2795. http://dx.doi.org/10.1007/s00221-014-3963-4.

Park, D.C., Lautenschlager, G., Hedden, T., Davidson, N.S., Smith, A.D., Smith, P.K., 2002. Models of visuospatial and verbal memory across the adult life span. Psychological Aging 17 (2), 299–320.

Pascual-Leone, A., Nguyet, D., Cohen, L.G., Brasil-Neto, J.P., Cammarota, A., Hallett, M., 1995. Modulation of muscle responses evoked by transcranial magnetic stimulation during the acquisition of new fine motor skills. Journal of Neurophysiology 74 (3), 1037–1045.

Ponti, G., Peretto, P., Bonfanti, L., 2008. Genesis of neuronal and glial progenitors in the cerebellar cortex of peripuberal and adult rabbits. PLoS One 3 (6), e2366. http://dx.doi.org/10.1371/journal.pone.0002366.

Puttemans, V., Wenderoth, N., Swinnen, S.P., 2005. Changes in brain activation during the acquisition of a multifrequency bimanual coordination task: from the cognitive stage to advanced levels of automaticity. The Journal of Neuroscience: the Official Journal of the Society for Neuroscience 25 (17), 4270–4278. http://dx.doi.org/10.1523/JNEUROSCI.3866-04.2005.

Resnick, S.M., Pham, D.L., Kraut, M.A., Zonderman, A.B., Davatzikos, C., 2003. Longitudinal magnetic resonance imaging studies of older adults: a shrinking brain. The Journal of Neuroscience: the Official Journal of the Society for Neuroscience 23 (8), 3295–3301.

Reuter-Lorenz, P.A., Cappell, K.A., 2008. Neurocognitive aging and the compensation hypothesis. Current Directions in Psychological Science 17 (3), 177–182. http://dx.doi.org/10.1111/j.1467-8721.2008.00570.x.

Reuter-Lorenz, P.A., Jonides, J., Smith, E.E., Hartley, A., Miller, A., Marshuetz, C., Koeppe, R.A., 2000. Age differences in the frontal lateralization of verbal and spatial working memory revealed by PET. Journal of Cognitive Neuroscience 12 (1), 174–187.

Reynolds, B.A., Weiss, S., 1992. Generation of neurons and astrocytes from isolated cells of the adult mammalian central nervous system. Science 255 (5052), 1707–1710.

Seo, T.B., Kim, B.K., Ko, I.G., Kim, D.H., Shin, M.S., Kim, C.J., Yoon, J.H., Kim, H., 2010. Effect of treadmill exercise on Purkinje cell loss and astrocytic reaction in the cerebellum after traumatic brain injury. Neuroscience Letters 481 (3), 178–182. http://dx.doi.org/10.1016/j.neulet.2010.06.087.

Slobounov, S., Hallett, M., Stanhope, S., Shibasaki, H., 2005. Role of cerebral cortex in human postural control: an EEG study. Clinical Neurophysiology 116 (2), 315–323. http://dx.doi.org/10.1016/j.clinph.2004.09.007.

Spirduso, W.W., Clifford, P., 1978. Replication of age and physical activity effects on reaction and movement time. Journal of Gerontology 33 (1), 26–30.

Stern, Y., 2009. Cognitive reserve. Neuropsychologia 47 (10), 2015–2028.

Sullivan, E.V., Pfefferbaum, A., 2007. Neuroradiological characterization of normal adult ageing. British Journal of Radiology 80 (Spec No 2), S99–S108. http://dx.doi.org/10.1259/bjr/22893432.

Szabo, Z., Ying, Z., Radak, Z., Gomez-Pinilla, F., 2010. Voluntary exercise may engage proteasome function to benefit the brain after trauma. Brain Research 1341, 25–31. http://dx.doi.org/10.1016/j.brainres.2009.01.035.

Szuhany, K.L., Bugatti, M., Otto, M.W., 2015. A meta-analytic review of the effects of exercise on brain-derived neurotrophic factor. Journal of Psychiatric Research 60, 56–64. http://dx.doi.org/10.1016/j.jpsychires.2014.10.003.

Taube, W., 2012. Neurophysiological adaptations in response to balance training. Deutsche Zeitschrift für Sportmedizin 63 (2012), 273–277.

Taubert, M., Lohmann, G., Margulies, D.S., Villringer, A., Ragert, P., 2011. Long-term effects of motor training on resting-state networks and underlying brain structure. NeuroImage 57 (4), 1492–1498. http://dx.doi.org/10.1016/j.neuroimage.2011.05.078.

ten Brinke, L.F., Bolandzadeh, N., Nagamatsu, L.S., Hsu, C.L., Davis, J.C., Miran-Khan, K., Liu-Ambrose, T., 2015. Aerobic exercise increases hippocampal volume in older women with probable mild cognitive impairment: a 6-month randomised controlled trial. British Journal of Sports Medicine 49 (4), 248–254. http://dx.doi.org/10.1136/bjsports-2013-093184.

Tremblay, S., Henry, L.C., Bedetti, C., Larson-Dupuis, C., Gagnon, J.F., Evans, A.C., Théoret, H., Lassonde, M., De Beaumont, L., 2014. Diffuse white matter tract abnormalities in clinically normal ageing retired athletes with a history of sports-related concussions. Brain 137 (Pt 11), 2997–3011. http://dx.doi.org/10.1093/brain/awu236.

Valenzuela, M.J., Sachdev, P., 2006. Brain reserve and dementia: a systematic review. Psychological Medicine 36 (4), 441–454. http://dx.doi.org/10.1017/S0033291705006264.

Van Impe, A., Coxon, J.P., Goble, D.J., Doumas, M., Swinnen, S.P., 2012. White matter fractional anisotropy predicts balance performance in older adults. Neurobiological Aging 33 (9), 1900–1912. http://dx.doi.org/10.1016/j.neurobiolaging.2011.06.013.

Voelcker-Rehage, C., Godde, B., Staudinger, U.M., 2010. Physical and motor fitness are both related to cognition in old age. European Journal of Neuroscience 31 (1), 167–176. http://dx.doi.org/10.1111/j.1460-9568.2009.07014.x.

Voelcker-Rehage, C., Godde, B., Staudinger, U.M., 2011. Cardiovascular and coordination training differentially improve cognitive performance and neural processing in older adults. Frontiers in Human Neuroscience 5, 26. http://dx.doi.org/10.3389/fnhum.2011.00026.

Wallace, M.T., Ramachandran, R., Stein, B.E., 2004. A revised view of sensory cortical parcellation. Proceedings of the National Academy of Sciences of the United States of America 101 (7), 2167–2172. http://dx.doi.org/10.1073/pnas.0305697101.

Warraich, Z., Kleim, J.A., 2010. Neural plasticity: the biological substrate for neurorehabilitation. PM & R 2 (12 Suppl. 2), S208–S219. http://dx.doi.org/10.1016/j.pmrj.2010.10.016.

Werner, C., Engelhard, K., 2007. Pathophysiology of traumatic brain injury. British Journal of Anaesthesia 99 (1), 4–9. http://dx.doi.org/10.1093/bja/aem131.

Wickens, C.D., 2008. Multiple resources and mental workload. Human Factors 50 (3), 449–455.

19

Update of Nutritional Antioxidants and Antinociceptives on Improving Exercise-Induced Muscle Soreness

N. Leelayuwat

Exercise and Sport Sciences Development and Research Group, and Department of Physiology, Faculty of Medicine, Khon Kaen University, Khon Kaen, Thailand

Abstract

Eccentric exercise and unaccustomed overload exercise were shown to cause muscle damage and soreness (DOMS). The phenomenon is still not completely understood. Many mechanisms are responsible for the soreness, including oxidative stress, inflammation, and mechanical stress disruption. DOMS reduces force production leading to reduced physical performances, e.g., endurance and strengthening performances. Among many modalities preventing and treating the DOMS, antioxidant and antinociceptic supplements are increasingly used for health promotion and sport competition. This chapter provided update of the information of these supplements for those purposes.

INTRODUCTION

Nowadays, exercise is promoted for improving health and sport competition worldwide. However, both beginners and athletes normally face exercise-induced muscle soreness or delayed onset of muscle soreness (DOMS) which occurs 1–3 days after the strenuous exercise. This makes the beginners not to continue their regular exercise or the athletes impaired their performances. Therefore, searching for supplement that can prevent or decrease DOMS gains more interest both for health promotion and sport competition. This chapter describes an updated scientific information about mechanism of DOMS and nutritional antioxidant and anti-nociceptive supplementations.

MECHANISMS RESPONSIBLE FOR THE DOMS

Free Radical Formation

Free radicals including reactive oxygen (ROS) and reactive nitrogen (RNS) species or both are called reactive oxygen and nitrogen species (RONS; Powers and Jackson, 2008) were demonstrated to play very important role in causing DOMS. The ROS production is often observed during aerobic exercise, in which one of the main source is the mitochondrial electron transport chain. The free radical promotes biochemical changes (damage to lipid, protein, and DNA) within the affected area, leading to generation of inflammatory cytokines and immune cell with more ROS that may further degrade muscle proteins, and contribute to signs and symptoms of injury (e.g., loss of muscle force, muscle soreness, leakage of cellular proteins into the blood).

Moreover, exercise-induced fatigue and muscle damage and impaired immune functions may be mediated via the regulation of mitochondrial dynamic remodeling, including the downregulation of mitochondrial biogenesis and upregulation of autophagy (Kerksick et al., 2008; Stupka et al., 2001). Mitochondrial mass is linked to mitochondrial capacity for aerobic energy production, which in muscles is an important determinant of endurance, because it is much more efficient than anaerobic energy metabolism in terms of moles ATP generated per mole glucose.

Eccentric exercise, however, (Nikolaidis et al., 2007; Paschalis et al., 2007) with high tension and relatively low oxygen demand, such as downhill running, really more causes DOMS than running with the same intensity on an even surface (Close et al., 2004). This implies that the main source of the generated free radicals is not the mitochondrial electron transport chain, but rather is due to secondary sources such as inflammatory agents (Camus et al., 1994). Eccentric contraction rapidly causes muscle damage in a fiber-specific manner evident and displays throughout individual fibers (i.e., focal injury).

Under exercise conditions, oxidative damage is mostly minimized by maintaining oxidative balance within physiological limits (Powers and Jackson, 2008). This is attributed to an antioxidant defense system which consists of antioxidants enzymes such as catalase (CAT), glutathione peroxidases (Gpx), superoxide dismutase (SOD), thioredoxins, peroxiredoxins, and glutathione (GSH) reductase which reduce ROS, and endogenous antioxidant substrates like GSH and uric acid that scavenge ROS and RNS (Powers and Jackson, 2008).

Exercise-Induced the Disruption of Contractile Protein

Friden et al. reported that DOMS-associated muscle damage included intermyofibrillar sarcoma disturbances, and Z-band streaming, especially in Type 2 fibers (Lieber et al., 1996). Eccentric exercise can trigger degradation of the cytoskeletal and contractile proteins (Armstrong et al., 1991) and disturb the desmin-negative muscle fibers appearance (Lieber et al., 1996). Therefore, the decline in post-exercise performance capacity are believed to result from damage of the cytoskeletal and contractile proteins and impairments of the excitation-contraction system (Murphy et al., 2013).

Exercise-Induced Nitric Oxide Generation

An increase in calcium concentration following the eccentric exercise in skeletal muscle a few days indicates the role of exercise in the regulation of activity of calcium-dependent cysteine proteases (calpains) and degradation of cytoskeletal and contractile proteins (Armstrong et al., 1991). The calpains activity can also be regulated by other mechanisms including endogenous calpain inhibitor calpastatin (Spencer and Mellgren, 2002; Carlin et al., 2006) and by nitric oxide (Barton et al., 2005). Moreover, one of the first studies to report a causative link between NO generation and decreased force generation showed that iNO inhibitions maintained force levels in the diaphragm. Andrade et al. (1998) concluded that NO can impair Ca^{2+} sensitivity, especially on actin filaments.

During exercise, muscle contraction generated nitric oxide (NO), as a result of neuronal NOS (nNO; Percival et al., 2010), inducible NO (iNO; Carmeli et al., 2010), and endothelial NO (eNO; Lee-Young et al., 2010) activation. It is shown that both inhibitors and donors of NO result in decreased force generation (Marechal and Beckers-Bleukx, 1998), which demonstrates that the dose response of NO follows a bell-shaped hormetic curve (Reid and Durham, 2002). In order to protect more damage, NO decreases force production and aggravate pain (by stimulating nociceptors of C-fibers). Moreover, it is also needed to the repair process. NO in skeletal muscle is known to influence force generation which includes cytochrome oxidase inhibition, which affects oxygen uptake (Finocchietto et al., 2009). In addition, NO could decrease ATP-ase activity via protein-nitrosylation of skeletal muscle (Nogueira et al., 2009), and produce an exaggerated exercise-induced fatigue (Kobayashi et al., 2008).

Furthermore, it is shown that sarcolemmal nNO is an important regulator of blood flow to exercising skeletal muscle (Percival et al., 2010). During eccentric exercise the induction of main mediators of the inflammatory process, nuclear factor kappa-B (Radak et al., 2004), reduces the NO transcription. This showed an important link between NO induction and DOMS-inflammation. Furthermore, the exercise induced NO generation seems to be important for the induction of heme oxygenase, HSP78, interleukin-6, and interleukin-8. Besides, NO can even affect the structure of skeletal muscle (Morrison et al., 1996).

Exercise-Induced Inflammation

Exercise-induced muscle damage stimulates immune cell which produces substances including cytokines and oxidants, such as hydrogen peroxide, free radicals, and hypochlorous acid. The immune cell products that accumulate in the interstitium, activate the group-IV sensory nerve endings and destroys invading organisms and damaged tissue, succeed recovery. However, oxidants and cytokines can harm healthy tissue. Excessive or uneven production of these substances is associated with mortality and morbidity after infection and trauma, and in inflammation. Oxidants enhance interleukin-1, interleukin-8, and tumor necrosis factor production in response to inflammatory stimuli by activating the nuclear transcription factor, NF kappa B. Many antioxidant defenses indirectly and directly protect the host against the damaging influence of cytokines and oxidants. Then, there is edema formation which has also been found in subjects suffering from DOMS (Bobbert et al., 1986).

Exercise-Induced Mechanical Stress

The strenuous exercise also contributes to mechanical stress which damages muscle fiber. Then, it produces bradykinin (which can produce NO) and neuro growth factor. These products activate nociceptors leading to DOMS (Murase et al., 2010).

ENDOGENOUS ANTIOXIDANTS AND EXERCISE-INDUCED MUSCLE SORENESS

An important role of integrated intracellular antioxidant system was to reduce free radical production and subsequent damage to lipid, amino acids, nucleic acids, cell membranes, and genetic material (Sen, 1995).

Normally, low and physiological levels of RONS are required for normal force production in skeletal muscle, but high levels of RONS promote contractile dysfunction resulting in muscle weakness fatigue and soreness. Therefore, antioxidant is important for reducing exercise-induced muscular damage and soreness. Muscle fibers contain antioxidants, i.e., enzymatic and nonenzymatic that work in combination to regulate RONS. These antioxidants are strategically compartmentalized within the fiber throughout the cytoplasm and within various organelles (e.g., mitochondria). In summary, these antioxidants protect muscle fibers from oxidative injury during periods of increased oxidative stress (e.g., streneous or prolonged exercise).

There are two types of antioxidants.

1. Non-enzyme antioxidant
   Non-enzyme antioxidant in cells includes GSH, uric acid, bilirubin, vitamin C, vitamin E, beta carotenoid, etc.
2. Enzyme antioxidant
   Enzyme antioxidant includes SOD, Gpx, and CAT. In addition, antioxidant enzymes such as glutaredoxin, peroxiredoxin, and thioredoxin reductase also protect cell against oxidation.

NUTRITIONAL ANTIOXIDANTS AND EXERCISE-INDUCED MUSCLE SORENESS

According to the major role of oxidative stress in producing DOMS and subsequent attenuated force production and impaired physical performance, antioxidant supplement gains more interest.

Nutritional antioxidants obtained from both antioxidant-rich foods and antioxidant supplements. Antioxidant-rich foods include fruits and vegetables that are high in nutrients such as vitamins A, C, and E, beta-carotene, lutein, lycopene, and selenium etc. Many antioxidant supplements include vitamins A, C, and E, beta-carotene, etc. This part describes only nutritional antioxidants that are mostly used to attenuate DOMS.

ANTIOXIDANT SUPPLEMENTS

Polyphenols

There are more than 10 classes of polyphenols, but the 4 major classes are the phenolic acids, flavonoids, stilbenes, and lignans (Bravo, 1998). Flavonoids are found in a wide variety of fruits and vegetables (de Vries et al., 1998).

Anthocyanin is one of the flavonoids which are shown to be beneficial in recovery from exercise, which is proposed to increase the capacity for the inhibition of inflammatory cyclooxygenase (COX-1 and COX-2) enzymes and oxidative stress (Wang et al., 1999; Seeram et al., 2001). Anthocyanins are glycosides of their aglycon, cyanidin, and have been shown (in vitro) to be superior to α-tocopherol and the commercially available antioxidants butylated hydroxyanisole and butylated hydroxytoluene in the attenuation of lipid peroxidation (Wang et al., 1999). Many kinds of fruits containing anthocyanin are montmorency cherries (MC), blueberries, cranberries, and bilberries.

In addition, a rat hepatocytes cell culture study anthocyanins were shown to inhibit hydrogen peroxide while upregulating the expression of endogenous antioxidants glutathione reductase, Gpx, and glutathione S-transferase.

Vitamin E, C, A

Important nutritional antioxidants include vitamin E, vitamin C, and carotenoids. Based on the previous study, receiving an 8-day dietary record from female soccer teams who then played 1 competition match the same week. Subjects who normally consumed balanced nutritional diet comprising important antioxidant vitamins, including vitamins A, C, and E had higher total antioxidant status, GPx, SOD, lactate dehydrogenase and the percent of lymphocytes were higher and the percent of neutrophils were lower immediately after the match than those who did not (Gravina et al., 2012). Zoppi et al. (2006) found that vitamin C and E supplementation in soccer players may reduce lipid peroxidation and muscle damage during high intensity efforts, but did not enhance performance (Khassaf et al., 2003).

Vitamin E is one of the most widely distributed antioxidants in nature. It is the primary chain-breaking antioxidant in cell membranes (Janero, 1991; Packer, 1991). Among eight structural isomers of tocopherols or tocotrienols (Janero, 1991; Schaffer et al., 2005), α-tocopherol is the best known and has the most antioxidant activity (Janero, 1991). Apart from its direct antioxidant activities, growing evidence suggests that some of the beneficial effects of intracellular vitamin E are its ability to regulate gene expression of proteins (Azzi et al., 2003, 2004; Han et al., 2004; Schulte et al., 2006). Vitamin E supplementation represents an important factor in the defense against oxidative stress and muscle damage but not against the inflammatory response in humans (Silva et al., 2010).

In contrast to both vitamin E and the carotenoids, vitamin C (ascorbic acid) is hydrophilic and functions better in an aqueous environment. Because the pK_a value of ascorbic acid is 4.25, the ascorbate anion is the predominant form existing at physiological pH (Yu, 1994). Ascorbate is widely distributed in mammalian tissues, and its role as an antioxidant is twofold. First, vitamin C can directly scavenge superoxide, hydroxyl, and lipid hydroperoxide radicals (Carr and Frei, 1999). Second, vitamin C plays an important role in the recycling of vitamin E, a process that results in the formation of a vitamin C (semiascorbyl) radical (Packer et al., 1979). Nonetheless, this semiascorbyl radical can be reduced back to vitamin C by NADH semiascorbyl reductase, or cellular thiols such as glutathione or dihydrolipoic acid (Packer, 1991).

The overall effect of vitamin C supplementation appeared to increase the baseline lymphocyte SOD and CAT activities and heat shock protein (HSP60) content, and to attenuate the increase in expression of these substances that normally follows exposure to oxidants. However, a study in young healthy men performing a bout of 240 maximal isokinetic eccentric muscle contractions (0.52 rad/s) after being supplemented for 30 d with either vitamin E (1200 IU/d). The results showed that vitamin E had no effect on indices of contraction-induced muscle damage nor inflammation (macrophage infiltration) as a result of eccentric exercise (Beaton et al., 2002).

In addition, well-trained athletes with suitable ultra-endurance training volume and intensity were reported that they do not require antioxidant vitamin supplements to adapt their endogenous antioxidant defenses to exercise-induced ROS (Leonardo-Mendonça et al., 2014).

Green Tea Catechins (Epigallocatechin Gallate, EGCG)

Green tea and its catechin components are known to stimulate antioxidant activity by scavenging free radicals, inhibiting pro-oxidant enzymes, and stimulating antioxidant enzymes. Moreover, Kerksick et al. (2010) investigated the effect of ingestion of either 1800 mg of green tea catechins (EGCG) or 1800 mg of NAC for 14 days following by 1 eccentric exercise bout (100 repetitions at 30 rounds/s) using the dominant knee extensors. The authors found that muscle soreness ratings were blunted in the two supplementation groups 24 h after exercise (Kerksick et al., 2010).

Quercetin

Quercetin (3,4,5,7-pentahydroxylflavone; molecular mass 302.236 g mol/L) has several physiological benefits including antioxidant, ergogenic properties, cardioprotective, anticarcinogenic, and antiapoptotic (Bischoff, 2008; Davis et al., 2009). Some studies have shown that quercetin supplementation improved exercise tolerance (Kressler et al., 2011; MacRae et al., 2006; Davis et al., 2010), but other studies did not find its effect on endurance capacity (Bigelman et al., 2010; Ganio et al., 2010). The antioxidative effect of quercetin feeding on endurance performance is also reported (Leelayuwat et al., 2012). Leelayuwat et al. suggested that ingestion of quercetin (150 mg/kg body weight) can improve endurance capacity, due probably to increase antioxidant activity and size of muscle fiber type 1 in mice.

Ubiquinone-10

Ubiquinone-10, a lipid soluble antioxidant, was found in high concentrations in meat and fish (Powers et al., 2004). Effect of ubiquinone-10 as an antioxidant in healthy individuals is not clear. It was reported to have a positive relationship with exercise capacity (Karlsson et al., 1996). Whereas, ubiquinone-10 supplementation may provide assistance to individuals with mitochondrial disease (Glover et al., 2010), most researches on healthy individuals show no effect (Braun et al., 1991) or a deleterious effect on exercise performance.

Polyphenolic Blend

Polyphenolic blend containing catechins and theaflavins (2000 mg/d) were shown to decrease oxidative stress and muscle stress, increase antioxidant, and promoted strength recovery after eccentric exercise (40 min downhill treadmill run; Herrlinger et al., 2015)

The Purple Mangosteen (*Garcinia mangostana*)

The purple mangosteen known as the "queen of fruit" is widely consumed and unique not only because of its outstanding appearance and flavor but also its remarkable and diverse pharmacological effects. A single oral administration of either 250 mL of the mangosteen-based juice (supplementation treatment; 305 mg of α-mangostin and 278 mg of hydroxycitric acid) 1 h before cycle ergometer exercise. Time to exhaustion was measured. It was concluded that acute mangosteen supplementation had no impact on a decrease in physical fatigue during exercise (Chang et al., 2016).

Hydroxytyrosol (HT)

Mediterranean diet consists of phenolic compounds such as HT, tyrosol, and oleuropein as its contents (Cicerale et al., 2009). HT may have potential of reducing the negative effects of ROS formation during exhaustive exercise. Moreover, HT supplementation may regulate dynamic remodeling of mitochondria and promote antioxidant defenses and thus improve exercise capacity (Feng et al., 2011).

L-arginine Supplementation

L-arginine supplementation after a single dose or repeated days improved subsequent exercise performance capacity tests, reduced numbers of damaged muscle fibers determined by the reduced loss of desmin content in the muscle and diminished *m*-calpain mRNA upregulation in RA rats (Lomonosova et al., 2014)

Docosahexaenoic Acid (DHA)

Supplementation with dietary DHA changed the erythrocyte membrane composition. This provided antioxidant defense and decreased protein peroxidative damage in the red blood cells of professional athletes after an 8-week training season and acute exercise (Martorell et al., 2015).

Taurine

Taurine is a sulfur-containing b-amino acid (2-aminoethane sulfonic acid) that is abundant in the cells of many tissues (Spriet and Whitfield, 2015). Classic work has implicated a role for taurine in many cellular processes, including cell development, cell signaling, membrane stability and receptor regulation, volume regulation, Ca^{2+} dependent excitation-contraction processes, antioxidant defense from stress responses, modulation of nerve excitement potential, and several metabolic effects related to improved glucose tolerance, insulin sensitivity, and substrate uptake, storage, and oxidation (Gomez-Cabrera et al., 2009).

N-acetylcysteine (NAC)

NAC is an antioxidant associated with glutathione production. Turnover of glutathione from its oxidized (GSSG) and reduced (GSH) forms is an important intracellular process that removes hydrogen peroxide from the cell structure and potential oxidative damage. Infusion of NAC in conjunction with a 90 min exhaustive treadmill run decreased oxidative stress and apoptosis (Quadrilatero and Hoffman-Goetz, 2005). In addition, supplementation of NAC; 20 mg/kg/day after muscle damaging exercise (300 eccentric contractions) attenuated the increase of inflammatory markers of muscle damage (creatine kinase activity, C-reactive protein, proinflammatory cytokines), nuclear factor kB phosphorylation, and the decrease in strength during the first 2 d of recovery. Although thiol-based antioxidant supplementation increases GSH availability in skeletal muscle, it disrupts the skeletal muscle inflammatory response and repair capability, potentially because of a blunted activation of redox-sensitive signaling pathways (Michailidis et al., 2013).

Green Tea Catechins (EGCG)

EGCG supplementation for 14 days contributed to lower levels of intramuscular oxidative stress and higher endogenous circulating antioxidants levels after electrical stimulation (Nagasawa et al., 2000).

Egg White Peptides (EWPs)

EWPs possessed the strongest antioxidant activity and showed an antifatigue effect and was safe (Sun et al., 2014).

FUNCTIONAL FOODS WITH HIGH ANTIOXIDANT CONCENTRATIONS

Fruits

Fruits contain many antioxidants such as melatonin, carotenoids, hydroxycinnamates, and several flavonoid groups including anthocyanins, as well as the flavonol quercetin (McCune et al., 2011). The antioxidant activities helps fruits in protecting muscular damage via avoiding mechanism mentioned in the first section the proliferation. In addition, MC have been reported to have similar anti-inflammatory properties to non-steroidal anti-inflammatory drugs (NSAID's), such as ibuprofen and naproxen (Seeram et al., 2001) and have highest anti-inflammatory property. MC both a single bout of exercise (Bell et al., 2014) and repeated days exercise (Bell et al., 2014) were shown to reduce oxidative stress and inflammatory responses to strenuous exercise (Connolly et al., 2006, p. 29; Vaile et al., 2008). Moreover, the ingestion of 30 mL of Montmorency tart cherry concentrate, twice per day for seven consecutive days decreased oxidative stress, inflammation, and muscle damage across 3 days simulated road cycle racing. Bell et al. (2014) also demonstrated that MC supplementation attenuated oxidative and inflammatory responses. This suggested that across 3 days simulated road cycle racing, MC can attenuate cellular disruption by combating post-exercise oxidative and inflammatory process.

Cashew Apple Juice

Prasertsri et al. (2013) showed that cashew apple juice supplementation (3.5 mL/kg body mass)/day for 4 weeks increased plasma vitamin C after the 4-week supplementations and all subjects performed cycling exercise at 85% of maximal oxygen consumption for 20 min high-intensity exercise in trained and untrained men (Prasertsri et al., 2013).

Phyllantus Amarus

Roengrit et al. demonstrated that Phyllantus Amarus decreased malondialdehyde and increased vitamin C concentrations 48 h after high-intensity exercise decreased pain in both legs 24 and 48 h after high-intensity exercise. There were no significant differences in creatine kinase, leukocyte counts or inflammation between groups (Roengrit et al., 2014).

Pomegranate Juice

Regular intake of pomegranate juice significantly modulates matrix metalloproteinases and serum levels of some inflammatory factors and thus protects against exhaustive exercise-induced oxidative injury in young healthy males (Mazani et al., 2014).

Spirulina

Spirulina supplementation induced a significant increase in exercise performance, fat oxidation, and GSH concentration and attenuated the exercise-induced increase in lipid peroxidation (Kalafati et al., 2010).

However, Traber (2006) found that both vitamins E and C supplementation only prevented increases in lipid peroxidation, but had no apparent effect on DNA damage, inflammation, or muscle damage. These findings suggest that the mechanism of oxidative damage is independent of the inflammatory and muscle damage responses. Moreover, in resistance trained men there seems to be no independent or combined effect of a prior bout of eccentric exercise or antioxidant supplementation (Bloomer et al., 2007)

Mixed Fruit and Vegetables

Bloomer et al. (2006) showed that ingestion of the three blend fruit, vegetable, and berry resulted in reduced exercise and induced increase of plasma protein carbonyl concentrations—a marker of RONS induced protein oxidation after 30 min treadmill running at 80% of VO_2. However, other studies suggested that antioxidant supplementation might contribute to muscle damage and hinder recovery (Close et al., 2006; Teixeira et al., 2009). These controversy are due to the diversity of different methods, subjects, surrogate endpoints, outcome measures, products.

ANTINOCICEPTIVE SUPPLEMENTS AND EXERCISE-INDUCED MUSCLE SORENESS

To date, not many researches reporting benefit effects of anti-nociceptive supplement on exercise-induced muscle soreness. Normally, endurance athletes used NSAIDs to prevent or reduce pain during competition (Gorski et al., 2009). However, known adverse effects include renal, gastrointestinal, and cardiovascular adverse events with the use of traditional oral NSAIDs (Howatson et al., 2008). Therefore, supplements which are natural and safe are increasingly used by both for health promotion and sport competition to reduce pain. The following supplements were investigated;

Tart Cherry (Kuehl et al., 2010)

Connolly et al. (2006) investigated anti-nociceptive effect of 12 fl oz of a cherry juice blend twice a day for eight consecutive days in male college students. On the fourth day of supplementation, a bout of eccentric exercise of elbow flexion (maximum contractions) was performed. The results showed that the cherry juice trial significantly decreased strength loss and pain including preserving muscle function. The specific anti-inflammatory activities of cherry juice supplementation on reduction in exercise-induced muscle damage is not clear (Jacob et al., 2003). However, it is likely that these effects of cherry juice may mediate this secondary response and avoid the proliferation of myofibrillar disruption (Connolly et al., 2003). The ingestion of tart cherry juice for 8 days decreased exercise-induced muscle pain among vigorous runners.

Phyllanthus amarus (PA)

PA is an herbal plant containing antioxidant compounds that scavenge free radicals. Acute ingestion of 2 PA capsules, 20 min before a single bout of cycling at high intensity for 20 min followed by 4 (2 capsules after lunch and dinner) and 6 capsules/day for the next 2 days reduced oxidative stress and muscle soreness induced by high-intensity exercise (Roengrit et al., 2014).

Resveratrol

Resveratrol is found in red wine, mulberries, the seeds and skins of grapes, peanuts, and rhubarb. It showed anti-inflammatory and immune-modulating actions via effective inhibition of cyclo-oxygenase activity (Markus and Morris, 2008; Naylor, 2009). However, Laupheimer et al. (2014) did not find the effect on inflammatory response and delayed onset muscle soreness after a marathon in male athletes (Laupheimer et al., 2014).

Polyphenolic Blend Containing Catechins and Theaflavins

Polyphenolic blend containing catechins and theaflavins were shown to decrease oxidative stress and muscle stress, increase antioxidant, and promoted strength recovery after eccentric exercise (40 min downhill treadmill run; Herrlinger et al., 2015). However, it had no effect on muscle soreness.

In future, the number of studies with these promising prevention and treatment on DOMS should increase. The results from those researches should be combined with practical observations and documentary reports to achieve sustainable health and performance of sporty people.

References

Andrade, F.H., Reid, M.B., Allen, D.G., Westerblad, H., 1998. Effect of nitric oxide on single skeletal muscle fibres from the mouse. Journal of Physiology 509, 577–586.

Armstrong, R.B., Warren, G.L., Warren, J.A., 1991. Mechanisms of exercise-induced muscle fibre injury. Sports Medicine 12, 184–207.

Azzi, A., Gysin, R., Kempna, P., Munteanu, A., Villacorta, L., Visarius, T., Zingg, J.M., 2004. Regulation of gene expression by alpha-tocopherol. Biological Chemistry 385, 585–591.

Azzi, A., Gysin, R., Kempna, P., Ricciarelli, R., Villacorta, L., Visarius, T., Zingg, J.M., 2003. The role of alpha-tocopherol in preventing disease: from epidemiology to molecular events. Molecular Aspects of Medicine 24, 325–336.

Barton, E.R., Morris, L., Kawana, M., Bish, L.T., Toursel, T., 2005. Systemic administration of L-arginine benefits mdx skeletal muscle function. Muscle and Nerve 32, 751–760.

Beaton, L.J., Allan, D.A., Tarnopolsky, M.A., Tiidus, P.M., Phillips, S.M., 2002. Contraction-induced muscle damage is unaffected by vitamin E supplementation. Medicine and Science in Sports and Exercise 34, 798–805.

Bell, P.G., Walshe, I.H., Davison, G.W., Stevenson, E., Howatso, G., 2014. Montmorency cherries reduce the oxidative stress and inflammatory responses to repeated days high-intensity stochastic cycling. Nutrients 6, 829–843.

Bigelman, K.A., Fan, E.H., Chapman, D.P., Freese, E.C., Trilk, J.L., Cureton, K.J., 2010. Effects of six weeks of quercetin supplementation on physical performance in ROTC cadets. Military Medicine 175, 791–798.

Bischoff, S.C., 2008. Quercetin: potentials in the prevention and therapy of disease. Current Opinion in Clinical Nutrition and Metabolic Care 11, 733–740.

Bloomer, R.J., Goldfarb, A.H., McKenzie, M.J., 2006. Oxidative stress response to aerobic exercise: comparison of antioxidant supplements. Medicine and Science in Sports and Exercise 38, 1098–1105.

Bobbert, M.F., Hollander, A.P., Huijing, P.A., 1986. Factors in delayed onset muscular soreness of man. Medicine and Science in Sports and Exercise 18, 75–81.

Braun, B., Clarkson, P.M., Freedson, P.S., Kohl, R.L., 1991. Effects of coenzyme Q10 supplementation on exercise performance, VO$_2$max, and lipid peroxidation in trained cyclists. International Journal of Sport Nutrition 1, 353–365.

Bravo, L., 1998. Polyphenols: chemistry, dietary sources, metabolism, and nutritional significance. Nutrition Reviews 56, 317–333.

Bloomer, R.J., Falvo, M.J., Schilling, B.K., Smith, W.A., 2007. Prior exercise and antioxidant supplementation: effect on oxidative stress and muscle injury. Journal of the International Society of Sports Nutrition 4, 9.

Camus, G., Deby-Dupont, G., Duchateau, J., Deby, J., Pincemail, J., Lamy, M., 1994. Are similar inflammatory factors involved in strenuous exercise and sepsis? Intensive Care Medicine 20, 602–610.

Carlin, K.R., Huff-Lonergan, E., Rowe, L.J., Lonergan, S.M., 2006. Effect of oxidation, pH, and ionic strength on calpastatin inhibition of mu- and mcalpain. Journal of Animal Science 84, 925–937.

Carmeli, E., Beiker, R., Maor, M., Kodesh, E., 2010. Increased iNOS, MMP-2, and HSP-72 in skeletal muscle following high-intensity exercise training. The Journal of Basic and Clinical Physiology and Pharmacology 21, 127–146.

Carr, A., Frei, B., 1999. Does vitamin C act as a pro-oxidant under physiological conditions? The Federation of American Societies for Experimental Biology Journal 13, 1007–1024.

Chang, C., Huang, T., Chang, W., Tseng, Y., Wu, Yu, Hsu, M., 2016. Acute Garcinia mangostana (mangosteen) supplementation does not alleviate physical fatigue during exercise: a randomized, double-blind, placebo-controlled, crossover trial. Journal of the International Society of Sports Nutrition 13, 20.

Cicerale, S., Conlan, X.A., Sinclair, A.J., Keast, R.S., 2009. Chemistry and health of olive oil phenolics. Critical Reviews in Food Science and Nutrition 49, 218–236.

Close, G.L., Ashton, T., Cable, T., Doran, D., Holloway, C., McArdle, F., MacLaren, D.P.M., 2006. Ascorbic acid supplementation does not attenuate postexercise muscle soreness following muscle-damaging exercise but may delay the recovery process. The British Journal of Nutrition 95, 976–981.

Close, G.L., Ashton, T., Cable, T., Doran, D., MacLaren, D.P., 2004. Eccentric exercise, isokinetic muscle torque and delayed onset muscle soreness: the role of reactive oxygen species. European Journal of Applied Physiology 91, 615–621.

Connolly, D.A.J., McHugh, M.P., Padilla-Zakour, O.I., 2006. Efficacy of a tart cherry juice blend in preventing the symptoms of muscle damage. British Journal of Sports Medicine 40, 679–683.

Connolly, D.A., Sayers, S.P., McHugh, M.P., 2003. Treatment and prevention of delayed onset muscle soreness. The Journal of Strength and Conditioning Research 17, 197–208.

Davis, J.M., Murphy, E.A., Carmichael, M.D., Davis, B., 2009. Quercetin increases brain and muscle mitochondrial biogenesis and exercise tolerance. American Journal of Physiology. Regulatory, Integrative and Comparative Physiology 296, R1071–R1077.

Davis, J.M., Carlstedt, C.J., Chen, S., Carmichael, M.D., Murphy, E.A., 2010. The dietary flavonoid quercetin increases VO(2max) and endurance capacity. International Journal of Sport Nutrition and Exercise Metabolism 20, 56–62.

Feng, Z., Bai, L., Yan, J., Li, Y., Shen, W., Wang, Y., Wertz, K., Weber, P., Zhang, Y., Chen, Y., Liu, J., 2011. Mitochondrial dynamic remodeling in strenuous exercise-induced muscle and mitochondrial dysfunction: regulatory effects of hydroxytyrosol. Free Radical Biology and Medicine 50, 1437–1446.

Finocchietto, P.V., Franco, M.C., Holod, S., Gonzalez, A.S., Converso, D.P., Arciuch, V.G., Serra, M.P., Poderoso, J.J., Carreras, M.C., 2009. Mitochondrial nitric oxide synthase: a masterpiece of metabolic adaptation, cell growth, transformation, and death. Experimental Biology and Medicine (Maywood) 234, 1020–1028.

Ganio, M.S., Armstrong, L.E., Johnson, E.C., Klau, J.F., Ballard, K.D., Michniak-Kohn, B., Kaushik, D., Maresh, C.M., 2010. Effect of quercetin supplementation on maximal oxygen uptake in men and women. Journal of Sports Sciences 28, 201–208.

Glover, E.I., Martin, J., Maher, A., Thornhill, R.E., Moran, G.R., Tarnopolsky, M.A., 2010. A randomized trial of coenzyme Q10 in mitochondrial disorders. Muscle and Nerve 42, 739–748.

Gomez-Cabrera, M.C., Vina, J., Ji, L.L., 2009. Interplay of oxidants and antioxidants during exercise: implications for muscle health. The Physician and Sportsmedicine 37, 116–123.

Gorski, T., Cadore, E.L., Pinto, S.S., da Silva, E.M., Correa, C.S., Beltrami, F.G., Kruel, L.F., 2009. Use of nonsteroidal anti-inflammatory drugs (NSAIDs) in triathletes: prevalence, level of awareness, and reasons for use. British Journal of Sports Medicine 45 (2), 85–90. http://dx.doi.org/10.1136/bjsm.2009.062166.

Gravina, L., Ruiz, F., Diaz, E., Lekue, J.A., Badiola, A., Irazusta, J., Gil, S.M., 2012. Influence of nutrient intake on antioxidant capacity, muscle damage and white blood cell count in female soccer players. Journal of the International Society of Sports Nutrition 9, 32.

Han, S.N., Adolfsson, O., Lee, C.K., Prolla, T.A., Ordovas, J., Meydani, S.N., 2004. Vitamin E and gene expression in immune cells. Annals of the New York Academy of Sciences 1031, 96–101.

Herrlinger, K.A., Chirouzes, D.M., Ceddia, M.A., 2015. Supplementation with a polyphenolic blend improves post-exercise strength recovery and muscle soreness. Food and Nutrition Research 59, 30034.

Howatson, G., van Someren, K.A., 2008. The prevention and treatment of exercise-induced muscle damage. Sports Medicine 38, 483–503.

Jacob, R.A., Spinozzi, G.M., Simon, V.A., Kelley, D.S., Prior, R.L., Hess-Pierce, B., Kader, A.A., 2003. Consumption of cherries lowers plasma urate in healthy women. Journal Nutrition 133, 1826–1829.

Janero, D.R., 1991. Therapeutic potential of vitamin E in the pathogenesis of spontaneous atherosclerosis. Free Radical Biology and Medicine 11, 129–144.

Kalafati, M., Jamurtas, A.Z., Nikolaidis, M.G., Paschalis, V., Theodorou, A.A., Sakellariou, G.K., Koutedakis, Y., Kouretas, D., 2010. Ergogenic and antioxidant effects of Spirulina supplementation in humans. Medicine and Science in Sports and Exercise 42, 142–151.

Karlsson, J., Lin, L., Sylven, C., Jansson, E., 1996. Muscle ubiquinone in healthy physically active males. Molecular and Cellular Biochemistry 156, 169–172.

Kerksick, C.M., Kreider, R.B., Willoughby, D.S., 2010. Intramuscular adaptations to eccentric exercise and antioxidant supplementation. Amino Acids 39, 219–232.

Kerksick, C., Taylor, L.T., Harvey, A., Willoughby, D., 2008. Gender related differences in muscle injury, oxidative stress, and apoptosis. Medicine and Science in Sports and Exercise 40, 1772–1780.

Khassaf, M., McArdle, A., Esanu, C., Vasilaki, A., McArdle, F., Griffiths, R.D., Brodie, D.A., Jackson, M.J., 2003. Effect of vitamin C supplements on antioxidant defence and stress proteins in human lymphocytes and skeletal muscle. Journal of Physiology 549.2, 645–652.

Kobayashi, Y.M., Rader, E.P., Crawford, R.W., Iyengar, N.K., Thedens, D.R., Faulkner, J.A., Parikh, S.V., Weiss, R.M., Chamberlain, J.S., Moorem, S.A., Campbell, K.P., 2008. Sarcolemma-localized nNOS is required to maintain activity after mild exercise. Nature 456, 511–515.

Kressler, J., Millard-Stafford, M., Warren, G.L., 2011. Quercetin and endurance exercise capacity: a systematic review and metaanalysis. Medicine and Science in Sports and Exercise 43, 2396–2404.

Kuehl, K.S., Perrier, E.T., Elliot, D.L., Chesnutt, J.C., 2010. Efficacy of tart cherry juice in reducing muscle pain during running: a randomized controlled trial. Journal of the International Society of Sports Nutrition 7, 17.

Laupheimer, M.W., Perry, M., Benton, S., Malliaras, P., Maffulli, N., 2014. Resveratrol exerts no effect on inflammatory response and delayed onset muscle soreness after a marathon in male athletes. A randomised, double-blind, placebo-controlled pilot feasibility study. Translational Medicine 10, 38–42.

Leelayuwat, N., Ladawan, S., Kanpetta, Y., Benja, M., Wongpan, D., Wattanathorn, J., Muchimapura, S., Yamauchi, J., 2012. Quercetin enhances endurance capacity via antioxidant activity and size of muscle fibre type I. Journal of the Peripheral Nervous System 2, 160–164.

Lee-Young, R.S., Ayala, J.E., Hunley, C.F., James, F.D., Bracy, D.P., Kang, L., Wasserman, D.H., 2010. Endothelial nitric oxide synthase is central to skeletal muscle metabolic regulation and enzymatic signaling during exercise in vivo. American Journal of Physiology. Regulatory, Integrative and Comparative Physiology 298, R1399–R1408.

Leonardo-Mendonça, R.C., Concepción-Huertas, M., Guerra-Hernández, E., Zabala, M., Escames, G., Acuña-Castroviejo, D., 2014. Redox status and antioxidant response in professional cyclists during training. European Journal of Sport Science 14, 830–838.

Lieber, R.L., Thornell, L.E., Friden, J., 1996. Muscle cytoskeletal disruption occurs within the first 15 min of cyclic eccentric contraction. Journal of Applied Physiology (1985) 80, 278–284.

Lomonosova, Y.N., Shenkman, B.S., Kalamkarov, G.R., Kostrominova, T.Y., Nemirovskaya, T.L., 2014. L-arginine supplementation protects exercise performance and structural integrity of muscle fibers after a single bout of eccentric exercise in rats. PLoS One 9, e94448.

MacRae, H.S.H., Mefferd, K.M., 2006. Dietary antioxidant supplementation combined with quercetin improves cycling time trial performance. International Journal of Sport Nutrition and Exercise Metabolism 16, 405–419.

Marechal, G., Beckers-Bleukx, G., 1998. Effect of nitric oxide on the maximal velocity of shortening of a mouse skeletal muscle. Pflugers Archiv 436, 906–913.

Martorel, M., Capó, X., Bibiloni, M.M., Sureda, A., Mestre-Alfaro, A., Batle, J.M., Llompart, I., Tur, J.A., Pons, A., 2015. Docosahexaenoic acid supplementation promotes erythrocyte antioxidant defense and reduces protein nitrosative damage in male athletes. Lipids 50, 131–148.

Markus, A., Morris, B.J., 2008. Resveratrol in prevention and treatment of common clinical conditions of aging. Clinical Interventions in Aging 2, 331–339.

Mazani, M., Fard, A.S., Baghi, A.N., Nemati, A., Mogadam, R.A., 2014. Effect of pomegranate juice supplementation on matrix metalloproteinases 2 and 9 following exhaustive exercise in young healthy males. Journal of Pakistan Medical Association 64, 785.

McCune, L.M., Kubota, C., Stendell-Hollis, N.R., Thomson, C.A., 2011. Cherries and health: a review. Critical Reviews in Food Science and Nutrition 51, 1–12.

Michailidis, Y., Karagounis, L.G., Terzis, G., Jamurtas, A.Z., Spengos, K., Tsoukas, D., Chatzinikolaou, A., Mandalidis, D., Stefanetti, R.J., Papassotiriou, I., Athanasopoulos, S., Hawley, J.A., Russell, A.P., Fatouros, I.G., 2013. Thiol-based antioxidant supplementation alters human skeletal muscle signaling and attenuates its inflammatory response and recovery after intense eccentric exercise. American Journal of Clinical Nutrition 98, 233–245.

Morrison, R.J., Miller, C.C., Reid, M.B., 1996. Nitric oxide effects on shortening velocity and power production in the rat diaphragm. Journal of Applied Physiology 80, 1065–1069.

Murase, S., Terazawa, E., Queme, F., Ota, H., Matsuda, T., Hirate, K., Kozaki, Y., Katanosaka, K., Taguchi, T., Urai, H., Mizumura, K., 2010. Bradykinin and nerve growth factor play pivotal roles in muscular mechanical hyperalgesia after exercise (delayed-onset muscle soreness). Journal of Neuroscience 30, 3752–3761.

Murphy, R.M., Dutka, T.L., Horvath, D., Bell, J.R., Delbridge, L.M., Lamb, G.D., 2013. Ca2+-dependent proteolysis of junctophilin-1 and junctophilin-2 in skeletal and cardiac muscle. Journal of Physiology 591, 719–729.

Nagasawa, T., Hayashi, H., Fujimaki, N., Nishizawa, N., Kitts, D.D., 2000. Induction of oxidatively modified proteins in skeletal muscle by electrical stimulation and its suppression by dietary supplementation of (-)-epigallocatechin gallate. Bioscience, Biotechnology, and Biochemistry 64, 1004–1010.

Naylor, A.J.D., 2009. Cellular effects of resveratrol in skeletal muscle. Life Sciences 84, 637–640.

Nikolaidis, M.G., Paschalis, V., Giakas, G., Fatouros, I.G., Koutedakis, Y., Kouretas, D., Jamurtas, A.Z., 2007. Decreased blood oxidative stress after repeated muscle-damaging exercise. Medicine and Science in Sports and Exercise 39, 1080–1089.

Nogueira, L., Figueiredo-Freitas, C., Casimiro-Lopes, G., Magdesian, M.H., Assreuy, J., Sorenson, M.M., 2009. Myosin is reversibly inhibited by S-nitrosylation. Biochemical Journal 424, 221–231.

Packer, L., 1991. Protective role of vitamin E in biological systems. American Journal of Clinical Nutrition 53, 1050S–1055S.

Packer, J.E., Slater, T.F., Willson, R.L., 1979. Direct observation of a free radical interaction between vitamin E and vitamin C. Nature 278, 737–738.

Paschalis, V., Nikolaidis, M.G., Fatouros, I.G., Giakas, G., Koutedakis, Y., Karatzaferi, C., Kouretas, D., Jamurtas, A.Z., 2007. Uniform and prolonged changes in blood oxidative stress after muscle-damaging exercise. In Vivo 21, 877–883.

Percival, J.M., Anderson, K.N., Huang, P., Adams, M.E., Froehner, S.C., 2010. Golgi and sarcolemmal neuronal NOS differentially regulate contraction-induced fatigue and vasoconstriction in exercising mouse skeletal muscle. Journal of Clinical Investigation 120, 816–826.

Powers, S.K., DeRuisseau, K.C., Quindry, J., Hamilton, K.L., 2004. Dietary antioxidants and exercise. Journal of Sports Science 22, 81–94.

Powers, S.K., Jackson, M.J., 2008. Exercise-induced oxidative stress: cellular mechanisms and impact on muscle force production. Physiological Reviews 88, 1243–1276.

Prasertsri, P., Roengrit, T., Kanpetta, Y., Tong-un, T., Muchimapura, S., Wattanathorn, J., et al., 2013. Cashew apple juice supplementation enhanced fat utilization during high-intensity exercise in trained and untrained men. Journal of the International Society of Sports Nutrition 10, 13.

Quadrilatero, J., Hoffman-Goetz, L., 2005. N-acetyl-L-cysteine inhibits exercise-induced lymphocyte apoptotic protein alterations. Medicine and Science in Sports and Exercise 37, 53–56.

Radak, Z., Chung, H.Y., Naito, H., Takahashi, R., Jung, K.J., Kim, H.J., et al., 2004. Age-associated increase in oxidative stress and nuclear factor kappaB activation are attenuated in rat liver by regular exercise. The Federation of American Societies for Experimental Biology Journal 18, 749–750.

Reid, M.B., Durham, W.J., 2002. Generation of reactive oxygen and nitrogen species in contracting skeletal muscle: potential impact on aging. Annals of the New York Academy of Sciences 959, 108–116.

Roengrit, T., Wannanon, P., Prasertsri, P., Kanpetta, Y., Sripanidkulchai, B., Leelayuwat, N., 2014. Antioxidant and anti-nociceptive effects of Phyllanthus amarus on improving exercise recovery in sedentary men: a randomized crossover (double-blind) design. Journal of the International Society of Sports Nutrition 11, 9.

Schaffer, S., Muller, W.E., Eckert, G.P., 2005. Tocotrienols: constitutional effects in aging and disease. Journal of Nutrition 135, 151–154.

Schulte, I., Bektas, H., Klempnauer, J., Borlak, J., 2006. Vitamin E in heart transplantation: effects on cardiac gene expression. Transplantation 81, 736–745.

Sen, C.K., 1995. Oxidants and antioxidants in exercise. Journal of Applied Physiology 79, 675–686.

Silva, L.A., Pinho, C.A., Silveira, P.C.L., Talita Tuon, T., De Souza, C.T., Dal-Pizzol, F., Pinho, R.A., 2010. Vitamin E supplementation decreases muscular and oxidative damage but not inflammatory response induced by eccentric contraction. The Journal of Physiological Sciences 60, 51–257.

Spencer, M.J., Mellgren, R.L., 2002. Overexpression of a calpastatin transgene in mdx muscle reduces dystrophic pathology. Human Molecular Genetics 11, 2645–2655.

Spriet, L.L., Whitfield, J., 2015. Taurine and skeletal muscle function. Current Opinion in Clinical Nutrition and Metabolic Care 18, 96–101.

Stupka, N., Tarnopolsky, M.A., Yardley, N.J., Phillips, S.M., 2001. Cellular adaptation to repeated eccentric exercise-induced muscle damage. Journal of Applied Physiology 91, 1669–1678.

Seeram, N.P., Momin, R.A., Nair, M.G., Bourquin, L.D., 2001. Cyclooxygenase inhibitory and antioxidant cyanidin glycosides in cherries and berries. Phytomedicine 8, 362–369.

Sun, S., Niu, H., Yang, T., Lin, Q., Luo, F., Ma, M., 2014. Antioxidant and anti-fatigue activities of egg white peptides prepared by pepsin digestion. The Journal of the Science of Food and Agriculture 94, 3195–3200.

Teixeira, V.H., Valente, H.F., Casal, S.I., Marques, A.F., Moreira, P.A., 2009. Antioxidants do not prevent postexercise peroxidation and may delay muscle recovery. Medicine and Science in Sports and Exercise 41, 1752–1760.

Traber, M.G., 2006. Relationship of vitamin E metabolism and oxidation in exercising human subjects. British Journal of Nutrition 96, S34–S37.

de Vries, J.H., Hollman, P.C., Meyboom, S., Buysman, M.N., Zock, P.L., van Staveren, W.A., Katan, M.B., 1998. Plasma concentrations and urinary excretion of the antioxidant flavonols quercetin and kaempferol as biomarkers for dietary intake. American Journal of Clinical Nutrition 68, 60–65.

Vaile, J., Halson, S., Gill, N., Dawson, B., 2008. Effect of hydrotherapy on recovery from fatigue. International Journal of Sports Medicine 29, 539–544.

Wang, H., Nair, M.G., Strasburg, G.M., Chang, Y.-C., Booren, A.M., Gray, J.I., et al., 1999. Antioxidant and antiinflammatory activities of anthocyanins and their aglycon, cyanidin, from tart cherries. The Journal of Natural Products 62, 294–296.

Yu, B.P., 1994. Cellular defenses against damage from reactive oxygen species. Physiological Reviews 74, 139–162.

Zoppi, C.C., Hohl, R., Silva, F.C., Lazarim, F.L., Joaquim, M.F., Neto, A., Stancanneli, M., Macedo, D.V., 2006. Vitamin C and E Supplementation effects in professional soccer players under regular training. Journal of the International Society of Sports Nutrition 3, 37–44.

CHAPTER

20

Effects of Exercise-Altered Immune Functions on Neuroplasticity

A.L. Aral, L. Pinar

Gazi University Faculty of Medicine, Ankara, Turkey

Abstract

Regular physical exercise affects many aspects of health, metabolism, mental capacity, and motivation by influencing the cytokine system and supporting neuroimmunological status. The beneficial effects of exercise on the mental capacity of the brain emerge through stimulation of neural plasticity, which is the basis for learning, memory, and neurogenesis. Regular exercise increases neurotrophic factors, such as nerve growth factors, and some immune mediators, such as interleukins. Because aging is a trigger for increased inflammation in the central nervous system, exercise may influence this process and facilitate the emergence of a beneficial anti-inflammatory state. In addition to preventing cognitive decline, an appropriate regular exercise program may also play a neuroprotective role in some neurodegenerative disorders.

INTRODUCTION

Regular physical exercise that is organized according to age and health status increases cardiovascular and pulmonary capacity, strengthens the musculoskeletal system, improves fitness and reshapes the body, and improves mental health, both in adults and in children (Pınar, 2015). Exercise affects many aspects of health, metabolism, mental capacity, and motivation. Recently, it was shown that exercise exerts plastic effects on the development of probiotic microbes in the intestine; thus, during the initial phases of life, it increases the gut bacterial species involved in promoting psychological and metabolic health (Mika and Fleshner, 2016). When designed appropriately, aerobic, isotonic exercises can be used even in the elderly, as well as in individuals of poor health (Guyton and Hall, 2006).

In this review, we first present a brief overview of the effects of exercise on immune function and an introduction to neuroplasticity, followed by a discussion regarding immunity of the central nervous system (CNS). Finally, we summarize the effects of exercise-altered immune function on neuroplasticity in the context of development, aging, and neurodegenerative disorders.

EFFECTS OF EXERCISE ON IMMUNE FUNCTION

It is now generally accepted that regular exercise is indicated in the treatment of many chronic disorders, and in several cases, is as effective as medical treatment (Pedersen and Saltin, 2006). However, some types exercise may be considered as a physical stressor because they induce a response of the immune system similar to subclinical inflammatory responses to pathological conditions (Rosa Neto et al., 2009). Long and strenuous exercise may disturb immune cell function due to increase in the levels of stress hormones and reactive oxygen species. In particular, acute and strenuous exercise may cause structural muscle damage through muscle fiber inflammation. It has been shown that moderate to severe exercise also stimulates the hypothalamo-pituitary-adrenal axis (HPA) and the release of cortisol, leading to an inflammatory state (Hill et al., 2008).

Although the most prominent cytokine produced during exercise is interleukin (IL)-6, which is known as myokine (Pedersen and Saltin, 2006), other proinflammatory cytokines, such as tumor necrosis factor (TNF)-α and IL-1β, may also appear in a cascade-like fashion (Mastorakos et al., 2005). The sources of cytokine production during exercise include muscle cells, peritendinous tissue, subcutaneous tissue, and the brain. These processes are closely related to the duration and intensity of exercise.

Regular exercise programs, however, stimulate the anti-inflammatory effects of IL-6, which inhibits TNF-α (Pedersen and Saltin, 2006) and IL-1 but stimulates the expression of TNF-receptor antagonist (ra), IL-10 receptor agonist, and IL-10 (Febbraio and Pedersen, 2002). In one of our recent studies, we found that strenuous exercise, a strong stressor, promoted IL-6 immunoreactivity in hippocampal slices of both regularly-trained and untrained rats compared with controls. However, IL-6 immunoreactivity in the hippocampus due to strenuous exercise-induced stress was milder in the trained group than in the untrained group (Aral et al., 2014). A group of researchers examined the link between exercise-induced increases in IL-6 and central fatigue, which was enhanced by hyperthermia, and found that an elevated core temperature during hyperthermic exercise in humans was not associated with altered cerebral IL-6 release compared with controls (Nybo et al., 2002).

The increase in IL-6 levels in the brain at the end of prolonged exercise may be related to excess post-exercise oxygen consumption, which persists for several hours (Gore and Withers, 1990). Cerebral release of IL-6 during exercise may be related to the effects of physical activity on the balance between energy expenditure and energy intake. Thus, an increase in brain IL-6 levels can also cause a sensation of fatigue during prolonged exercise (Davis and Bailey, 1997). In our study, we observed that the rats with the highest IL-6 levels in the brain showed the lowest exercise performance and became exhausted much more quickly. One day after strenuous exercise, the highest levels of the proinflammatory cytokine IL-6 were found in both the trained and the untrained animals but were higher in the untrained subjects than in the trained subjects (Aral et al., 2014). In our related previous study, we also observed that maximum muscle damage, IL-6 immunoreactivity and oxidant levels increased 1 day after strenuous exercise in both trained and untrained rats but were higher in the untrained group. We hypothesized that several factors, particularly cortisol, prevented the proinflammatory actions of IL-6 in muscle immediately after strenuous exercise. However, 1 day after exercise, the acute effects of cortisol had decreased, and the effect of IL-6 became more prominent. In the trained animals, compared with the untrained animals, the decreases in IL-6 and oxidants and increases in antioxidants and the regeneration process in histological samples became apparent on the 3rd day after strenuous exercise. However, in the acutely running untrained group, although IL-6 activity decreased, tissue oxidant levels were still found to be significantly higher, and antioxidant levels were lower than in the controls on the 3rd day after exercise (Deveden et al., 2013). These results were similar to those regarding IL-6 levels in the brains of rats.

Although acute strenuous exercise is shown to cause oxidative stress, cytokine expression, and damage in related tissues, the physiopathologic effects of acute exercise on resident immune cells in the CNS remain unclear. In a recent study that investigated the effects of a single bout of strenuous exercise on the hippocampus of healthy mice, IL-6 levels were found to be significantly increased, whereas TNF-α levels were decreased (Pervaiz and Hoffman-Goetz, 2012). Under inflammatory conditions such as viral infection, the levels of proinflammatory cytokines increase, and a particular type of neuronal death may occur depending on TNF-α receptor activation. Following exercise, on the other hand, the increase in IL-6 levels in the hippocampus may act as an anti-inflammatory mediator by inhibiting TNF-α, and this regulatory effect may protect neurons against cell death (Harry et al., 2008).

Macrophages are one of the primary cells responsible for innate immunity and may be grouped into tissue- and circulating-macrophages. Resident macrophages in the CNS are called microglia, and their distinct types are found in different locations in the CNS, with different morphologies and functions (David and Kroner, 2011). Exercise may polarize the microglial cells from the proinflammatory M1 type to the anti-inflammatory M2 type. It may also lead to a decrease in Toll-like receptor (TLR) expression in macrophages. In a recent study, it was shown that following brain ischemia in rats, treadmill running decreased TLR-2 and TLR-4 levels in the brain. These are stimulating receptors for production of other proinflammatory cytokines (Ma et al., 2013). Exercise may stimulate another alternative pathway to induce microglia using insulin-like growth factor (IGF)-1 in the prefrontal cortex and hippocampus. IGF-1 has some anti-inflammatory effects and stimulates the polarization of macrophages from M1 to M2 (Eyre and Baune, 2012). Although it is clear that the positive effects of exercise include increased levels of neurotrophic factors, elevated expression of anti-inflammatory cytokines, reduced levels of proinflammatory cytokines and activated microglia, the parameters influencing these positive effects, such as exercise intensity and duration, must be investigated further (Svensson et al., 2014).

ROLE OF EXERCISE IN ENHANCING BRAIN CAPACITY THROUGH NEUROPLASTICITY

Neuroplasticity: Learning, Memory, and Neurogenesis

Plasticity is a neural mechanism for improving our brain abilities (Kandel and Siegelbaum, 2013). From early postnatal life to older age, the brain has the ability to undergo axonal growth, and various cellular mechanisms promote the formation and strengthening or weakening and elimination of synapses. Under these conditions, circuits can undergo fundamental changes in their architecture and biochemistry in response to repetitive activity. Plasticity is the basis for learning, memory, and neurogenesis.

Learning is a reflection of the effect of acquired experiences on behavior. For any type of permanent learning, an *engram (connections between neurons)* should be formed related to this information. Learning something and transforming it to permanent memory may be performed with either a very intensive sensory stimulus or many repetitive stimuli.

Memory is the ability to store learned information in the CNS and recall it when necessary. The learning center of the brain is the hippocampus and its nearby areas, the entorhinal cortex and subiculum.

Memory traces are located in the cortical areas related to visual, auditory, olfactory, and other senses. There are strong neuronal links between these components (Kandel and Siegelbaum, 2013).

In the formation of long-term memory, structural changes occur in the presynaptic and postsynaptic neurons that convey information. For this, new protein synthesis is required. By means of the glutamate and long-term potentiation (LTP) mechanisms, immediate early gene expression and new protein synthesis occur in presynaptic and postsynaptic cells (Di Filippo et al., 2008). New protein structures cause the formation of new axonal branches in presynaptic neurons and new receptors and dendrites in postsynaptic neurons, which increases the numbers of neuronal connections.

The constitutive process of memory begins with the activation of the glutamatergic N-methyl-D-aspartate (NMDA) and α-amino-3-hydroxy-5-methyl-4-isoxazolepropionic acid (AMPA) receptors in the hippocampus, amygdala, and medial septum. Activation of the AMPA receptors, followed by the NMDA receptors, with glutamate opens Ca^{++} and Na^+ channels. Ca^{++} activates Ca^{++}/calmodulin kinase II (CaMKII), which phosphorylates AMPA receptors and triggers their increased conductance and movement from cytoplasmic storage sites into synaptic cell membranes. Ca^{++} also triggers protein kinase-C, arachidonic acid, and nitric oxide (NO). Protein kinase-C activates the protein synthesis necessary for the production of new proteins. NO and arachidonic acid are thought to move to the presynaptic terminal by retrograde transport and facilitate longer neurotransmitter release (Kandel and Siegelbaum, 2013).

Synaptic connections that are not used frequently may be inhibited by long-term depression (LTD). In this mechanism, the presynaptic neurotransmitter is also glutamate but affects the GluR2 subunits of AMPA receptors. LTD causes a decrease in synaptic strength. Stimulation of a presynaptic neuron by weak, low frequency (<20 Hz) impulses causes less Ca^{++} entry into the postsynaptic neuron. Low Ca^{++} levels activate protein phosphatases instead of protein kinases and inactivate CaMKII. This mechanism causes weakening and then death of synaptic connections. It has been shown that in addition to unused neural links, long-term stress also causes LTD (Kandel and Siegelbaum, 2013).

Another plastic feature of the brain, neurogenesis, generates new nerve cells in the brain. This feature was first described in the 1990s, when neuronal stem cells (neurogenerator cells) were reported in the subventricular areas, olfactory bulb, and hippocampus in human and animal brains. These neuronal stem cells can proliferate, differentiate and migrate to other regions of the brain. The factors responsible for increasing the neurogenesis that can be seen even in adulthood include exercise, which causes the release of neurotrophic hormones; dynamic life style, stress, and glucocorticoids; and lesions, including global ischemia of the brain. However, destruction of the hippocampus decreases neurogenesis (Sanes and Jessell, 2013).

There are numerous signaling molecules that can potentiate or inhibit neural plasticity. Some of the best known growth factors are nerve growth factor (NGF), brain-derived neurotrophic factor (BDNF), neurotrophins (NT-3, 4/5), leukemia inhibitory factor (LIF), IGF-1, and glial cell derived neurotrophic factor (GDNF). Growth factors ensure neuronal proliferation, development of growth cones at the axon terminal, and neuronal survival. In addition, cell adhesion molecules, including netrins, integrins, cadherins, selectins, and IgG-superfamily members, play roles in cell movement, adhesion of cells to one another and to the basal lamina, embryonic development of the nervous system, inflammation and wound healing, tumor metastasis, and signal conduction (Pınar, 2015). Stress and regular exercise should be particularly emphasized for enhancing neurogenesis among the factors listed earlier. However, it has been shown that higher stress levels can even suppress consciousness in addition to inhibiting neurogenesis.

Some types of psychological stress increase the release of proinflammatory cytokines, such as IL-1β, IL-6, and TNF-α, which may lead to cognitive disorders, especially in the elderly (Simpson et al., 2015). Permanent changes related to learning and memory mechanisms require activation of some genetic transcription and translation mechanisms, which are affected by sterile inflammatory conditions in the brain (Di Filippo et al., 2008). The factors that affect brain plasticity in a positive or negative manner are discussed in the next section, "Immunological Factors Effecting Neuroplasticity."

IMMUNITY OF THE CNS

Although the CNS has been accepted as an "immune-privileged" area for a long time, we currently know that there is bidirectional cross-talk between these systems. Cytokines produced by neurons and glial cells are the key players in these interactions. In addition to cytokines, there are several molecules that also take part in brain-immune system communication, including major histocompatibility complexes (MHC), NO, and cyclo-oxygenase (Di Filippo et al., 2008).

It is now accepted that cytokines that are classically known as immunomodulatory agents exert some neuro-modulatory effects in the developing and adult nervous system. They can affect cellular and molecular pathways that play a role in hippocampal-dependent long-term memory consolidation including synaptic plasticity, synaptic scaling, and neurogenesis (Sheridan et al., 2014). Previous studies have shown that the proinflammatory cytokines in particular exert some detrimental effects on neuronal function, cell viability, and plasticity (Allan and Rothwell, 2001). In contrast, there are also studies that show that basal levels of some pro- and anti-inflammatory cytokines are necessary for glial regulation, bidirectional interaction, and regulation of synaptic plasticity in the healthy brain (Avital et al., 2003). These different results may be related either to the amount of cytokines or to their homeostatic balance in the synaptic cleft.

Cytokines can be classified as cytokines that inhibit or stimulate LTP and those that increase synaptic transmission. In addition, there are also several cytokines that are members of the "neuropoietic cytokine family," including ciliary neurotrophic factor, LIF, neurotrophins, oncostatin-M, and IL-6, all of which support neuronal survival or inhibit neuronal apoptosis.

Neuropoietic cytokines may exert their effects on behavior through neural stem cells and regulate glial and immune cell functions via neuronal excitability. These cytokines play an important role in the response to pain sensations, and they may regulate stress, feeding, and depressive behaviors. Their diurnal rhythmicity may also regulate daily motor activity (Bauer et al., 2007).

IL-6 is a proinflammatory cytokine that exerts pleiotropic effects after exercise and is known as a myokine because, in addition to its other sources, it is also released from trained muscles. Like other members of the neuropoietic cytokine family, IL-6 stimulates the development of neurons in the central and peripheral nervous systems, affects their function, and plays a role in degeneration/regeneration processes. The binding of IL-6 to its receptor carries the signal into the cell and activates many kinases, followed by phosphorylation of transcription factors that play a role in neuronal survival and differentiation (Jüttler et al., 2002). IL-6 may also regulate neuronal excitability (Bauer et al., 2007).

Data from studies in mice suggest that the hippocampus is the likely source of IL-6 in the brain (Rasmussen et al., 2011). IL-6 levels increase in several pathologies of the CNS, including depression, encephalitis, seizures, neurodegenerative disorders, stroke, and injury. The overexpression of IL-6 also interferes with the integrity of the blood–brain barrier (Jüttler et al., 2002).

In a healthy brain after LTP induction, IL-6 is upregulated in hippocampal astrocytes. Treatment of hippocampal slices with low levels of IL-6 caused inhibition of LTP, and use of anti-IL-6 antibodies after treatment increased the duration of LTP and improved long-term memory (Li et al., 1997). In another study, IL-6 knockout (KO) mice were more successful in cognitive tests, whereas injection or overexpression of IL-6 caused retention in avoidance learning tests and affiliative social interactions (Bauer et al., 2007). Increased IL-6 levels during endotoxemia have negative effects on memory and emotion in humans. Neurons that play a role in endocrine and behavioral stress may use IL-6 as an extracellular signaling molecule (Jüttler et al., 2002). IL-6 *trans*-signaling is increased in the senescent brain following peripheral LPS challenge. Inhibition of this *trans*-signaling pathway may have protective effects against infection-related neuroinflammation and cognitive dysfunction in the senescent mouse (Burton and Johnson, 2012). It is well known that sleep is another physiologic process for memory consolidation. In particular, IL-6 signaling enhances the late nocturnal sleep period. It was shown that intranasal IL-6 specifically enhanced slow wave activity and related sleep-associated emotion but did not affect other types of memory (Benedict et al., 2009).

IL-1β is a member of the IL-1 proinflammatory cytokine family. Under healthy conditions, IL-1β is constitutively expressed in brain tissue and may increase rapidly after injury. The first study regarding the effects of IL-1β on mice hippocampal mossy fibers in the CA3 pathway (Katsuki et al., 1990) showed an inhibitory effect of this proinflammatory cytokine on LTP and was followed by other studies that verified these results (Vereker et al., 2000).

Both in vitro and in vivo studies showed a significant increase in IL-1β gene expression during LTP and that blocking its receptor impaired LTP (Schneider et al., 1998). Studies with IL-1β receptor KO mice showed impairment in hippocampal-related memory tests and a decline in LTP generation in the dentate gyrus (Avital et al., 2003). Under stressful conditions and with aging, it has been shown that there is a significant increase in the levels of IL-1β, which is an important player in the impairment of LTP in the hippocampus (Murray and Lynch, 1998).

Altogether, these data show that IL-1β is a necessary cytokine for LTP generation under physiological conditions, but its concentration is also one of the key players in LTP impairments caused by several pathological conditions, especially aging (Di Filippo et al., 2008). Physiological levels of IL-1β are also necessary for memory consolidation. In a study with an elderly population, genetic variations of IL-1β converting enzyme (ICE) expression, which is related to decreased levels of IL-1β, resulted in improved cognitive function. Low levels of IL-1β may be a protective factor against impaired learning and memory function. In elderly patients, testing for genetic variation among cytokines and their receptors has tremendous value. Blocking ICE may be a therapeutic target for preserving cognitive functionality (Trompet et al., 2008).

The IL-1β-related local inflammatory process is another player in the impairment of LTP-related β-amyloid protein (Aβ) in Alzheimer's Disease. This impairment can be inhibited via IL-1ra (Schmid et al., 2009). In the same study, it was also shown that under healthy conditions, using IL-1ra causes a significant depression in LTP, which is evidence for the link between physiologic levels of IL-1β and LTP and synaptic plasticity.

TNF-α is another member of the proinflammatory cytokine family that participates in communication between neurons and astrocytes. In hippocampal slices prepared from the brains of TNF-α KO or TNF-αR KO mice, it has been shown that there was no impairment in LTP or LTD generation either in TNF-α incubated slices or in the control group. These data suggest that TNF-α is not one of the necessary cytokines for these types of plasticity (Beattie et al., 2002). However, it is an important cytokine for several forms of homeostatic plasticity (Stellwagen and Malenka, 2006).

In addition to IL-1β and IL-6, IL-1 ra and IL-18 (del Rey et al., 2013), CX3CL1 (fractalkine) (Sheridan et al., 2014) and IL-15 (Li et al., 2010) play different roles in LTP maintenance and the generation of hippocampal-dependent memory. In several studies with MHC-Class I mutant mice, an increase in LTP generation and the disappearance of LTD have been observed (Boulanger, 2004). Although there are studies in the literature regarding the effects of several cytokines or molecules of the immune system on LTP or LTD, the mechanisms underlying these effects need to be investigated further.

EFFECTS OF EXERCISE-ALTERED IMMUNE FUNCTION ON NEUROPLASTICITY

Physical exercise has favorable effects on the balance between hippocampal pro- and anti-inflammatory cytokines during aging and is thought to play preventive and curative roles in various inflammatory nervous system disorders through these compensatory effects (Fischer, 2006). Regular physical activity reduces the risk of developing several age-related disorders, such as Alzheimer's and Parkinson's disease (PD) (Fischer, 2006). In addition to its preventive effects, physical exercise also slows down the progression and attenuates the symptoms of these neurodegenerative disorders (Svensson et al., 2014). Elderly people with a high level of aerobic fitness capacity have a larger hippocampal volume and improved spatial memory compared with elderly individuals with a low level of physical activity (Fischer, 2006). Exercise-induced changes in immune function are one of the most important effects of regular physical activity (Fischer, 2006). It is well known that exercise increases the efficiency of the immune system response to infection by changing the cytokine profile. Exercise primarily increases pleiotropic cytokine IL-6 levels (Fischer, 2006), downregulates TNF-α levels and TLR-4 expression and alters the differentiation of monocytes into an anti-inflammatory mode, thereby supporting brain plasticity (Svensson et al., 2014). TLR-4 activation has been implicated in memory impairment, but the underlying molecular mechanism is still not fully understood.

Exercise-induced effects of the immune system on neuroplasticity include positive regulation of neural circuit remodeling, neurogenesis promotion, memory consolidation, and hippocampal function (Yirmiya and Goshen, 2011). These effects include interactions of microglia, astrocytes, and neurons with immune function and decreased levels of proinflammatory cytokines and other mediators. In addition to these effects, glial cells are also known as modulatory cells for synaptic scaling, homeostatic plasticity, and metaplasticity via changes in synaptic coverage and release of cytokines and transmitters (Ben Achour and Pascual, 2010). It has been shown that glial hypertrophy increases synaptic numbers via synaptogenesis and leads to improvement in motor-skill learning (Anderson et al., 1994). However, whether repetitive exercise alone induces prominent glial hypertrophy remains unknown (Foster et al., 2011).

Regular exercise has some beneficial effects both on the fetus and on the mother during pregnancy (Marques et al., 2015). Because prenatal stress impacts an offspring's mental progress, HPA axis function (Entringer et al., 2009) and neurogenesis (Korosi et al., 2012), exercise during pregnancy improves maternal brain health and mood and prevents fatigue, increasing serum levels of IGF-1 and BDNF (Vega et al., 2011). In addition to decreasing the fetal complications related to pre-eclampsia (such as intrauterine growth restriction), regular exercise induces an anti-inflammatory state, improves endothelial function and enhances vasodilatory responses by reducing TNF-α levels and increasing NO bioavailability (Lee et al.). When mothers exercise regularly, their babies have higher APGAR scores (Haakstad and Bø, 2011), higher general intelligence, and higher oral language scores at age 5 (Clapp, 1996). Even in adolescence, regular exercise increases neuroplasticity-related growth factors, such as BDNF and IGF-1, and exerts a significant impact during development (Pareja-Galeano et al., 2013).

Uncontrolled increase of proinflammatory conditions may cause an impaired ability to maintain hippocampal-LTP in the aged brain. Because of this impairment, enhanced activation of stress-activated protein kinases and reactive oxygen species may occur (O'Donnell et al., 2000). It was previously shown that intracerebroventricular injection of an anti-inflammatory cytokine, such as IL-10, reversed LTP impairment in the aged brain (Lynch et al., 2004). In another study, an aerobic exercise program increased anti-inflammatory cytokine levels during hippocampal formation (Gomes da Silva et al., 2013). Interestingly, in the same study, proinflammatory cytokine levels were not significantly different between the study groups. These findings indicate that physical exercise is necessary to regulate the balance between hippocampal anti- and proinflammatory cytokines during aging (Gomes da Silva et al., 2013). A negative correlation was recently reported between exercise-induced IL-1β levels and performance on aversive memory tests in aged rats (Lovatel et al., 2013). These data supported previous findings that an IL-1β blockade in the dorsal hippocampus facilitated inhibitory avoidance tasks (Depino et al., 2004). Exercise-induced decreases in IL-4 levels also significantly contributed to impairment in inhibitory avoidance models in healthy aged rats. In addition to restoring cytokine balance, exercise may ameliorate aging-related memory decline in rats through an epigenetic mechanism involving histone acetylation (Lovatel et al., 2013).

There are studies suggesting that a low level of inflammation is also related to cognitive decline in healthy older adults (Kohman, 2012). Aerobic exercise may be an effective way of attenuating neuroinflammation in the aged brain. In addition to its effects on cytokine production, exercise stimulates changes in microglia that play a key role in brain aging. In the aged brain, the normal functions of microglia, including regulation of plasticity and repair of the brain, are reduced (Harry, 2013). Exercise exerts different effects on microglia number and function depending on its duration and intensity and the brain regions affected (Fischer, 2006). Macrophage polarization is another factor that may play an important role in enhancing neuroplasticity and repairing the sites of injury and disease. Although it has been shown that exercise induces M1 to M2 polarization and inhibits M1 infiltration into the injured area in adipose tissue, it is still unknown whether this type of exercise-induced polarization occurs in the CNS in neurodegenerative disorders (Petzinger et al., 2013).

PD is a neurodegenerative disorder with strong immune system components in its pathophysiologic mechanisms. Cycling improves motor performance by increasing anti-inflammatory cytokine levels in the plasma of PD patients (Scalzo et al., 2010). Although IL-6 is known as a proinflammatory cytokine in PD pathophysiology and is correlated with decreased walking speed, it plays an anti-inflammatory role after exercise. Increased IL-6 levels after exercise increase IL-10 and IL-1ra levels and decrease TNF-α levels in PD patients (Steensberg et al., 2006).

In addition to PD pathophysiology, increased proinflammatory cytokines and glial activation are also associated with cognitive decline in elderly patients with Alzheimer's disease. Neuroinflammation stimulates the production of pathologic isoforms of the tau protein by activating microglia, produces nuclear factor (NF)-KB, and induces cell apoptosis-promoting signals. These increased signals promote over activation of some cell cycle enzymes in addition to tau hyperphosphorylation (Maccioni et al., 2009). Exercise may play a neuroprotective role in patients with Alzheimer's Disease by stimulating neuroplastic responses via the creation of an anti-inflammatory milieu (Foster et al., 2011).

Exercise can also be used to enhance neuroplasticity and facilitate motor recovery after a stroke. In a rat stroke model, treadmill running reduced brain damage, enhanced the expression of midkine as a reparative neurotrophic factor and NGF, increased angiogenesis via Platelet endothelial cell adhesion molecule, and decreased the expression of caspase-3. In addition to motor improvement, exercise also attenuated neurological deficits and infarct volume (Matsuda et al., 2011).

In conclusion, the adult brain has a greater plastic capacity than previously known. A minimum level of inflammation that can be produced by a moderate level of exercise can improve learning, memory, and neurogenesis in the brain during life, both in development and in aging. An appropriately-designed regular exercise program that increases neurotrophic and neuroinflammatory factors is one of the most important ways of increasing brain capacity by increasing neurotrophic and neuroinflammatory factors. Thus, exercise also plays a role in protection against neurodegenerative diseases, in addition to maintain physical and mental health, both in younger and in older people.

References

Anderson, B.J., Li, X., Alcantara, A.A., Isaacs, K.R., Black, J.E., Greenough, W.T., 1994. Glial hypertrophy is associated with synaptogenesis following motor-skill learning, but not with angiogenesis following exercise. Glia 11 (1), 73–80.

Allan, S.M., Rothwell, N.J., 2001. Cytokines and acute neurodegeneration. National Reviews Neuroscience 2, 734–744.

Aral, L.A., Pınar, L., Göktaş, G., Deveden, E.Y., Erdoğan, D., 2014. Comparison of hippocampal interleukin-6 immunoreactivity after exhaustive exercise in both exercise-trained and untrained rats. Turkish Journal of Medical Sciences 44 (4), 560–568.

Avital, A., Goshen, I., Kamsler, A., Segal, M., Iverfeldt, K., Richter-Levin, G., Yirmiya, R., 2003. Impaired interleukin-1 signaling is associated with deficits in hippocampal memory processes and neural plasticity. Hippocampus 13, 826–834.

Bauer, S., Kerr, B.J., Patterson, P.H., 2007. The neuropoietic cytokine family in development, plasticity, disease and injury. National Reviews Neuroscience 8, 221–232.

Beattie, E.C., Stellwagen, D., Morishita, W., Bresnahan, J.C., Ha, B.K., Von Zastrow, M., Beattie, M.S., Malenka, R.C., 2002. Control of synaptic strength by glial TNFα. Science 295, 2282–2285.

Ben Achour, S., Pascual, O., 2010. Glia: the many ways to modulate synaptic plasticity. Neurochemistry International 57 (4), 440–445.

Benedict, C., Scheller, J., Rose-John, S., Born, J., Marshall, L., 2009. Enhancing influence of intranasal interleukin-6 on slow-wave activity and memory consolidation during sleep. FASEB Journal 23 (10), 3629–3636.

Boulanger, L.M., 2004. MHC class I in activity-dependent structural and functional plasticity. Neuron Glia Biology 1 (3), 283–289.

Burton, M.D., Johnson, R.W., 2012. Interleukin-6 trans-signaling in the senescent mouse brain is involved in infection-related deficits in contextual fear conditioning. Brain, Behavior, and Immunity 26 (5), 732–738.

Clapp 3rd, J.F., 1996. Morphometric and neurodevelopmental outcome at age five years of the offspring of women who continued to exercise regularly throughout pregnancy. The Journal of Pediatrics 129 (6), 856–863.

David, S., Kroner, A., 2011. Repertoire of microglial and macrophage responses after spinal cord injury. National Reviews Neuroscience 12 (7), 388–399.

Davis, J.M., Bailey, S.P., 1997. Possible mechanisms of central nervous system fatigue during exercise. Medicine and Science in Sports and Exercise 29, 45–57.

Depino, A.M., Alonso, M., Ferrari, C., del Rey, A., Anthony, D., Besedovsky, H., Medina, J.H., Pitossi, F., 2004. Learning modulation by endogenous hippocampal IL-1: blockade of endogenous IL-1 facilitates memory formation. Hippocampus 14 (4), 526–535.

Deveden, E., Pınar, L., Göktaş, E., Aral, A.L., Özer, Ç., Erdoğan, D., 2013. After an exhaustive exercise the most prominent muscle damage occurs a day later. Turkish Journal of Physical Medicine and Rehabilitation 59, 229–235.

Entringer, S., Kumsta, R., Hellhammer, D.H., Wadhwa, P.D., Wüst, S., 2009. Prenatal exposure to maternal psychosocial stress and HPA axis regulation in young adults. Hormones and Behavior 55 (2), 292–298.

Eyre, H., Baune, B.T., 2012. Neuroimmunological effects of physical exercise in depression. Brain, Behavior, and Immunity 26, 251–266.

Di Filippo, M., Sarchielli, P., Picconi, B., Calabresi, P., 2008. Neuroinflammation and synaptic plasticity: theoretical basis for a novel, immune-centred, therapeutic approach to neurological disorders. Trends in Pharmacological Sciences 29 (8), 402–412.

Febbraio, M.A., Pedersen, B.K., 2002. Muscle-derived interleukin-6: mechanisms for activation and possible biological roles. FASEB Journal 16, 1335–1347.

Foster, P.P., Rosenblatt, K.P., Kuljis, R.O., 2011. Exercise induced cognitive plasticity, implications for mild cognitive impairment and Alzheimer's disease. Frontiers in Neurology 2, 28.

Fischer, C.P., 2006. Interleukin-6 in acute exercise and training: what is the biological relevance? Exercise Immunology Review 12, 6–33.

Gomes da Silva, S., Simões, P.S., Mortara, R.A., Scorza, F.A., Cavalheiro, E.A., da Graça Naffah-Mazzacoratti, M., Arida, R.M., 2013. Exercise-induced hippocampal anti-inflammatory response in aged rats. Journal of Neuroinflammation 10, 61.

Gore, C.J., Withers, R.T., 1990. The effect of exercise intensity and duration on the oxygen deficit and excess post-exercise oxygen consumption. European Journal of Applied Physiology and Occupational Physiology 60, 169–174.

Guyton, A.C., Hall, J.E., 2006. Textbook of Medical Physiology, eleventh ed. Elsevier Inc., Philadelphia (Chapter 57).

Haakstad, L.A., Bø, K., 2011. Exercise in pregnant women and birth weight: a randomized controlled trial. BMC Pregnancy and Childbirth 11, 66.

Harry, G.J., 2013. Microglia during development and aging. Pharmacology & Therapeutics 139 (3), 313–326.

Harry, G.J., d'Hellencourt, C., McPherson, C.A., Funk, J.A., Aoyama, M., Wine, R.N., 2008. Tumor necrosis factor p55 and p75 receptors are involved in chemical-induced apoptosis of dentate granule neurons. Journal of Neurochemistry 106, 281–298.

Hill, E.E., Zack, E., Battaglini, C., Viru, M., Viru, A., Hackney, A.C., 2008. Exercise and circulating cortisol levels: the intensity threshold effect. Journal of Endocrinological Investigation 31, 587–591.

Jüttler, E., Tarabin, V., Schwaninger, M., 2002. IL-6: a possible neuromodulator induced by neuronal activity. The Neuroscientist 8 (3), 268–275.

Katsuki, H., Nakai, S., Hirai, Y., Akaji, K., Kiso, Y., Satoh, M., 1990. Interleukin-1 beta inhibits long-term potentiation in the CA3 region of mouse hippocampal slices. European Journal of Pharmacology 181, 323–326.

Kohman, R.A., 2012. Aging microglia: relevance to cognition and neural plasticity. Methods in Molecular Biology 934, 193–218.

Korosi, A., Naninck, E.F., Oomen, C.A., Schouten, M., Krugers, H., Fitzsimons, C., Lucassen, P.J., 2012. Early-life stress mediated modulation of adult neurogenesis and behavior. Behavioural Brain Research 227 (2), 400–409.

Kandel, E.R., Siegelbaum, S.,A., 2013. Cellular mechanisms of implicit memory involves changes in the effectiveness of synaptic transmission. In: Kandel, E.R., Schwartz, J.H., Jessell, T.M., Siegelbaum, S.A., Hudspeth, A.J. (Eds.), Principles of Neuroscience, fifth ed. The Mc-Graw Hill Companies Inc., New York, pp. 1461–1486.

Li, A.J., Katafuchi, T., Oda, S., Hori, T., Oomura, Y., 1997. Interleukin-6 inhibits long-term potentiation in rat hippocampal slices. Brain Research 748 (1–2), 30–38.

Li, Z., Guo, X., Pan, W., 2010. Interleukin-15 receptor is essential to facilitate GABA transmission and hippocampal-dependent memory. The Journal of Neuroscience 30 (13), 4725–4734.

Lovatel, G.A., Elsner, V.R., Bertoldi, K., Vanzella, C., Moysés Fdos, S., Vizuete, A., Spindler, C., Cechinel, L.R., Netto, C.A., Muotri, A.R., Siqueira, I.R., 2013. Treadmill exercise induces age-related changes in aversive memory, neuroinflammatory and epigenetic processes in the rat hippocampus. Neurobiology of Learning and Memory 101, 94–102.

Lynch, A.M., Walsh, C., Delaney, A., Nolan, Y., Campbell, V.A., Lynch, M.A., 2004. Lipopolysaccharide-induced increase in signalling in hippocampus is abrogated by IL-10-a role for IL-1 beta? Journal of Neurochemistry 88 (3), 635–646.

Ma, Y., He, M., Qiang, L., 2013. Exercise therapy downregulates the overexpression of TLR4, TLR2, MyD88, and NF-kB after cerebral ischemia in rats. International Journal of Molecular Sciences 14, 3718–3733.

Maccioni, R.B., Rojo, L.E., Fernández, J.A., Kuljis, R.O., 2009. The role of neuroimmunomodulation in Alzheimer's disease. Annals of the New York Academy of Sciences 1153, 240–246.

Marques, A.H., Bjorke-Monsen, A., Teixeira, A.L., Silverman, M.N., 2015. Maternal stress, nutrition and physical activity: impact on immune function, CNS development and psychopathology. Brain Research 1617, 28–46.

Mastorakos, G., Pavlatou, M., Diamanti-Kandarakis, E., Chrousos, G.P., 2005. Exercise and the stress system. Hormones 4, 73–89.

Matsuda, F., Sakakima, H., Yoshida, Y., 2011. The effects of early exercise on brain damage and recovery after focal cerebral infarction in rats. Acta Physiologica 201 (2), 275–287.

Mika, A., Fleshner, M., 2016. Early-life exercise may promote lasting brain and metabolic health through gut bacterial metabolites. Immunology & Cell Biology 94, 151–157.

Murray, C.A., Lynch, M.A., 1998. Evidence that increased hippocampal expression of the cytokine interleukin-1 beta is a common trigger for age- and stress-induced impairments in long-term potentiation. The Journal of Neuroscience 18, 2974–2981.

Nybo, L., Nielsen, B., Pedersen, B.K., Møller, K., Secher, N.H., 2002. Interleukin-6 release from the human brain during prolonged exercise. The Journal of Physiology 542, 991–995.

O'Donnell, E., Vereker, E., Lynch, M.A., 2000. Age-related impairment in LTP is accompanied by enhanced activity of stress-activated protein kinases: analysis of underlying mechanisms. The European Journal of Neuroscience 12 (1), 345–352.

Pareja-Galeano, H., Brioche, T., Sanchis-Gomar, F., Montal, A., Jovaní, C., Martínez-Costa, C., Gomez-Cabrera, M.C., Viña, J., 2013. Impact of exercise training on neuroplasticity-related growth factors in adolescents. Journal of Musculoskeletal & Neuronal Interactions 13 (3), 368–371.

Pedersen, B.K., Saltin, B., 2006. Evidence for prescribing exercise as therapy in chronic disease. Scandinavian Journal of Medicine & Science in Sports 16, 3–63.

Pervaiz, N., Hoffman-Goetz, L., 2012. Immune cell inflammatory cytokine responses differ between central and systemic compartments in response to acute exercise in mice. Exercise Immunology Review 18, 142–157.

Petzinger, G.M., Fisher, B.E., McEwen, S., Beeler, J.A., Walsh, J.P., Jakowec, M.W., 2013. Exercise-enhanced neuroplasticity targeting motor and cognitive circuitry in Parkinson's disease. The Lancet Neurology 12 (7), 716–726.

Pınar, L., 2015. Sinir Ve Kas Fizyolojisi, third ed. Akademisyen, Ankara (Chapter 3).

del Rey, A., Balschun, D., Wetzel, W., Randolf, A., Besedovsky, H.O., 2013. A cytokine network involving brain-borne IL-1β, IL-1ra, IL-18, IL-6, and TNFα operates during long-term potentiation and learning. Brain, Behavior, and Immunity 33, 15–23.

Rasmussen, P., Vedel, J.C., Olesen, J., Adser, H., Pedersen, M.V., Hart, E., Secher, N.H., Pilegaard, H., 2011. In humans IL-6 is released from the brain during and after exercise and paralleled by enhanced IL-6 mRNA expression in the hippocampus of mice. Acta Physiologia 201, 475–482.

Rosa Neto, J.C., Lira, F.S., Oyama, L.M., Zanchi, N.E., Yamashita, A.S., Batista Jr., M.L., Oller do Nascimento, C.M., Seelaender, M., 2009. Exhaustive exercise causes an anti-inflammatory effect in skeletal muscle and a pro-inflammatory effect in adipose tissue in rats. European Journal of Applied Physiology 106, 697–704.

Scalzo, P., Kümmer, A., Cardoso, F., Teixeira, A.L., 2010. Serum levels of interleukin-6 are elevated in patients with Parkinson's disease and correlate with physical performance. Neuroscience Letters 468 (1), 56–58.

Schneider, H., Pitossi, F., Balschun, D., Wagner, A., del Rey, A., Besedovsky, H.O., 1998. A neuromodulatory role of interleukin-1β in the hippocampus. Proceedings of the National Academy of Sciences of the United States of America 95, 7778–7783.

Steensberg, A., Dalsgaard, M.K., Secher, N.H., Pedersen, B.K., 2006. Cerebrospinal fluid IL-6, HSP72, and TNF-α in exercising humans. Brain, Behavior, and Immunity 20 (6), 585–589.

Simpson, R.J., Kunz, H., Agha, N., Graff, R., 2015. Exercise and the regulation of immune functions. Progress in Molecular Biology and Translational Science 135, 355–380.

Schmid, A.W., Lynch, M.A., Herron, C.E., 2009. The effects of IL-1 receptor antagonist on beta amyloid mediated depression of LTP in the rat CA1 in vivo. Hippocampus 19 (7), 670–676.

Stellwagen, D., Malenka, R.C., 2006. Synaptic scaling mediated by glial TNF-α. Nature 440, 1054–1059.

Sanes, R.S., Jessell, T.,M., 2013. Repairing the damaged brain. In: Kandel, E.R., Schwartz, J.H., Jessell, T.M., Siegelbaum, S.A., Hudspeth, A.J. (Eds.), Principles of Neuroscience, fifth ed. The Mc-Graw Hill Companies Inc., New York, pp. 1284–1305.

Svensson, M., Lexell, J., Deierborg, T., 2014. Effects of physical exercise on neuroinflammation, neuroplasticity, neurodegeneration, and behavior: what we can learn from animal models in clinical settings. Neurorehabilitation and Neural Repair 29 (6), 577–589.

Sheridan, G.K., Wdowicz, A., Pickering, M., Watters, O., Halley, P., O'Sullivan, N.C., Mooney, C., O'Connell, D.J., O'Connor, J.J., Murphy, K.J., 2014. CX3CL1 is up-regulated in the rat hippocampus during memory-associated synaptic plasticity. Frontiers in Cellular Neuroscience 12 (8), 233.

Trompet, S., de Craen, A.J., Slagboom, P., Shepherd, J., Blauw, G.J., Murphy, M.B., Bollen, E.L., Buckley, B.M., Ford, I., Gaw, A., Macfarlane, P.W., Packard, C.J., Stott, D.J., Jukema, J.W., Westendorp, R.G., PROSPER Group, 2008. Genetic variation in the interleukin-1 beta-converting enzyme associates with cognitive function. The PROSPER study. Brain 131, 1069–1077.

Vega, S.R., Kleinert, J., Sulprizio, M., Hollmann, W., Bloch, W., Strüder, H.K., 2011. Responses of serum neurotrophic factors to exercise in pregnant and postpartum women. Psychoneuroendocrinology 36 (2), 220–227.

Vereker, E., O'Donnell, E., Lynch, M.A., 2000. The inhibitory effect of interleukin-1beta on long-term potentiation is coupled with increased activity of stress activated protein kinases. The Journal of Neuroscience 20, 6811–6819.

Yirmiya, R., Goshen, I., 2011. Immune modulation of learning, memory, neural plasticity and neurogenesis. Brain, Behavior, and Immunity 25 (2), 181–213.

Index

'*Note*: Page numbers followed by "f" indicate figures and "t" indicate tables.'

A

Active Brains Project, 17
Adeno-associated-virus (AAV), 112
Aerobic exercise, 190–191
  brain activity, 16
    executive functions, 16
    learning and memory, 16
  brain structure
    DTI, white matter microstructure using, 15–16
    gray matter, 14
    subcortical gray matter, 15
  cognition, 17
  defined, 14–16
  future directions, 17–18
  magnetic resonance imaging (MRI), 13–14
  measuring physical activity levels, 13
Aging brain
  brain remodeling, 165–168
  circuitries, 166
  connection-moving, 162
  contradictory findings, 165
  defined, 161–162
  exercise, 162
    age-related cognitive decline, 162–165, 163t
    attention and processing speed, 164
    BDNF, 167–168
    episodic memory, 163
    executive function, 163–164
    memory consolidation, 165
    synaptic plasticity, 166–167
  memories, 166
  molecular and cellular building blocks, 165–168
  neurons, 166
ALS. *See* Amyotrophic lateral sclerosis (ALS)
Alzheimer's disease (AD), 123, 176
  physical exercise
    bio-markers, 146–147
    cognitive functions, 142–145
    defined, 141
    functional capacity, 145–146
    neuropsychiatric symptoms, 145
    physical activity level, 141–142
    physical activity programs, 142
Amyotrophic lateral sclerosis (ALS), 71
Anterior cingulate cortex (ACC), 123
Antioxidant supplements
  docosahexaenoic acid (DHA), 203
  egg white peptides (EWP), 204
  functional foods, 204–205

    cashew apple juice, 204
    fruits, 204
    mixed fruit and vegetables, 205
    phyllantus amarus, 204
    pomegranate juice, 204
    spirulina, 204–205
  green tea catechins, 202, 204
  hydroxytyrosol (HT), 203
  L-arginine supplementation, 203
  N-acetylcysteine (NAC), 203–204
  polyphenolic blend, 203
  polyphenols, 201
  purple mangosteen, 203
  quercetin, 202
  taurine, 203
  ubiquinone-10, 203
  vitamin E, C and A, 202
Apolipoprotein E (APOE), 179
Apoptosis, 87–88
Arylalkylamine-N-acetyltransferase (AANAT), 95–96
Astrocytes, 89
Attention deficit hyperactivity disorder (ADHD), 18

B

BDNF. *See* Brain-derived neurotrophic factor (BDNF)
Bilirubin, 98–99
Bio-markers, 146–147
Brain-derived neurotrophic factor (BDNF), 4–5, 7–8, 46–47, 68–69, 86, 112, 145
Brain temperature (T$_{BRAIN}$)
  defined, 29–30
  exercise effects, 30–37, 31t
    ambient temperature, 32
    brain site measured, 33–35, 35f
    exercising humans, 36–37
    intensity and protocol, 32–33, 33f–34f
    performance, 35–36, 36f
  measuring during exercise, 30

C

Caffeine, 61
Calcitonin-gene-related peptide (CGRP), 109–110
Cannabinoid receptor 1 (CB1), 66–68
Cannabinoid receptor 2 (CB2), 66–67
Cardiorespiratory fitness (CRF), 123
Cardiovascular diseases (CVD), 4, 126
Catecholamines, 54, 56, 57f
CBF. *See* Cerebral blood flow (CBF)
Central fatigue, 155

Cerebral blood flow (CBF)
  defined, 77–78
  positron emission tomography (PET), 79–80
  regional CBF (rCBF), 79–80, 81f
    brain beneficial effects, 82
    exercise, 80–82
    transcranial Doppler (TCD) method, 78, 79f, 79t
Cerebral blood volume (CBV), 82
Cerebral networks
  ageing brain, 8
  cognitive ageing, 3–6, 6f
  cognitive reserve, 3–4, 7–8
  molecular basis exercise, 8
  neuroplasticity, 7–8
  physical activity, 7–8
  physical exercise and health, 4–5
Cerebral vasomotor reactivity (CVR), 82
Chaperones, 25–26
Cognition, 17
  central nervous system diseases, 128–129
  effective connectivity (EC), 122–123
  functional connectivity (FC), 122–123
  neuroimaging studies
    brain structure training intervention, 126
    cerebral blood flow and FC training intervention, 126–127
    CRF levels and cognitive performances, 124–126
    structural studies, 123–124
  overview, 121–129
  physiological mechanisms, 122
Cognitive functions, 142–145
Combined physical/mental activities
  cognition, 176–178, 177t
  mechanisms, 178–180
    human brain changes identification, 179–180
    molecular and cellular level changes identification, 178–179
Concussion, 194–195
Conditioned place preference (CPP), 43
Core body temperature (T$_{CORE}$), 29–30
Cortical-abdominal temperature, 34
Cortical adaptations, 110–111
Cortical reorganization
  brain reorganization after stroke, 156–157
  exercising brain, 152–155
  fatigue-related brain reorganization, 155–156, 156f
  overview, 151–152

D

Default mode network (DMN), 5, 7, 123
Delayed onset of muscle soreness (DOMS)
　mechanisms
　　contractile protein disruption, 200
　　free radical formation, 199–200
　　inflammation, 200–201
　　mechanical stress, 201
　　nitric oxide generation, 200
Dementia, 176, 193–194
Dentate gyrus (DG), 122
Depression, 68–69
Dickkopf-related protein 1 (DKK-1), 90
3,4-dihydroxyphenylacetic acid (DOPAC),
　56, 58–59
Dihydroxypheylalanine (DOPA), 56

E

Electroencephalogram (EEG), 147
End-diastolic velocity (EDV), 78
Endocannabinoid system
　Alzheimer's disease, 70–71
　amyotrophic lateral sclerosis (ALS), 71
　brain-derived neurotropic factor (BDNF),
　　68–69
　chronic conditions, 68
　chronic pain, 69
　depression, 68–69
　epilepsy, 69–70
　musculoskeletal disorders, 70
　overview, 65
　runners high, 65–66
　stimulation effects, 66–68
　stress-related disorders, 71–72
Energy metabolism, 25
Epigenetics, 86–87
Epilepsy, 69–70
Exercise-induced hyperthermia, 29–30, 33
Exercise-induced muscle soreness, 201
　anti-nociceptive supplements, 205–206
　　phyllanthus amarus, 205
　　polyphenolic blend containing catechins
　　　and theaflavins, 205–206
　　resveratrol, 205
　　tart cherry, 205
　endogenous antioxidants, 201
　nutritional antioxidants, 201
Exercise-induced neuroprotection
　age-related neurodegenerative diseases, 90
　apoptosis, 87–88
　epigenetics, 86–87
　neurogenesis, 88–89
　neurotrophic factors, 86
　overview, 85–86
　oxidative stress, 88
　synaptogenesis, 89–90

F

FITKids, 17
Functional magnetic resonance imaging
　(fMRI), 7

G

Glial-cell-derived-neurotrophic factor
　(GDNF), 86, 108–109
Glucocorticoid receptors (GRs), 8

Glyceraldehyde-3-phosphate dehydrogenase
　(GAPDH), 25
Gray matter (GM), 14, 123
GRP78, 25–26

H

Heme oxygenase 1 (HO-1) activity, 100
Hippocampal neurogenesis, 89
Hippocampus, 162
Homovanillic acid (HVA), 56
Hyperthermia-mediated changes, 33

I

Inclined ladder stepping apparatus, 113
inducible nitric oxide synthase
　(iNOS), 98
Inflammatory signaling, 97–98, 98f
Insulin-like growth factor 1 (IGF-1), 122,
　178–179

L

Locus coeruleus (LC), 57
Long-term potentiation (LTP), 162

M

Magnetic resonance imaging (MRI), 13–14,
　180
Major histocompatibility complex II (MHC
　II), 89
MASCOT program, 23
Mass spectrometry, 23
Mean arterial pressure (MAP), 81–82
Medial temporal gyri (MTG), 124–125
Medial temporal lobe (MTL), 5, 121
Medium spiny neurons (MSN), 134
Melatonin
　biosynthesis, 95–96
　induced inflammatory signaling,
　　96–97
　inflammatory signaling, 97–98, 98f
　oxidative stress, 96–97
　physiological effects, 95–96
　sources, 95–96
　strenuous exercise, 98–100
Methamphetamine
　addiction, 47–48
　animal models
　　drug reinforcement, 42–43
　　illicit drugs reward, 42–43
　　self-administration, 43–44, 45f
　　sustained physical activity, 43–44,
　　　44f–45f
　defined, 41–42
　exercise, 47–48
　wheel running. *See* Wheel running
Methylphenidate (MPH), 60
1-methyl-4-phenyl-1,2,3, 6-tetrahydropuridine
　(MPTP), 136
Middle frontal gyrus (MFG), 124
Mild cognitive impairment
　(MCI), 123
MRI. *See* Magnetic resonance
　imaging (MRI)
Multivariate analysis of variance
　(MANOVA), 5–6

N

N-acetyl serotonin is O-methylated by
　hydroxyindole-O-methyltransferase,
　95–96
National Institutes on Drug Abuse (NIDA),
　41–42
Neural plasticity, 188–190
Neurological changes
　exercises, 190–193
　　aerobic exercise, 190–191
　　balance and strength training exercise,
　　　192–193
　　concussion, 194–195
　　dementia, 193–194
　　therapy, 193–195
Neuronal circuitry, 88–89
Neuroplasticity
　exercise-altered immune functions
　　CNS immunity, 212–213
　　defined, 213–215
　　enhancing brain capacity, 211–212
　　immune function, 209–210
　　learning, 211–212
　　memory, 211–212
　　neurogenesis, 211–212
Neuropsychiatric symptoms (NPS), 145
Neurotransmission
　central nervous system (CNS), 53
　　structure and function, 53–54
　monoamines
　　caffeine, 61
　　DA/noradrenaline reuptake inhibitor, 62
　　DA receptor agonist, 60–61
　　DA reuptake inhibitor, 60
　　dopaminergic system, 55–56, 56f–57f,
　　　56t, 58–59
　　drugs manipulating and exercise
　　　performance, 59–62
　　exercise, 57–59
　　noradrenaline reuptake inhibitor, 62
　　noradrenergic system, 57, 58f, 58t, 59
　　physiological properties, 54–57
　　selective DA receptor antagonist, 61
　　selective serotonin receptor agonist, 60
　　selective serotonin receptor
　　　antagonist, 60
　　selective serotonin reuptake inhibitor
　　　(SSRI), 59–60
　　serotoninergic system, 54, 54f–55f, 55t,
　　　57–58
Neurotrophic-3 (NT3), 108–109
Neurotrophic factors, 136
Non-aerobic physiological processes, 17
Nuclear factor-kB (NF-kB), 98

O

Optic dominant atrophy 1 (OPA1), 88
Oscillatory activities, 155
Oxidative stress, 8, 96–97
Oxygen uptake (VO2), 77–78, 79f

P

P300, 147
Palmitoylethanolamide (PEA), 71
Parahippocampal gyri (PHG), 124–125

Parkinson's disease (PD)
  brain-animal models, 135–137
    dopamine metabolism, 136
    dopamine receptor functions, 136
    functional changes, 136–137
    neurotrophic factors, 136
  brain-human studies, 137–138
    brain networks, functional and
      structural changes, 138
    dopamine receptor changes, 137
    neurotrophic factors, 137
  defined, 133–134
  exercise interventions, 135
  overview, 133
Partial least squares analysis (PLS), 5–6
PDIA3, 25–26
Positron emission tomography (PET),
  79–80
Post-traumatic stress disorder (PTSD), 71–72
Potassium-chloride co-transporter (KCC2),
  110
Prefrontal cortex (PFC), 121
Protein identification, 23–24, 24f, 24t
  CC and HC regions, 23–24, 25t
Proteomics
  chaperones, 25–26
    miscellaneous proteins, 26
  defined, 21–22
  exercise training regimens, 22
  sample preparation, 22–23
  swimming exercise, 22
  treadmill running, 22
  two-dimensional polyacrylamide gel
    electrophoresis (2D-PAGE), 23–26
    energy metabolism, 25
    mass spectrometry, 23
    protein identification, 23–24
    signal transduction, 25
    synaptic plasticity, 25
  voluntary exercise (VE), 21–22
  voluntary wheel running, 22

R
Reactive oxygen species (ROS), 88, 96–97, 161
Retrosplenial cortex (RSC), 123

S
Selective brain cooling (SBC), 30–32, 34–35
Signal transduction, 25
Sodium-potassium-chloride co-transporter
  (NKCC1), 110
Spinal cord injury (SCI)
  defined, 107–108
  mechanisms, 108–112
    cell membrane proteins, 110
    cell signalling pathways, 110
    Hoffman Reflex (H-reflex), 109–110
    intraspinal circuitry, 109–110
    motor and somatosensory cortex
      adaptations, 110–111
    trophic factors, 108–109
  rehabilitation programs, 112–115
    frequency and duration, 113–115
    motor skill transfer, 113, 114t
    onset, 115
  skill training
    descending tract plasticity, 112
    motor cortex plasticity, 111–112
    spinal networks, 111
Strenuous exercise, 98–100
Subcortical gray matter, 15
Subgranular zone (SGZ), 89
Subsequent memory effect paradigm, 16
Superior frontal gyrus (SFG), 124
Supplementary motor area (SMA), 125
Swimming exercise, 22
Synaptic cleft, 53
Synaptic plasticity, 25

T
Δ9(−)-tetrahydrocannabinol (THC), 66
Transcranial Doppler (TCD) method, 78, 79f,
  79t

Transcranial magnetic stimulation (TMS),
  138
Treadmill running, 22
Two-dimensional polyacrylamide gel
    electrophoresis (2D-PAGE),
    23–26
  energy metabolism, 25
  mass spectrometry, 23
  protein identification, 23–24
  signal transduction, 25
  synaptic plasticity, 25
Tyrosine Hydroxylase (TH), 136

V
Vascular endothelial growth factor (VEGF),
  146–147, 178–179
VEGF. See Vascular endothelial growth
  factor (VEGF)
Vertebral arteries (VA), 80
Voluntary exercise (VE), 21–22
Voluntary wheel running, 22

W
Wheel running
  brain reward circuitry, 45
  methamphetamine-induced neurotoxicity,
    45–47
    factors, 46–47
  methamphetamine self-administration
    developmental effects, 43–44
    reward substitution, 44
  neural mechanisms underlying reinforcing
    effects, 45
  neuroprotection, 45–47
  neurotransmission, 45, 46t
White adipose tissue (WAT) genes,
  96–97
White matter (WM), 124
Wisconsin Card Sorting Task (WCST),
  124–125

Printed in the United States
By Bookmasters